Differential Diagnosis in SURGERY

Differential Diagnosis in SURGERY

Mahmoud Sakr MD PhD FACS
Professor of Surgery
Chief of Head and Neck and Endocrine Surgery Unit
Faculty of Medicine
University of Alexandria
Egypt

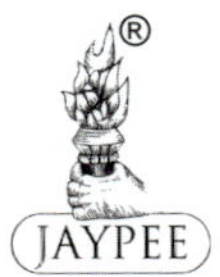

JAYPEE BROTHERS MEDICAL PUBLISHERS (P) LTD

New Delhi • London • Philadelphia • Panama

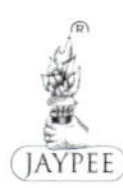

Jaypee Brothers Medical Publishers (P) Ltd

Headquarters

Jaypee Brothers Medical Publishers (P) Ltd
4838/24, Ansari Road, Daryaganj
New Delhi 110 002, India
Phone: +91-11-43574357
Fax: +91-11-43574314
Email: jaypee@jaypeebrothers.com

Overseas Offices

J.P. Medical Ltd
83, Victoria Street, London
SW1H 0HW (UK)
Phone: +44-2031708910
Fax: +02-03-0086180
Email: info@jpmedpub.com

Jaypee-Highlights Medical Publishers Inc
City of Knowledge, Bld. 237, Clayton
Panama City, Panama
Phone: + 507-301-0496
Fax: + 507-301-0499
Email: cservice@jphmedical.com

Jaypee Medical Inc
The Bourse
111 South Independence Mall East
Suite 835, Philadelphia, PA 19106, USA
Phone: + 267-519-9789
Email: joe.rusko@jaypeebrothers.com

Jaypee Brothers Medical Publishers (P) Ltd
17/1-B Babar Road, Block-B, Shaymali
Mohammadpur, Dhaka-1207
Bangladesh
Mobile: +08801912003485
Email: jaypeedhaka@gmail.com

Jaypee Brothers Medical Publishers (P) Ltd
Shorakhute, Kathmandu
Nepal
Phone: +00977-9841528578
Email: jaypee.nepal@gmail.com

Website: www.jaypeebrothers.com
Website: www.jaypeedigital.com

Inquiries for bulk sales may be solicited at: jaypee@jaypeebrothers.com

Differential Diagnosis in SURGERY

First Edition: **2014**
ISBN 978-93-5090-982-9
Printed at: Samrat Offset Pvt.Ltd

Dedicated to
My family, my professors, my colleagues
and my students

Preface

In these days, when there is a tendency for ward rounds to be sometimes recitals of biochemical, radiological and endoscopic findings, the patient's bedclothes unruffled and the patient a silent witness, the importance of signs and symptoms cannot be overemphasized.

In clinical medicine, sins of omission are more common than sins of commission. It is the disorders one does not think of and the conditions one forgets that leads to misdiagnosis or no diagnosis. This book aims to help the medical student and clinician to be sure that he has considered all the disorders that might lie behind his patient's particular symptoms or physical signs.

It is my collective hope that this book will be as useful and popular as its predecessors.

Mahmoud Sakr

Contents

1. Differential Diagnosis of Swellings **1**

- *Swellings of the scalp 1*
  - *Congenital swellings 2*
  - *Acquired swellings 5*
- *Swellings of the face 13*
  - *Diffuse swellings 13*
  - *Localized swellings 14*
- *Swellings of the lips 18*
  - *Surgical anatomy 18*
  - *Localized swellings 19*
- *Swellings of the tongue 21*
  - *Causes of acute swellings of the tongue 21*
  - *Causes of chronic or persistent swelling of the tongue 21*
- *Swellings of the oral cavity 23*
  - *Swellings in the floor of the mouth 23*
  - *Swellings in the palate 26*
- *Swellings of the jaw 28*
  - *Epulides 28*
  - *Odontomas 32*
  - *Tumors arising from the bone 35*
- *Swellings of salivary glands 43*
  - *Parotid gland 43*
  - *Clinical classification 44*
  - *Acute swellings in the parotid region 45*
  - *Chronic swellings in the parotid region 46*
  - *Submandibular gland 54*
  - *Minor salivary glands 58*
- *Cervical lymphadenopathy 60*
  - *Causes of cervical lymphadenopathy 60*
- *Swellings of the thyroid gland 69*
- *Swellings of midline of the neck 91*
  - *Classification according to anatomical region 91*
  - *Classification according to consistency 92*
  - *Midline cystic swellings of the neck 92*

Swellings in lateral side of the neck 97
- *Solid swellings 97*
- *Cystic swellings 103*

Swellings of the chest wall 110
- *Swellings from the chest wall 110*
- *Swellings from within the chest 112*

Swellings of the axilla 115
- *Swellings from the walls of the axilla 115*
- *Swellings from contents of the axilla 118*

Swellings of the breast 121
- *Classification 121*
- *Swellings of the whole breast 121*
- *Swellings in the breast 122*
- *Swellings pushing the breast forward 134*
- *Male breast diseases 134*
- *Benign breast conditions that mimic breast cancer 136*
- *Breast lesions in children and adolescents 137*
- *Nipple discharge 141*

Abdominal masses 144
- *Mass in the right iliac fossa 147*
- *Parietal swellings (Abscess pointing in the RIF) 148*
- *Intra-abdominal swellings 148*
- *Retroperitoneal swellings 153*
- *Most common causes of a swelling in the RIF 155*
- *Mass in the right hypochondrium 156*
- *Parietal swellings 156*
- *Intra-abdominal swellings 156*
- *Retroperitoneal swellings 168*
- *Mass in the epigastric region 170*
- *Mass in the umbilical region 174*
- *Mass in the suprapubic region 176*
- *Mass in the left iliac fossa 178*
- *Retroperitoneal swellings 180*
- *Mass in the left hypochondrium 181*
- *Mass in the lumbar region 183*

Swelling in the groin 190
- *Inguinal swellings 190*
- *Femoral swellings 197*
- *Inguinal-femoral swellings 201*

- *Inguinoscrotal swellings 203*
  - *Causes 203*
- *Scrotal swellings 210*
  - *Swellings affecting the skin 210*
  - *Swellings of the connective tissue coverings 210*
  - *Swellings of the tunica vaginalis 212*
  - *Swellings of the testicle/epididymis 214*
  - *Swellings of the spermatic cord (Lower end) 220*
  - *Urethral conditions 220*
- *Swellings of the popliteal fossa 224*
  - *Chronic cystic swellings 224*
  - *Chronic solid swellings 227*
- *Cystic swellings of skin and SC tissues 230*
  - *Sebaceous cyst 230*
  - *Inclusion dermoid cyst (Sequestration dermoid) 231*
  - *Implantation dermoid cyst (Acquired) 232*
  - *Ganglion 233*
  - *Subcutaneous bursa 234*
- *Solid swellings of the skin 235*
  - *Classification (Ackermann) 235*
  - *Benign tumors of the skin 236*
  - *Malignant tumors of the skin 243*
- *Solid swellings of SC tissues 253*
  - *Benign tumors 253*
  - *Soft tissue sarcoma 256*
- *Bone swellings 259*
  - *Swellings at the end of long bones 259*
  - *Swellings at the mid-shaft of long bones 269*
  - *Multiple bone swellings 271*

2. Differential Diagnosis of Organomegaly 277

- *Hepatomegaly 277*
  - *Etiologic classification of hepatomegaly 277*
  - *Clinical classification of hepatomegaly 278*
  - *Characteristic clinical features according to cause 279*
- *Splenomegaly 283*
  - *Causes of splenic enlargement 283*
  - *Characteristic features of common causes of splenomegaly 285*

3. Differential Diagnosis of Lymphadenopathy 287
- *Clinical approach 287*
- *Localized lymph node enlargement 289*
  - *Infections 289*
  - *Malignancy 292*
- *Generalized lymph node enlargement 294*
  - *Infections 294*
  - *Malignancy 295*
  - *Other causes 297*

4. Differential Diagnosis of Ulcers 299
- *Classification of ulcers 299*
  - *Definition 299*
  - *Pathological classification 299*
  - *Non-specific ulcers 300*
  - *Specific ulcers 302*
  - *Malignant ulcers 305*
- *Ulcers of the face 310*
  - *Classification 310*
  - *Ulcerating infective lesions 310*
  - *Ulcerating tumors 312*
- *Ulcers of the lips 314*
  - *Cracked or fissured lips 314*
  - *Malignant ulcer 314*
  - *Syphilitic ulcer 315*
  - *Dyspeptic (aphthous) ulcers 315*
  - *Traumatic (dental) ulcers 316*
- *Ulcers of the tongue 317*
  - *Causes of tongue ulcers 317*
  - *Traumatic ulcers 317*
  - *Inflammatory ulcers 318*
  - *Dyspeptic (aphthous) ulcers 320*
  - *Malignant ulcers 320*
- *Scrotal and penile ulcers 323*
  - *Scrotal ulcers 323*
  - *Penile ulcers (Sores) 325*
- *Ulcers of the leg 328*
  - *Causes of chronic leg ulcer 328*
  - *Diagnostic approach 329*

- *Venous ulcer 330*
- *Arterial ulcer 333*
- *Traumatic ulcer (Footballer's ulcer) 335*
- *Tuberculous ulcer 335*
- *Gummatous ulcer (Syphilis—third stage) 336*
- *Meleney's ulcer (Meleney's gangrene; pyoderma gangrenosum) 336*
- *Parasitic ulcer (Oriental sore—leishmaniasis) 337*
- *Leg ulcers in the tropics 337*
- *Neuropathic ulcers (Trophic—perforating ulcers) 339*
- *Malignant ulcers 340*
- *Leg ulcer complicating blood diseases 342*
- *Leg ulcer in rheumatoid arthritis 342*
- *Leg ulcer associated with osteitis deformans 342*
- *Artefact ulcer (factitious ulcer; automutilation ulcer) 343*

5. Differential Diagnosis of Pain 344

- *Pain in the tongue 344*
  - *Pain underneath the tongue or deeper 344*
  - *Pain upon the surface of the tongue 345*
- *Pain in the breast 347*
  - *Pregnancy 347*
  - *Menstruation 347*
  - *The onset of puberty 347*
  - *Lactation 347*
  - *Cracked/inflamed nipple 347*
  - *Breast abscess (Acute suppurative mastitis) 348*
  - *Other causes of mastitis 348*
  - *Tuberculosis of the breast 348*
  - *Other inflammatory lesions of the breast 349*
  - *Galactocele (milk cyst) 349*
  - *Fibrocystic disease 349*
  - *Acute cancer of pregnancy and lactation (Mastitis carcinomatosa) 349*
  - *After effects of a blow or injury 349*
  - *Lesions outside the breast 350*
  - *Anxiety state 350*

- *Pain in the abdomen 351*
  - *Inflammation 352*
  - *Perforation 355*
  - *Torsion/volvulus 356*
  - *Abdominal colic 358*
  - *Intestinal obstruction 359*
  - *Ischemia 361*
  - *Internal hemorrhage 362*
  - *Extra-abdominal disease 363*
  - *Medical causes 364*
- *Epigastric pain 367*
  - *Sudden severe epigastric pain 367*
  - *Chronic or recurrent epigastric pain 367*
- *Pain in the umbilical region 371*
  - *Pain arising in the umbilicus 371*
  - *Pain referred to the umbilicus 372*
- *Chronic back pain 376*
  - *Acute back pain 376*
  - *Chronic back pain 376*
- *Pain in the perineum 381*
- *Pain in the testicle 387*
  - *Diseases of body of testis or epididymis 387*
  - *Diseases of coverings of the testis 392*
  - *Diseases of the spermatic cord 393*
  - *Retained or misplaced (ectopic) testis 393*
  - *Testicular pain from extra-testicular lesions 394*
- *Pain in the penis 395*
  - *Causes of pain in the penis during micturition 395*
  - *Penile pain following micturition 396*
  - *Pain in the penis apart from micturition 396*
- *Pain in the lower limbs 398*
  - *Sciatica 398*
  - *Pain in the front and sides of the thigh 399*
  - *Pain in the foot 400*
  - *Tabes dorsalis 401*
  - *Vascular causes 402*
- *Pain in the upper limbs 405*
  - *Local causes 405*
  - *Referred pain 405*

6. Differential Diagnosis of Dyspepsia **407**

- *Dyspepsia 407*
  - *Simulation of symptoms of dyspepsia by other conditions 407*
  - *Organic versus functional dyspepsia 410*
  - *Causes of organic dyspepsia 410*
  - *Causes of functional dyspepsia 414*

7. Differential Diagnosis of Dysphagia **416**

- *Dysphagia 416*
  - *Functional grades of dysphagia 416*
  - *Causes of dysphagia 416*
  - *Differential diagnosis 418*
  - *Mechanical obstruction to the esophagus 418*
  - *Dysphagia due to nervous causes 422*
  - *Mechanical defects of mouth and pharynx 425*
  - *Pain - but no mechanical obstruction 426*

8. Differential Diagnosis of Constipation **427**

- *Constipation 427*
  - *Definition 427*
  - *Common complications of constipation 428*
  - *Pathophysiology 428*
  - *Etiology 429*
  - *Evaluation of patients with severe chronic constipation 430*
  - *Pertinent questions that may aid in diagnosis of constipation 432*
  - *Individual causes of constipation 434*

9. Differential Diagnosis of Jaundice **439**

- *Jaundice 439*
  - *Unconjugated hyperbilirubinemia—prehepatic (hemolytic) 439*
  - *Unconjugated hyperbilirubinemia—hepatic 441*
  - *Conjugated hyperbilirubinemia—hepatic 441*
  - *Conjugated hyperbilirubinemia—posthepatic 445*
  - *Surgical jaundice 445*
  - *Calcular obstructive jaundice 447*
  - *Malignant obstructive jaundice 448*
  - *Postoperative jaundice 453*

10. Differential Diagnosis of Bleeding 456

- *Hematemesis 456*
  - *Causes of hematemesis 456*
  - *Swallowed blood 458*
  - *Diseases of the esophagus 459*
  - *Diseases of the stomach 461*
  - *Diseases of the duodenum 464*
  - *Portal obstruction 465*
  - *Blood diseases 466*
  - *Acute febrile diseases 467*
  - *Miscellaneous diseases 468*
- *Melena 470*
  - *Definition 470*
  - *Causes (Source) 470*
  - *Other causes of black stools 471*
- *Bleeding per rectum 472*
  - *Definition 472*
  - *Frank red blood passed per anus 474*
  - *Passage of blood per anus in a child 478*
- *Hematuria 479*
  - *Definitions 479*
  - *Pathogenesis of hematuria 479*
  - *Other causes of red coloration of urine 480*
  - *Causes of hematuria 480*
  - *Hematuria from neighboring viscera involving the urinary tract 483*
  - *Hematuria in general disease 483*
  - *General causes of hematuria 484*
- *Menorrhagia 491*
  - *Definitions 491*
  - *Diagnosis 491*
  - *Causes of menorrhagia 491*
- *Hemoptysis 493*
  - *Definitions 493*
  - *Sources of hemoptysis 493*

11. Differential Diagnosis of Urinary Retention 496

- *Urinary retention 496*
  - *Definitions 496*

- *Acute urinary retention 496*
- *Chronic urinary retention 501*

12. Differential Diagnosis of Swollen Limb 504

- *Swollen limb 504*
  - *Differential diagnosis 504*
  - *History taking 508*
  - *Clinical examination 509*
  - *Special investigations 510*

13. Differential Diagnosis of Gangrene 511

- *Gangrene 511*
  - *Definition 511*
  - *Cardinal signs of gangrene 511*
  - *Types of gangrene 511*
  - *Classification of gangrene according to etiology 512*
  - *Causes of gangrene 512*
  - *Cardiovascular gangrene 513*
  - *Neuropathic gangrene 521*
  - *Traumatic gangrene 522*
  - *Infective gangrene 523*

14. Differential Diagnosis of Testicular Atrophy and Impotence 526

- *Testicular atrophy 526*
  - *Definition 526*
  - *Causes of atrophy of a normally situated testis 526*
- *Impotence 529*
  - *Definitions 529*
  - *Temporary impotence 529*
  - *Causes of impotence 529*

15. Differential Diagnosis of Gynecomastia 531

- *Gynecomastia 531*
  - *Definitions 531*
  - *Causes of gynecomastia 532*
  - *Physiological gynecomastia 532*
  - *Pathological gynecomastia 534*

Bibliography 539

Index 541

CHAPTER

1

Differential Diagnosis of Swellings

1. SWELLINGS OF THE SCALP

Classification of Swellings of the Scalp

I. Congenital	1. Meningocele/ Encephalocele 2. Inclusion (Sequestration) Dermoid Cyst 3. Circoid Aneurysm	
II. Acquired		
A. Traumatic	Cephalohematoma: 1. Subcutaneous 2. Subgalial or subaponeurotic 3. Subperiosteal	
B. Inflammatory	1. Infected granuloma 2. Osteomyelitis 3. Cock's peculiar tumor 4. Suppuration (Abscess) 5. Cellulitis and erysipelas	
C. Sebaceous Cyst	1. Single cyst - Multiple cysts 2. Cock's peculiar tumor	

Contd...

Contd...

D. Neoplastic	*Benign Tumors*	*Malignant Tumors*
	1. Papilloma 2. Hemangioma 3. Lymphangioma 4. Circoid aneurysm 5. Neurofibroma 6. Lipoma 7. Osteoma 8. Chondroma	*Primary Tumors* 1. Squamous cell carcinoma 2. Basal cell carcinoma 3. Malignant melanoma 4. Multiple myeloma 5. Fibrosarcoma *Secondary Tumors From* 1. Thyroid 2. Breast 3. Bronchogenic 4. Kidneys 5. Suprarenal glands 6. Prostate
E. Pott's Puffy Tumor		

I. CONGENITAL SWELLINGS

Meningocele/Encephalocele

- It is a protrusion of the meninges through a defect in the skull (**Figure 1.1**) (or spinal canal). It contains cerebrospinal fluid (CSF).
- The commonest site is the occipital region. The other 3 sites are all

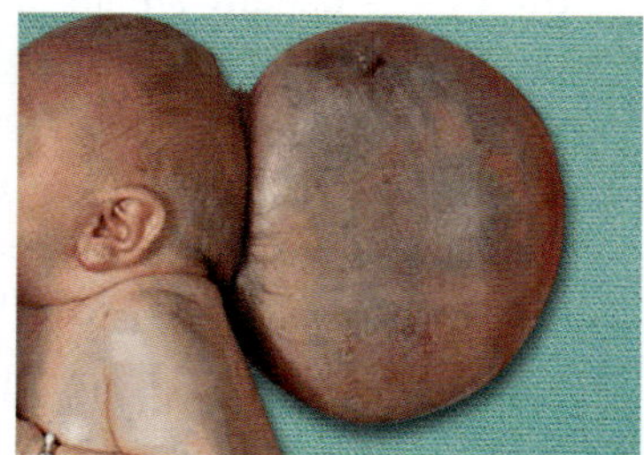

Fig. 1.1: Encephalocele

extremely rare, through the root of the nose, the pterion, and the mastoid region.

- Meningocele is translucent, but encephalocele is not. It is tense, rounded, fluctuant, not adherent to the skin and yields an impulse on straining (crying).

Inclusion Dermoid Cyst (Sequestration Dermoid)

- *Duration:*
  It may be noticed at birth, but usually first seen a few years later when it begins to fill up.
- *Symptoms*:
  Parental distress at the cosmetic disfigurement and concern about diagnosis.
- *Sites (Position):*
  Midline of scalp. Very rarely, it may have an *intracranial extension* through a defect in the underlying bone forming a dumbbell-shaped swelling known as "hour-glass dermoid".
- *Clinical Examination*:
  The cyst is usually single. It is small (1-2 cm) and ovoid or spherical, with a smooth surface and well-defined borders. Consistency is cystic or soft. The cyst may fluctuate but will *not* transilluminate (*opaque*). It is *not* pulsatile, compressible or reducible. The skin overlying is normal unless it is inflamed. They lie in the SC tissue and unlike sebaceous cysts, are not attached to the overlying skin.
- *Investigations*:
  Plain X-ray of the skull may show the defect in the bone.

Differences between Dermoid Cyst and Sebaceous Cyst

Criteria	Dermoid Cyst	Sebaceous Cyst
Age	Childhood and adolescence	Middle and old age
Site	At lines of embryonal fusion	Anywhere especially in scalp and face
Punctum	-ve	+ve
Pinching skin	+ve (SC location)	-ve (intradermal)
Consistency	Cystic or soft	Cystic or doughy (indented)
Multiplicity	Usually single	Commonly multiple
Extension	± intracranial	-ve

Circoid Aneurysm

- It is a painful and tender, pulsating swelling, which is formed of arterial malformation (hamartoma).
- The commonest site is the side of the scalp (superficial temporal artery).
- It is elongated and irregular in shape (**Figure 1.2**).
- It is *not* attached to the skin or the skull
- It empties easily on pressure and refills very rapidly on releasing the pressure.

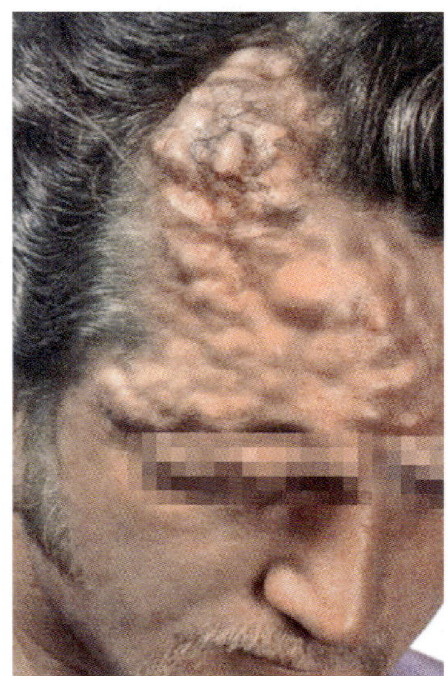

Fig. 1.2: Circoid aneurysm

- *A thrill* may be *felt* and a *bruit* may be *heard.*
- The *skull* may show a bone defect on Plain X-ray (PXR).
- An *angiogram* is essential as it may show an intracranial extension, i.e. the feeding artery may be an intracerebral vessel.

II. ACQUIRED SWELLINGS

A. Traumatic

Cephalhematoma

- It usually occurs in *neonates* following traumatic labor, and in infants following direct trauma.
- It may be *subcutaneous, subgalial* (*subaponeurotic) or subperiosteal.*
  - *Subcutaneous Hematoma*:
    It is always small and limited because the SC of the scalp is dense and fibrous and does not allow effusion of much blood.
  - *Subaponeurotic Hematoma*:
    It is always diffuse because the aponeurosis of the occipito-frontalis muscle (galea aponeurotica) is loosely attached to the underlying periosteum by a very loose areolar layer. The hematoma will be limited by the attachment of the aponeurosis to the superior nuchal line behind, and to the superior temporal lines on either side. However, anteriorly, the hematoma can extend into the 2 upper eyelids causing black eyes.
  - *Subperiosteal Hematoma:*
    It spreads under the pericranium (periosteum) taking the shape of the bones underneath because it is limited by the attachment of the periosteum at the suture lines. As a general rule, it is accompanied by a fissure fracture of the bone and may act as a "safety valve hematoma",

i.e. instead of the blood accumulating inside the skull, it escapes through the fracture to the outside of the skull, thus, preventing compression of the brain. The hematoma is soft and fluctuant (cystic as it contains fluid). If left for a few days, the edges become raised and hard. It may then be mistaken for a *depressed fracture*, but the lip is above the level of the rest of the skull. In addition, the edges of a fracture are sharp, while those of a hematoma are firm and smooth. A plain X-ray is diagnostic.

Difference between Subperiosteal Hematoma and Depressed Fracture

Subperiosteal Hematoma	Depressed Fracture
The center of the hematoma lies on the same level of the skull	The center of the Hematoma lies below the level of the skull
Hematoma edge is firm and smooth	Fracture edge is hard, sharp and ragged
X-ray is diagnostic	X-ray is diagnostic

- Absence of signs of inflammation excludes *abscess*, and the lack of increase in its size with crying excludes *meningocele.*

B. Inflammatory

1. Infected Granuloma

- Repeated injury of the scalp by a sharp comb, or scratching by a nail causes abrasions which result in infection and a reaction in the skin with granulation tissue and fibrous tissue formation so that it becomes more subjected to trauma, ending in a small swelling which is soft, strawberry colored, and covered by clots and dirty crusts. It is not malignant (sure diagnosis is by biopsy).

- Painting it with a silver nitrate solution causes it to shrink and disappear.

2. Osteomyelitis of Skull Bones

- It is common in the mastoid region, reaching it from the middle ear due to otitis media.
- It is also common in skull bones close to sinuses where infection occurs, and at any site of trauma (e.g. fracture which causes bone infection).

3. Cock's Peculiar Tumor

- It is *not* actually a tumor, but a *big sebaceous cyst* in the scalp, which has been traumatized by a sharp comb causing injury and infection, thus forming "*an ulcer on top of the sebaceous cyst*". Repeated injury and infection causes elevation and the overlying skin ulcerates simulating a malignant ulcer (epithelioma). The edges are *raised* and not everted, and there is dry sebaceous material, necrotic tissue and pus. In addition, hair is attached to it.

4. Suppuration (Abscess)

- *SC Abscess*: Small and tense because of the dense fibrous tissue septae in the SC layer of the scalp.
- *Subaponeurotic (Subgalial) Abscess*: It may extend from the forehead to the occiput. It may also extend to the intracranial contents via the emissary veins.
- *Subperiosteal (Subepicranial) Abscess*: Due to infection of cranial bone.

5. Cellulitis and Erysipelas

- These commonly affect the scalp.

C. Sebaceous Cyst

It is an acquired retention cyst caused by obstruction of the duct of a sebaceous gland by dried sebum, or inflammatory scarring. *It is the commonest swelling in the scalp, usually multiple.*

- *Age*: All age groups, mostly in adulthood and middle age, and rarely before adolescence (slow-growing).
- *Sex*: Males > Females.
- The swelling is painless (unless infected), smooth, well defined and cystic or doughy in consistency.
- There is a *punctum,* which is the opening of the occluded sebaceous duct.
- The swelling may be *indented* due to its doughy sebaceous material inside.
- You *cannot* pinch the skin over it (it is intradermal), but it is mobile over the underlying structures.
- Squeezing causes the sebaceous material to come out through the punctum. Sometimes a cyst will discharge its contents through its punctum spontaneously and then regress or even disappear.
- It may present by any of its complications, which include: *infection* (abscess formation), *sebaceous horn, Cock's peculiar tumor* (ulcer on top of the sebaceous cyst simulating epithelioma), *malignant transformation* (into sebaceous adenocarcinoma), and atrophy of the hair follicles and baldness of the scalp.
- *It should be differentiated from* other diseases of the sebaceous gland such as sebaceous adenoma or adenocarcinoma, and from a dermoid cyst (refer to the Table before).

D. Neoplastic

1. Soft Tissue Swellings

a. ***Lipoma***:

   It may be subcutaneous, subaponeurotic, or subperiosteal.

b. ***Neurofibroma***:

A firm nodule along one of the scalp nerves. It may occur in the skin and SC tissues and has a soft knotty feeling. Overlying skin may be redundant (=plexiform neuroma or pachydermatocele).

Lipoma of the Scalp	Neurofibroma
Flat deep surface and a spherical superficial one	Fusiform with the long axis along the nerve
It causes dimpling of the skin	Not attached to skin and does not dimple it
It moves in all directions	It moves from side-to-side only
Soft or pseudocystic in consistency	Firm or soft in consistency

c. ***Hemangioma:***

It is bluish and compressible.

d. ***Turban Tumor:***

It is an irregular mass that covers the whole scalp, looking like a "turban".

It is a descriptive term and may be caused by:

1. *Multiple Cylindromata*: Turban tumor is most often used to describe multiple cylindromata, which present as firm pink nodules in the scalp.
2. *Nodular Multiple Basal Cell Carcinoma*: Firm and retain their pearly white appearance and covering of fine blood vessels.
3. *Multiple Hidradenomata*: Multiple sweat gland tumors form soft boggy swellings in the scalp. Although soft, they are not fluctuant and cannot be compressed or indented.
4. *Plexiform Neurofibroma*: It is the rarest of all and is usually associated with neurofibromata in other sites and "cafe au lait" patches.

2. Bony Swellings

Bony lesions of the skull are characterized by having no mobility whatsoever, and the surrounding or underlying bone may be eroded or thickened.

a. *Ivory Osteoma*:
   - This is an osteoma of the cortical bone that forms the outer table of the skull, particularly the frontal, parietal, or occipital bones. It appears during adolescence and young adult life as a well defined, hard swelling, but causes no symptoms. It is more or less stationary in course.
   - Its onset is not related to trauma (excludes encysted hematoma), and was not accompanied by constitutional manifestations (rule out a chronic abscess).

b. *Multiple Myeloma:*
   The plain X-ray is diagnostic. It shows multiple radiolucent bone defects without reaction around **(Figure 1.3).**

c. *Secondaries*:
   They are the most common tumors of the skull.
   - Primary tumors that give bone metastases (blood-borne and start in the diploe) are those of the thyroid, breast, bronchi, kidneys, adrenal glands, and prostate.

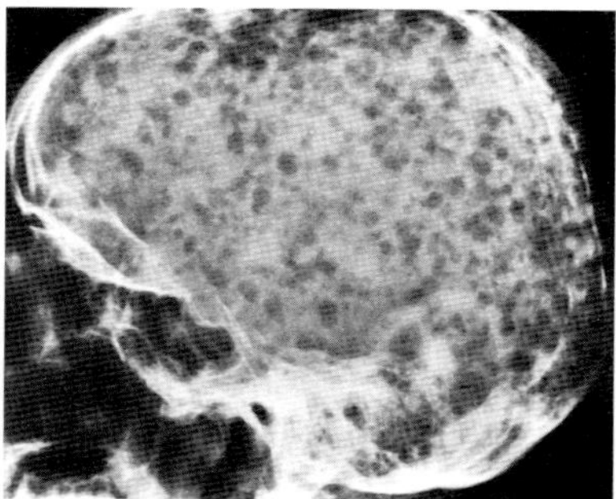

Fig. 1.3: Multiple myeloma

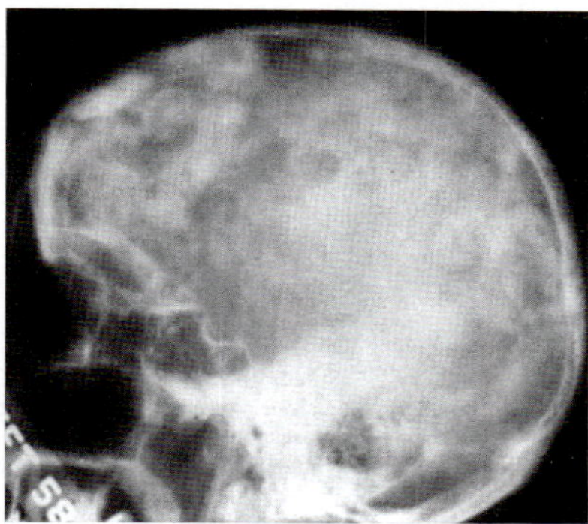

Fig. 1.4: Osteoblastic metastases multiple sclerotic lesions due to metastases from cancer of the breast

- The swellings are painful, tender, with ill-defined edges and hard consistency (or soft depending on vascularity). Some extremely vascular metastases show pulsations.
- *PXR* shows multiple lesions that are usually osteolytic but may be osteoblastic as from the prostate or the breast **(Figure 1.4).**

E. Pott's Puffy Tumor

- It *is not* really, a tumor. It is simply "*edema*" of the overlying skin and SC tissue, over an area of *osteomyelitis* of the skull, or in front of an intracranial lesion such as a *chronic intracranial abscess* in a "silent" area, so that it presents only on the outside of the skull.
- In the frontal region, it is due to imperfectly treated *acute frontal sinusitis*. About 10 days after the onset, considerable pyrexia with severe pain and tenderness over the sinus strongly suggests osteomyelitis.

Clinical Key Points— Swelling in the Scalp

The Following Signs are Helpful Diagnostic Guides

- Movement of the swelling over the underlying bone rules out a bony swelling.
- Transillumination is observed in meningocele.
- A useful approach for Diagnosis of a swelling in the scalp is to determine whether it is *cystic, pulsating, or solid:*

Cystic Swellings	Pulsating Swellings	Solid Swellings
1. Sebaceous cyst	1. Circoid aneurysm	***A. Soft Tissue Swellings:***
2. Inclusion dermoid cyst	2. Sarcoma of the skull	1. Lipoma
3. Cephalohematoma	3. Encephalocele	2. Turban tumor
4. Hemangioma		***B. Bony Swellings:***
5. Lymphangioma		1. Ivory osteoma
6. Abscess		2. Multiple myeloma
		3. Secondaries

2. SWELLINGS OF THE FACE

I. DIFFUSE SWELLINGS

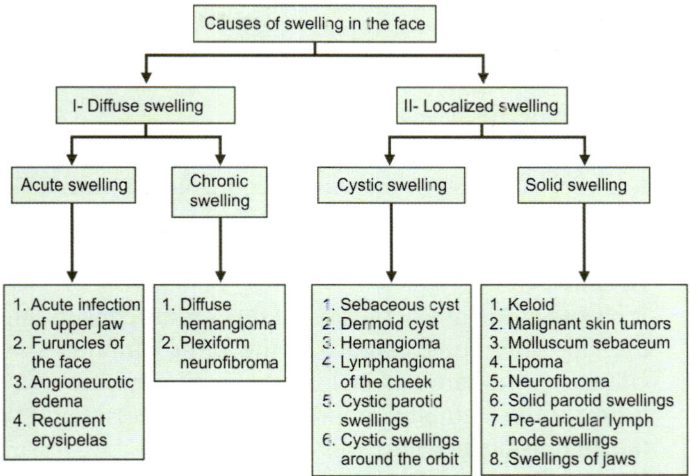

A. Acute Diffuse Swellings

1. *Acute infection of the upper jaws:* It is the commonest as a result of apical infection or after tooth extraction. Pain is marked, temperature is high, the swelling is diffuse and edema may close the eyes.
2. *Multiple furuncles of the face (furunculosis)* may lead to diffuse edema of the face.
3. *Angioneurotic edema* of the face is allergic in nature.
4. *Recurrent erysipelas:* It causes repeated attacks of swelling of the face particularly in the upper lip. The rosy red color, absence of lymph nodes, raised margins with vesicles at the periphery and desquamation may help to reach a diagnosis.

B. Chronic Diffuse Swellings

1. *Diffuse hemangioma.*
2. *Plexiform neurofibroma.*

II. LOCALIZED SWELLINGS

A. Cystic Swellings

1. **Sebaceous Cyst:**
   It is very common in the face of young adults with acne vulgaris, usually multiple. It is like a sebaceous anywhere else (page 7).
2. **Dermoid Cyst:**
   It occurs at the lines of fusion of the 5 parts constituting the face. The outer canthus is the most common site. Other sites are rare and include the inner canthus, at the fusion of the mandibular and maxillary processes and in the midline of the chin.
3. **Hemangioma:**
   It is either capillary or cavernous, in the skin and SC tissue, or mixed. Early onset, bluish coloration and compressibility are characteristic.
4. **Lymphangioma:**
   Uncommon. It causes thickening of the tissues of the cheek. It is translucent and does not empty on pressure.
5. **Cystic Swellings of the Parotid Gland (**Look later**).**
6. **Cystic Swellings Around the Orbit (Figure 1.5):**
   a. *External Angular (Sequestration) Dermoid Cyst*: The outer end of the eyebrow characteristically extends over the swelling, which distinguishes it from a swelling of the lacrimal gland. The skin is mobile over the swelling, which is partly mobile on the underlying structures. There is evident indentation of bones beneath the swelling. It is no compressible and its size does not $\uparrow$ on straining.

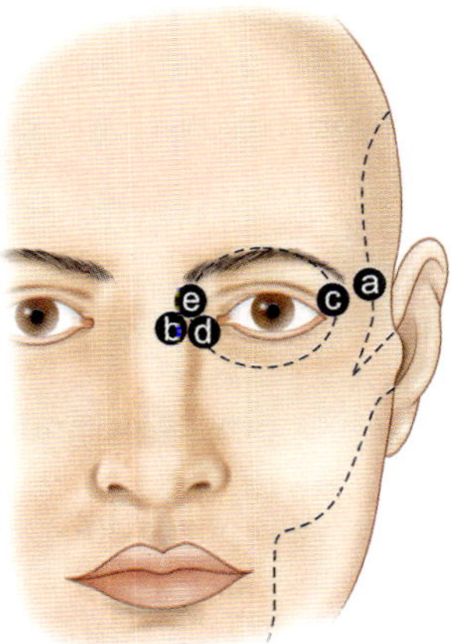

Fig. 1.5: Cystic swellings around the orbit

b. *Inner Angular Dermoid Cyst*: It is less common than the external angular dermoid. It lies over the root of the nose, in a more or less central position.
c. *Swellings of Lacrimal Glands*: The lacrimal gland may be the seat of a tumor (similar to salivary gland tumors) or Mickulicz disease. Its position is more medial to the site of the external angular dermoid.
d. *Swellings of the Lacrimal Sac*:
    - *Dacryocystitis* (lacrimal sac inflammation) causes swelling below and medial to the inner canthus.
    - *Mucocele of the lacrimal* sac is the result of blockage of the nasolacrimal duct. It results in a cystic swelling between the root of the nose and the inner canthus, accompanied by lacrimation. There is usually a history of recurrent inflammation.
e. *Mucocele of the Frontal Sinus*:
    - It results from frontonasal duct blockage and lies just above and medial to the inner canthus.
    - If it enlarges more, it displaces the globe.

B. Solid Swellings

1. **Keloid**
   - The lesion is elevated above the skin surface and is devoid of hair.
   - It is unsightly, tender and usually itchy.
   - Firm in consistency.
   - Pinkish in color in its early states, but later on it becomes pale.
   - May give claw-like processes and the margin is ill defined.
   - Usually occurs at sites of previous scars, abscesses, or tuberculous sinuses.
   - It is more common in Negroes, tuberculous patients, and pregnant women.
2. **Malignant Skin Tumors (**look later)
   - Basal cell carcinoma (BCC).
   - Squamous cell carcinoma (SCC).
   - Malignant melanoma.
   - Mycosis fungoides.
   - Metastatic carcinoma.
   - Malignant skin adnexal tumors.
3. **Lipoma:**
   - It is subcutaneous and is similar to lipoma elsewhere
   - It is usually attached to the overlying skin by strands causing dimpling of the skin
   - Freely mobile and soft in consistency
   - Surface is lobulated and the edge is slippery.
4. **Neurofibroma:**
   - Common in the supraorbital region and the face
   - It may be a firm nodule, fusiform in shape, along the course of a nerve, or it may occur in the form of a plexiform neuroma involving the skin and subcutaneous tissue

- The skin may be redundant, overhanging and pigmented
- Other neurofibromata and cafe au lait patches may be present (Neurofibromatosis).

5. **Solid Swellings of the Parotid Gland** (look later):
   - Chronic parotitis
   - Parotid tumors (benign - malignant)
   - Autoimmune diseases (Mikulicz and Sjogren's syndromes).
6. **Swellings of the Preauricular Lymph Nodes** (look later):
   - Inflammatory
   - Neoplastic
   - Miscellaneous.
7. **Swellings of the Jaw** (look later):
   - Epulides (tumors arising from the mucoperiosteum)
   - Odontomas (swellings derived from epithelial or mesothelial elements)
   - Bone swellings (Inflammatory—Neoplastic).

3. SWELLINGS OF THE LIPS

SURGICAL ANATOMY

- The lips are rich in connective tissue and massive edema can occur in some disorders such as trauma and cellulitis. They are also rich in mucus glands, and so mucus cysts can result from duct obstruction.
- Elasticity of the lip tissues allows removal of a large part of the lip and suturing the remaining parts with minimal postoperative deformity.
- **Arteries**: The labial arteries are branches of the facial arteries (they are closer to the mucus membrane rather than the skin). Wounds of the lips bleed massively and heal quickly because of their rich blood supply.
- **Veins**: They drain into the facial veins. Infections of the lips may be complicated with cavernous sinus thrombosis since facial veins are connected to veins of the pterygoid plexus, which are connected to the cavernous sinus.
- **Lymphatics**: Those of the upper lip pass to the submandibular nodes, while those from the lower lip pass to both the submandibular and submental nodes. Some lymphatics from the angles of the lips pass to the pre-auricular lymph nodes (**Figure 1.6**)

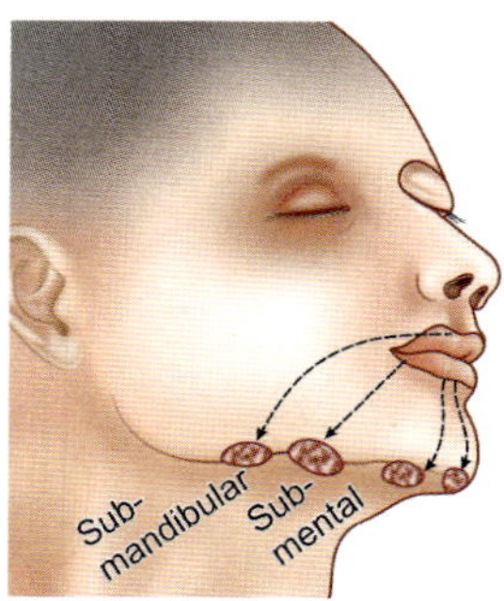

Fig. 1.6: Lymphatic drainage of the lips

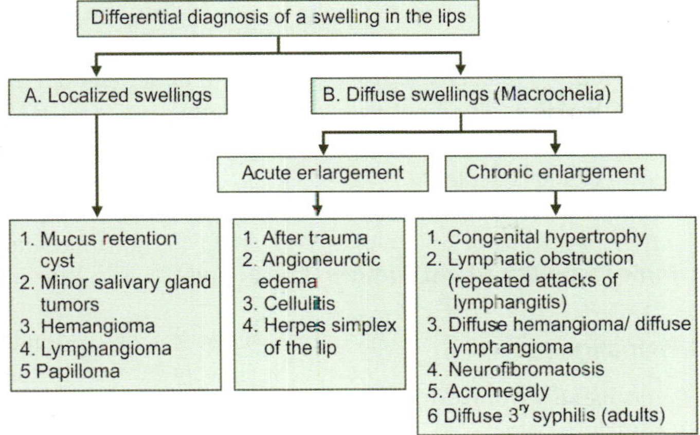

LOCALIZED SWELLINGS

1. Mucus Retention Cyst

- *Etiology*: It results from duct obstruction of one of the mucus glands or minor salivary glands.
- *Complaints*: Painless lump on the inner side of the lip. It may interfere with eating and may get bitten.
- *Site*: Most common on the lower lip (**Figure 1.7**) and in the buccal mucus membranes at the level of the bite of teeth.

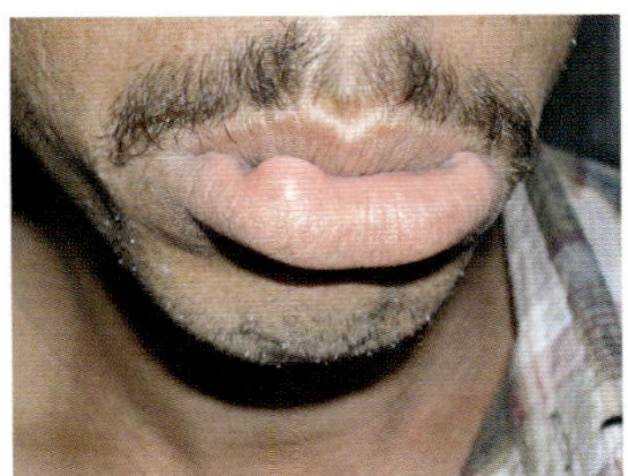

Fig. 1.7: Mucus retention cyst of the lower lip

- *Color*: Pale pink, but if the overlying epithelium has been frequently damaged, it looks white and scarred.
- *Shape and Size:* Spherical, approximately 0.5-2 cm in diameter.

- *Surface*: Smooth.
- *Consistency*: Soft or tense.
- *Fluctuation and Transillumination:* Can be detected if the cyst can be grasped between the 2 fingers.
- *Relations*: Not fixed to the overlying mucus membrane or underlying muscle.
- *Lymph Nodes:* Not enlarged (and local tissues are normal).

2. Minor Salivary Gland Tumors (Look Later)

3. Hemangioma

- It is usually a cavernous hemangioma.
- Bluish in color.
- Compressible.

4. Lymphangioma

- Uncommon.
- It causes thickening of the tissues of the lips.
- Translucent but does not empty on pressure.

5. Papilloma

- A benign lesion covered with mucus membrane.
- Pedunculated.
- Soft or firm in consistency.

4. SWELLINGS OF THE TONGUE

CAUSES OF ACUTE SWELLINGS OF THE TONGUE

1. A bite or sting.
2. Injury, for instance by a fish-bone, or by biting during an epileptic fit.
3. Corrosion or acute irritant applications.
4 Acute edema secondary to:
    - Inflammatory conditions such as glossitis, or stomatitis.
    - The effect of certain drugs such as mercury, and rarely, aspirin.
    - Erythema bullosum or pemphigus.
    - Serum injections and other conditions liable to cause giant urticaria.
    - Angioneurotic edema of the tongue (rare but important because it may, rarely, prove fatal due to suffocation).
    - Hemorrhage into the tongue substance, as in scurvy, leukemia and other hemorrhagic states.

CAUSES OF CHRONIC OR PERSISTENT SWELLING OF THE TONGUE

Localized Swellings	Diffuse Swellings (Macroglossia)
A. Cystic Swellings:	
1. Retention mucus cyst 2. Sublingual (dermoid cyst - ranula) 3. Thyroglossal cyst (at foramen cecum) 4. Hemangioma 5. Chronic abscess	1. Diffuse cavernous hemangioma 2. Arteriovenous fistula 3. Multiple lymphangiomas 4. Multiple neurofibromatosis 5. Congenital Causes: a. Cretinism (muscle hypertrophy) b. Mongolism c. Glycogen storage disease

Contd...

Contd..

6. Softened gumma or TB nodule 7. Hydatid cyst 8. Blood cyst	6. Endocrinal Causes: a. Myxedema b. Acromegaly 7. Primary Amyloidosis (amyloid infiltration) 8. Diffuse carcinoma 9. Chronic diffuse syphilitic glossitis
B. Solid Swellings: 1. Neurofibroma 2. Papilloma 3. Lingual thyroid 4. Carcinoma (usually an ulcer) 5. Sarcoma (if degenerated it → cystic)	

Tumors of the Tongue

Origin	Benign Tumors	Malignant Tumors
A. *Epithelial*	*Papilloma* Small elevated or pedunculated firm swelling, which is precancerous and\ should be excised and biopsied.	1. Epithelioma (SSC) 2. Lymphoepithelioma 3. Adenocarcinoma 4. Basal cell carcinoma (BCC)
B. Mesenchymal	1. Cavernous hemangioma 2. Lymphangioma 3. Neurofibroma 4. Fibroma 5. Lipoma (very rare)	1. Fibrosarcoma 2. Lymphosarcoma 3. Hemangioendothelioma 4. Rhabdomyosarcoma
C. *Salivary Glands*	Mixed salivary gland tumor	Malignant salivary gland tumors
D. *Thyroid Origin*	Lingual thyroid	Malignancy in remnants of thyroid tissue

5. SWELLINGS OF THE ORAL CAVITY

SWELLINGS IN THE FLOOR OF THE MOUTH

A. Cysts of the Floor of the Mouth

1. **Retention Mucus Cysts:**
   - Result from obstruction of the ducts of the sublingual salivary glands.
   - Multiple.
   - Small.
   - Translucent.

2. Ranula:
   - It is a large mucus retention cyst in the floor of the mouth (In Latin, ranula = a small frog).
   - *Age:* It affects children and young adults.
   - *Sex*: Both sexes are equally affected.
   - *Complaints*: A swelling in the floor of the mouth. It usually ruptures and refills again.
   - *Clinical Examination*:

     Physical examination of the ranula reveals the following characteristic features that differentiates it from "subligual dermoid cyst":
     - A small spherical cyst (only the top 1/2 is seen), about 1–5 cm in size, in the floor of the mouth, between the symphysis menti and the tongue, just to one side of the midline (**Figure 1.8**).
     - It may extend into the submandibular triangle (*plunging or deep cervical ranula*).
     - The cyst is characteristically translucent and has a bluish tinge.
     - It is smooth and covered by tortuous veins, and the submandibular duct is displaced and stretched over it.

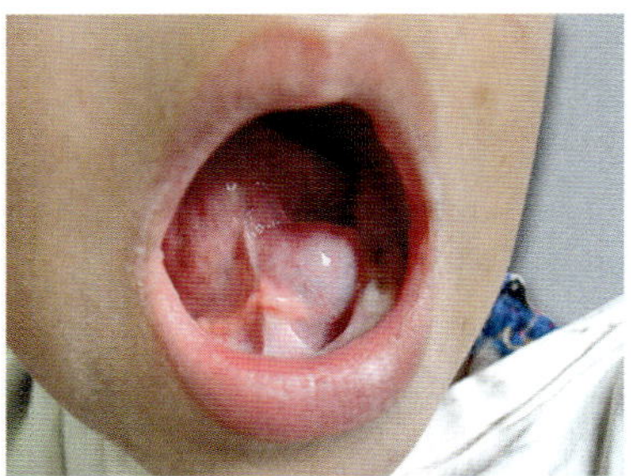

Fig. 1.8: Ranula between the symphysis menti and tongue

- The edge is difficult to feel and the cyst is soft but cannot be compressed or reduced.

3. **Sublingual Dermoid Cyst:**

- *Age:* Usually between 10–25 years.
- *Sex:* Both sexes are equally affected.
- *Complaints:*
  A swelling under the tongue, which becomes painful and tender if it gets infected.
- *Clinical Examination:*
  Physical examination reveals the following characteristic features:
  - A smooth, clearly defined, spherical swelling.
  - About 2–5 cm in size
  - Lying in the midline between the tongue and the inner surface of the chin **(Figure 1.9)**
  - It may bulge into the submental triangle of the neck below the chin (**Figure 1.10**)
  - The mucous membrane appears normal
  - It can be felt bimanually (with one finger in the mouth and the other beneath the chin)
  - It is characteristically opaque and fluctuant.

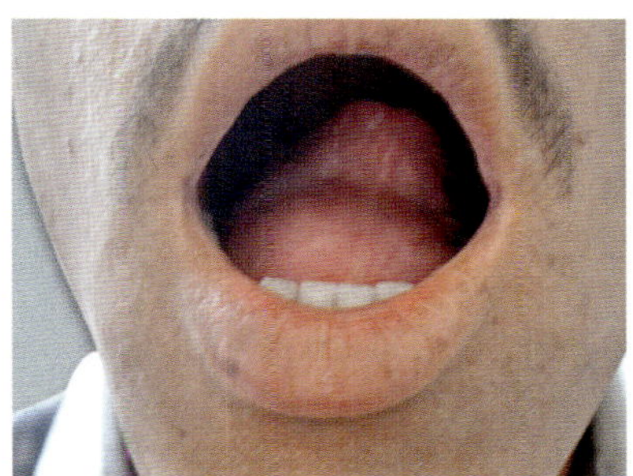

Fig. 1.9: Sublingual dermoid cyst in the midline

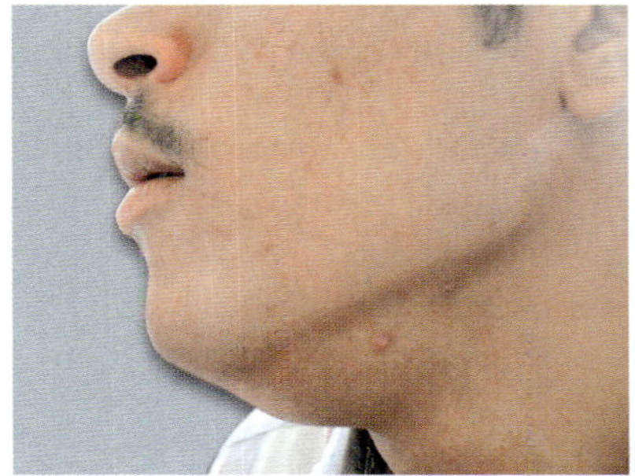

Fig. 1.10: It is bulging into the submental triangle

B. Solid Swellings of the Floor of the Mouth

1. **Minor Salivary Gland Tumors:**
   - Firm, lobulated mass that increases in size with eating.
2. **Stone in the Submandibular Salivary Duct:**
   - Felt as a hard swelling along the line of the edematous duct.
   - The patient C/O of a swelling in the submandibular region during meals (which is the distended gland).

3. Papilloma:
- It occurs in relation to a bad tooth in children.
- Sessile, or pedunculated, with a smooth surface.

4. Epithelioma of the Floor of the Mouth:
- Swelling (or ulcer) with bloody salivation and foul discharge.
- Cervical lymph nodes may be enlarged and hard.

SWELLINGS IN THE PALATE

A. From the Mucosa

1. *Ectopic Salivary Gland Tumor:*
   - The palate is the most frequent site **(Figure 1.11)**.
   - At first it is symptomless, but when it ulcerates it becomes painful.
   - A large portion of these tumors is of low-grade malignancy (cylindroma) and may ultimately metastasize to regional lymph nodes, viscera and skeleton.
   - Locally, it may invade the base of the skull and affect certain cranial nerves causing severe pain in their distribution.
   - Mixed tumors also occur.

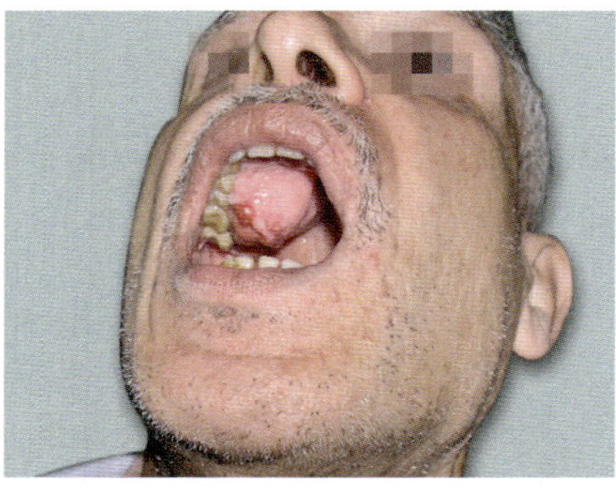

Fig. 1.11: Mixed salivary tumor of the hard palate

2. *Squamous Cell Carcinoma:*
   It can arise in the epithelium of the hard palate, or the soft palate. Inability to wear an upper denture is sometimes the first symptom.
3. *Retention mucus Cyst:*
   It is bluish in color and translucent.
4. *Gumma (Syphilis):*
   A firm, painless swelling, which ulcerates, resulting in the typical gummatous ulcer.
5. *Rare Tumors:*
   Neurofibroma.
   Lipoma.
   Hemangioma.

B. Extension From

1. *Carcinoma of the Maxillary Sinus* invading (or depressing) the palate.
2. *Cyst of the Jaw,* example dental cysts bulging medially into the palate close to the alveolar border.

6. SWELLINGS OF THE JAW

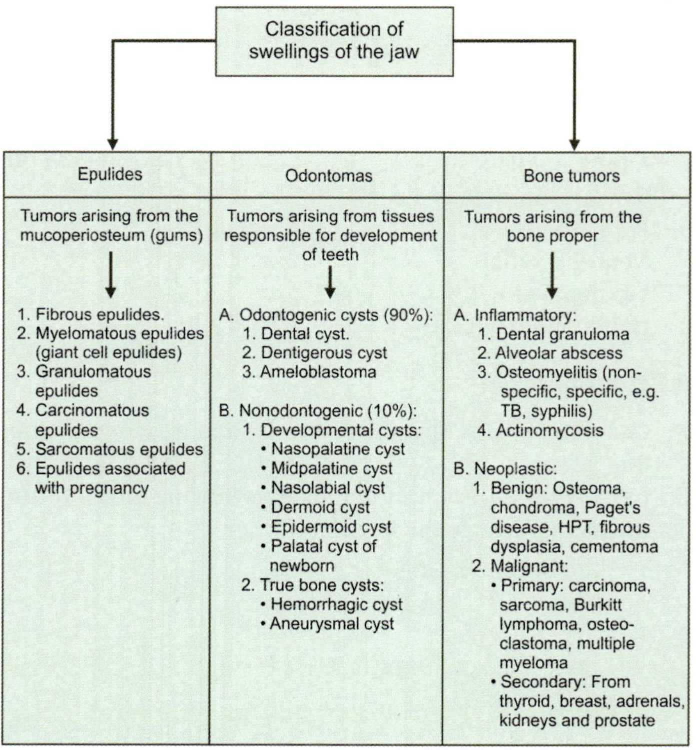

Classification of swellings of the jaw

Epulides	Odontomas	Bone tumors
Tumors arising from the mucoperiosteum (gums)	Tumors arising from tissues responsible for development of teeth	Tumors arising from the bone proper
1. Fibrous epulides. 2. Myelomatous epulides (giant cell epulides) 3. Granulomatous epulides 4. Carcinomatous epulides 5. Sarcomatous epulides 6. Epulides associated with pregnancy	A. Odontogenic cysts (90%): 1. Dental cyst. 2. Dentigerous cyst 3. Ameloblastoma B. Nonodontogenic (10%): 1. Developmental cysts: • Nasopalatine cyst • Midpalatine cyst • Nasolabial cyst • Dermoid cyst • Epidermoid cyst • Palatal cyst of newborn 2. True bone cysts: • Hemorrhagic cyst • Aneurysmal cyst	A. Inflammatory: 1. Dental granuloma 2. Alveolar abscess 3. Osteomyelitis (non-specific, specific, e.g. TB, syphilis) 4. Actinomycosis B. Neoplastic: 1. Benign: Osteoma, chondroma, Paget's disease, HPT, fibrous dysplasia, cementoma 2. Malignant: • Primary: carcinoma, sarcoma, Burkitt lymphoma, osteoclastoma, multiple myeloma • Secondary: From thyroid, breast, adrenals, kidneys and prostate

I. EPULIDES

Definition

Swellings arising from the mucoperiosteum are known as epulides (Any solid swelling situated in the gums). It may affect the lower jaw or upper jaw **(Figure 1.12)** and may reach a huge size as shown in **Figure 1.13**.

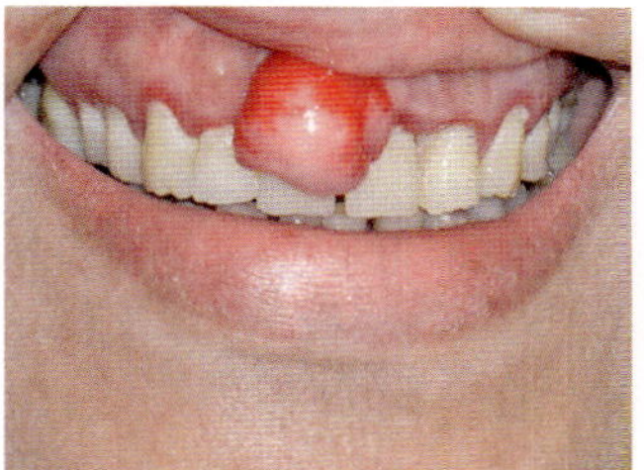

Fig. 1.12: Epulides between incisors of the upper jaw

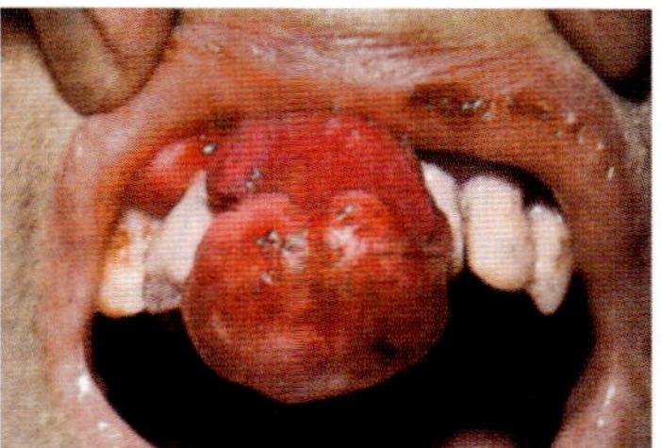

Fig. 1.13: Epulides between incisors of the upper jaw reaching a large size

Fibrous Epulides

- *Site:* Usually between incisor teeth of the lower jaw **(Figure 1.14)**.
- *Age and Sex:* Middle age - Females > males (3:1).
- *Clinical Picture*:
  - It is first sessile and then becomes pedunculated.
  - Whitish in color (diminished vascularity simulating fibroma).
  - Firm in consistency and covered by intact mucosa.
- *Types:*
  1. Fibroangiomatous: It bleeds easily on touch.
  2. Fibrosarcomatous: Due to malignant transformation.
  3. Congenital epulides: Present since birth.

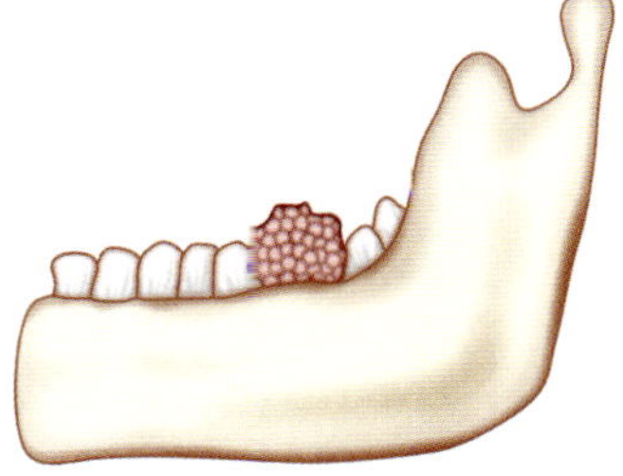

Fig. 1.14: Fibrous epulides between incisor teeth of the lower jaw

Myelomatous Epulides (Giant Cell Epulides)

- *Site:* Peripherally, in the jaw (mandible and maxilla) (**Figure 1.15**).

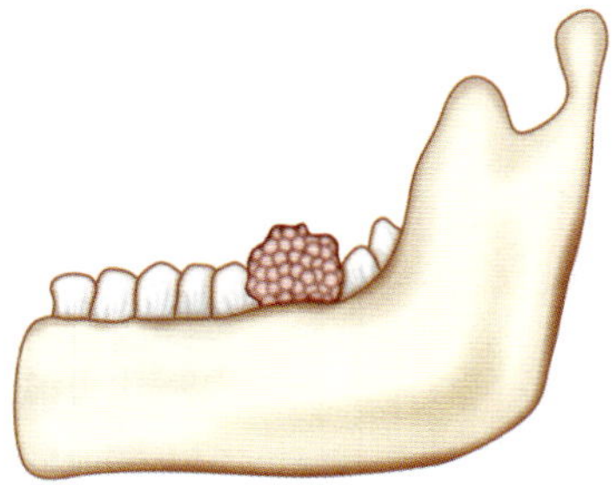

Fig. 1.15: Myelomatous epulides situated peripherally in the lower jaw

- *Age:* 30–40 years, but can occur at any age.
- *Clinical Picture*:
  - Rapidly growing, bulky, red mass.
  - Sessile and lobulated.
  - Painless.
  - Covered with intact mucosa that bleeds on touch (very vascular).
  - Fixed to the underlying tissues.
- Liable to necrosis, ulceration, cyst formation and malignant transformation.
- *Plain X-ray:*
  Eating up of the jaw under the tumor.

Granulomatous Epulides

- It is a mass of granulation tissue formed around a carious tooth or gingivitis **(Figure 1.16)**.
- *Clinical Picture:*
  - Soft.
  - Red
  - Lobulated mass

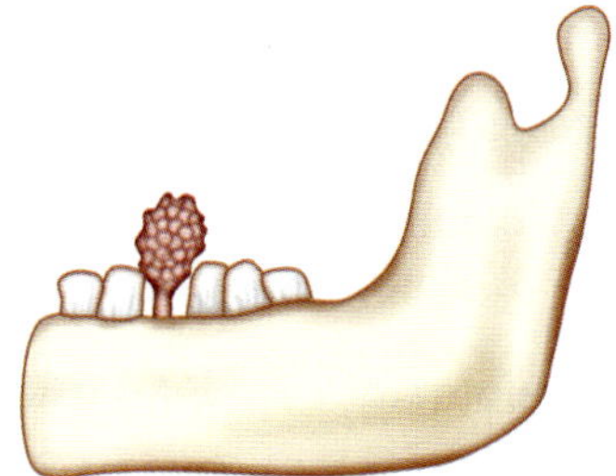

Fig. 1.16: Granulomatous epulides

- Bleeds easily on touch.
- It is not covered with mucosa.

Carcinomatous Epulides

- *Origin:* It is now considered as an "alveolar carcinoma" arising from the mucus membrane covering the gum (squamous epithelium).
- *Clinical Picture and Diagnosis:*
  - Painful, infected, fungating or ulcerating mass with indurated base and hard cervical lymph nodes. It invades the bone.
  - *Biopsy* is a must for diagnosis.

Sarcomatous Epulides

- *Age:* Middle age.
- *Sex:* Males > Females.
- *Clinical Picture*:
  - A sessile mass which may be fixed to the underlying jaw.
  - It may be hard, firm or soft (denotes degeneration or high-grade malignancy).
  - Ulceration and bleeding occur later.
- *Plain X-ray*: May show bone infiltration.

Epulides Associated with Pregnancy

- *Cause:* Increased estrogen + bad oral hygiene (in 25% of pregnant women).
- *Site:* In relation to the posterior teeth, especially the upper jaw.
- *Clinical Picture:* There is hypertrophy of the gums, with tendency to bleed.

II. ODONTOMAS

Definition

- Odontomas are swellings derived from epithelial or mesothelial elements which take part in the development of teeth.
- They are either *odontogenic* (90%) or *nonodontogenic* (10%).

Main Types

1. Dental (Radicular or Subapical) Cysts.
2. Dentigerous (Follicular) Cysts.
3. Ameloblastoma (Adamantinoma).

1. Dental (Radicular or Subapical) Cysts

2. Dentigerous (Follicular) Cysts

Both types show a slowly growing, painless swelling, hard in consistency (covered by bone), expanding the bone internally and externally resulting in an *"egg-shell crackling sensation"*.

Criteria	1. Dental (Radicular) Cysts (Figure 1.17)	2. Dentigerous (Follicular) Cysts (Figure 1.18)
Site	Upper jaw > lower jaw.	Lower jaw > upper jaw
Age	Middle age (30–40 years)	Younger age (7–25 years)
Clinical Picture	Smaller in size Clear fluid inside rich in cholesterol Overlying tooth is present	Larger in size. Viscid fluid inside + missed tooth Overlying tooth is absent
Plain X-ray	Clear cavity with evident outline + cholesterol crystals. No tooth inside the cavity.	No cholesterol crystals. Tooth inside the cavity.

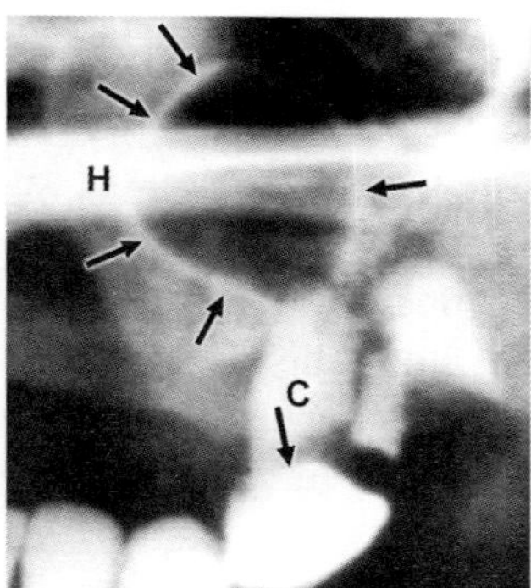

Fig. 1.17: Regular, well-circumscribed lucent lesion (arrows). The involved tooth has growth caries (C). The shadow of the hard palate (H) is superimposed across the cyst

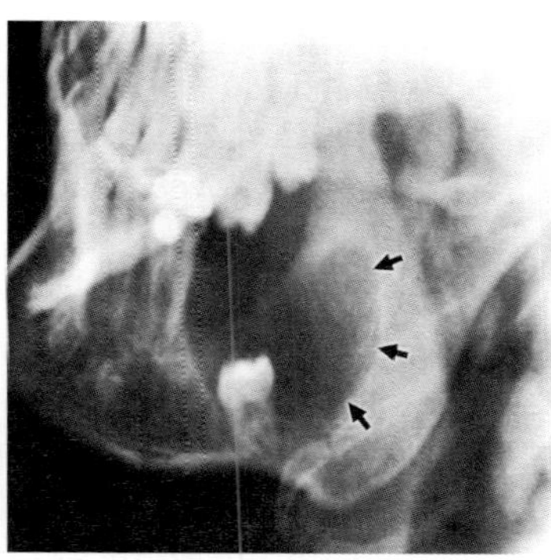

Fig. 1.18: Smooth, well-circumscribed lucent cavity (arrows) containing the crown of an unerupted tooth

3. Adamantinoma (Ameloblastoma = Multilocular Cyst):

- *Origin*: It is an epithelial tumor arising from the ameloblasts (epithelial debris of Malassez) or it is a sort of BCC from the basal cells of the dental epithelium.
- *Sites*: The angle of the mandible is the commonest site, but it grows forwards to the body of the mandible, and/or upwards to the ascending ramus of the mandible.
- *Age and Sex:* Adults (30-40 years), but may occur at a younger age - *Sex:* Females > Males (9:1).
- *Clinical Picture:*
  1. A chronic *painless* swelling at the angle of mandible (or maxilla) (5:1).
  2. Well-defined, lobulated, expanding the jaw externally > internally ± ulceration of the mucus membrane and loosening of the overlying tooth or teeth.

3. Hard in consistency, but may have an egg-shell crackling sensation due to degeneration.
   - *Investigations*:
   - *Plain X-ray:* Fine soap and bubble or honey-comb appearance.
   - *Biopsy* is essential for diagnosis.
   - *Differential Diagnosis*: It should be differentiated from "osteoclastoma" which has a fine and coarse soap and bubble appearance on X-ray (**Figure 1.19**).
   - *Complications*: Ulceration, loosening of teeth, pathological fracture and recurrence after removal.

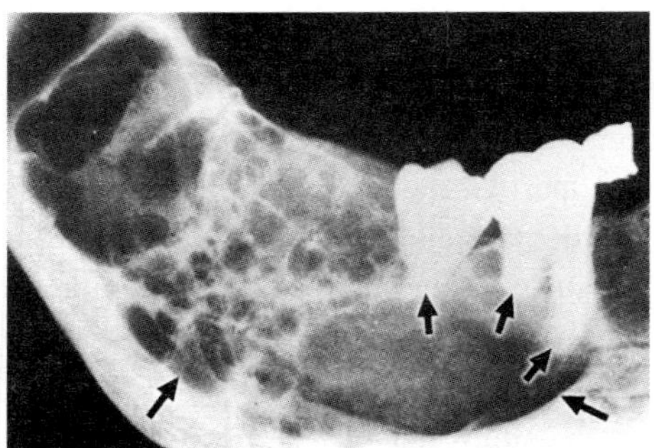

Fig. 1.19: PXR of an excised specimen showing a lesion extending from the molar region to the superior portion of the ramus (upper left). Note multilocularity of the lesion, the well-defined margins (large arrows), and resorption of tooth root (small arrows).

III. TUMORS ARISING FROM THE BONE

A. Inflammatory		B. Neoplastic	
	(a) Benign Tumors	(b) Malignant Tumors (M.Ts)	
		Primary M.Ts.	Secondary M.Ts
1. Dental granuloma. 2. Alveolar abscess. 3. Osteomyelitis (specific, non-specific). 4. Actinomycosis.	1. Osteoma 2. Chondroma 3. Paget's disease 4. Hyperparathyroidism 5. Benign fibro-osseous lesions (Fibrous dysplasia, cementoma) 6. Others (Hemangioma, peripheral nerve tumors, fibroma).	1. Carcinoma: (adenocarcinoma, SSC, lympho-epithelioma) 2. Sarcoma: (Osteogenic sarcoma, Chondro-sarcoma, Fibro-sarcoma, Ewings sarcoma,..) 3. Lymphoma (Burkitt's) 4. Osteoclastoma 5. Multiple myeloma	From cancer: 1. Thyroid 2. Breast 3. Adrenal glands 4. Kidneys 5. Prostate

A. INFLAMMATORY

Dental Granuloma

- It may occur in the form of a giant cell granuloma, which represents a failure of an attempt at repair of a hematoma of the jaw.
- It affects females > males, below the age of 20 years.
- PXR (occlusal view) demonstrates an expansile radiolucency in the anterior portion of the mandible producing even, regular swelling of the buccal cortical plate (arrows) and intrusion of a canine tooth (C) **(Figure 1.20)**.

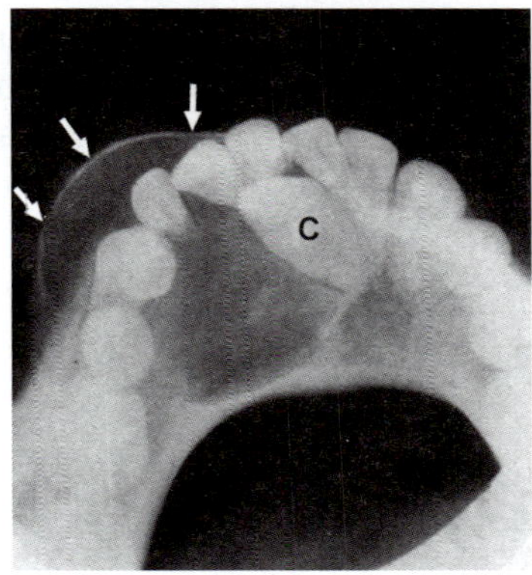

Fig. 1.20: Giant cell granuloma

Alveolar (Dental) Abscess

- It is an abscess that occurs in the socket of the tooth (alveolus).
- *Age:* It can develop at any age, with the 1st or 2nd dentition (common in childhood and early adult life).
- *Symptoms:* Pain (throbbing) + swelling (painful) + malaise, sweating and anorexia.
- *Examination:* Hot, tender, reddish (hyperemic) swelling with an ill-defined edge (merging into the surrounding tissues). Large abscesses may fluctuate. The mass is clearly fixed to, and feels as if it is part of the underlying bone. Upper cervical lymph nodes are enlarged and tender.
- Plain X-ray shows rarefaction of the bone around the apex of the affected tooth.

Osteomyelitis

- *Types*: It may be acute, or chronic (specific or non-specific).
- *Clinical Picture*:
  - *History* of tooth extraction - long duration.
  - *Swelling*: Painful, warm bony in consistency, nodular surface, border gradually merges into normal bone, expansion may affect one side only or both.
  - Tenderness ± edema, redness and hotness.
  - Trismus may be present.
  - Draining lymph nodes are enlarged and painful.
  - Sinus and/or abscess may be present. Delayed sequestrum formation and delayed healing result from improper rest (continuous motility of the jaw) and recurrent infection from the mouth.

Cervicofacial Actinomycosis

- Very long history, in an adult male.
- Common at the angle of the jaw.

- Nodular, tender, warm, and fixed to the skin, with multiple sinuses and sulfur granules.
- Trismus is commonly present.

B. NEOPLASTIC

Benign Tumors (Osteoma, Chondroma)

- Tumors of this group are composed of varying proportions of fibrous tissue and bone.
- It is hard in consistency if made mainly of bone, or firm if made mainly from fibrous tissue. Myxomatous degeneration causes softening in some parts.
- The condition can be localized or diffuse.
- Osteoma and chondroma are hard, well-defined swellings that grow slowly.
- *PXR:* Dense well-defined bone (osteoma) or a mottled appearance (chondroma).

Paget's Disease

- It occurs in elderly patients.
- It is characterized by preliminary softening and bending of the bones, followed by recalcification.
- Bones become enormously thickened. The jaw may be the first site of bone thickening.

Hyperparathyroidism (HPT) (Generalized Osteitis Fibrosa)

- It is a rare condition sometimes associated with HPT due to adenoma or hyperplasia.
- There is widespread resorption of the skeleton resulting in softening and bending of bones.
- PXR shows ↓ density, areas of fibrocystic formation, and presence of bone cysts.
- Diagnosis is clinched by ↑ serum Ca^{++} and urinary Ca^{++} output, ↓ plasma phosphorus and ↑ plasma phosphatase.

Carcinoma of the Maxilla

Origin and Anatomy: It arises from the "*Maxillary Antrum*", which is *pyramidal* in shape:

- *Base*: Lateral wall of the nose.
- *Apex*: Zygomatic process of the maxilla.
- *Floor*: Alveolar part of the maxilla.
- *Roof*: Floor of the orbit.

Clinical Picture

- The clinical presentation depends on the site and direction of growth of the tumor:
  - Anterior and Lateral Wall → Swelling of the face and cheek.
  - Medial Wall → Nasal obstruction, anosmia, epiphora (infiltration of the naso-lacrimal duct).
  - Posterior Wall → Nasopharynx → dyspnea and change of voice.
  - Roof → Proptosis + diplopia.
  - Floor → Bulging of the hard palate.
- It may present with pain in the region of the maxilla (referred to upper teeth) due to blockage and infection of the antrum, and lately due to involvement of branches of the trigeminal nerve.
- The primary tumor may be occult and present with enlarged lymph nodes in the neck.

Investigations

- Plain X-ray: Soft tissue shadow in the antrum and signs of bone destruction.
- Biopsy.

Sarcoma of the Maxilla

Characteristics

It differs from carcinoma in the following:

- It affects a younger age group and females > males.
- It has a shorter history with more pain.
- It causes worse general condition and has a worse prognosis.

Clinical Features

- Painful swelling in the face + loosening of teeth.
- Blocking of the nose + epistaxis.
- Fetor oris and increased salivation.
- Skin overlying the swelling is stretched, glistening, and shows dilated veins.

Investigations

- Plain X-ray shows clouding of the sinuses + bone destruction.
- Chest X-ray for detection of secondaries.

Burkitt's Lymphoma

Age: 2–14 years.

Geographical Distribution

- Children of the "equatorial" regions of Africa.

Clinical Picture

- Jaw tumors (50%) in the mandible or maxilla (**Figure 1.21**) (osteolytic lesions).
- Abdominal tumor (in the 2nd most common presentation).
- Renal involvement (usually bilateral).
- In girls, involvement of the ovaries is characteristic.
- Involvement of the nervous system.

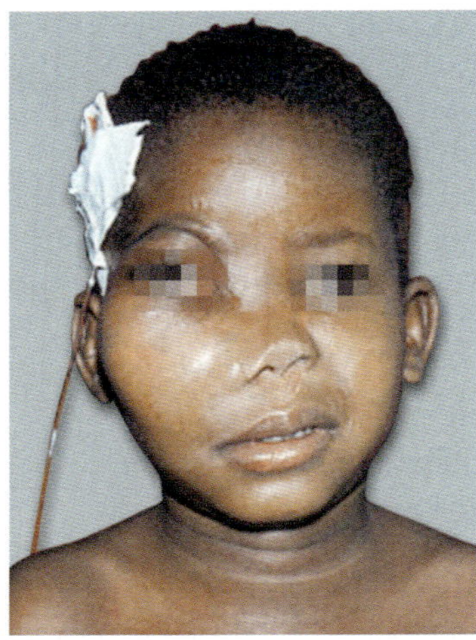

Fig. 1.21: Burkitt's lymphoma

Plain X-ray

- It shows multiple osteolytic deposits with bone destruction.

Osteoclastoma (Giant Cell Tumor)

- It is a *locally malignant tumor*.
- *Age:* It usually affects adults (20–40 years).
- *Sex:* Men are more affected than women.
- *Site*
  - Lower end of the femur.
  - Upper end of the humerus.
  - Lower end of the radius.
  - Upper end of the tibia.
  - Clavicle.
  - It may also affect the ***mandible***, and rarely the ***maxilla***.
- It does not cross the midline (symphysis menti).
- It grows gradually with *no metastases*.

- It may attain a large size causing dull aching pain. On examination, it may be hot and tender.

Differential Diagnosis

It should be differentiated from:

1. Ameloblastoma (Adamantinoma):
   It is similar to adamantinoma, with the following differences:

Criteria	Adamantinoma	Osteoclastoma
Site of origin	Near the angle of the mandible	Near the symphysis menti
Growth Direction	Upwards and forwards, and may cross the symphysis menti	Backwards in the body of mandible, but never crosses the S. menti
Rate of Growth	Slowly growing	Rapidly growing
Age	4th and 5th decades	Adolescents or 20–40 years
Sex	Females > males (9:1)	Males > Females
Clinical Findings	Not hot and not tender	Hotter, more tender and painful
Shape of Tumor	Lobulations (may be equal)	Variable lobulations (coarse and fine)
Jaw Expansion	External > Internal	Equal on both sides
Color	Pale or pink	Reddish or brownish (more vascular)
Plain X-ray	Fine soap bubbles	Coarse and fine soap bubbles
Special Character	Radioresistant	Radiosensitive (post-operative radiotherapy)

2. Other Giant Cell Lesions

- Giant Cell Granuloma:
  - It represents a failure of an attempt at repair of a hematoma of the jaw.

- It affects females > males, below the age of 20 years.
- Perforation of the cortex is very rare.

- Brown Tumor of Hyperparathryroidism:
  - The jaw may be affected due to generalized bone affection (*von Recklinghausen's Disease*).
  - The *brown* coloration is due to hemorrhage inside the lesion.

7. SWELLINGS OF SALIVARY GLANDS

I. PAROTID GLAND

Swelling in the Parotid Region

Tissue of Origin	Causes of the Swelling
1. Skin	1. Benign tumor, e.g. papilloma 2. Cyst, e.g. sebaceous cyst 3. Malignant tumor, e.g. SCC, BCC, malignant melanoma, etc.
2. SC Tissues	1. Benign tumor: Lipoma - Fibroma - Neurofibroma - Hemangioma 2. Cyst, e.g. dermoid cyst 3. Malignant tumor: sarcomas
3. Parotid L.Ns	1. Chronic Nonspecific Lymphadenitis 2. Chronic Specific Lymphadenitis, e.g. T.B 3. Malignancy, e.g. secondaries or lymphoma
4. Parotid Gland	1. Chronic parotitis 2. Parotid cyst 3. Parotid tumor (Benign - Malignant) 4. Autoimmune diseases (Mikulicz and Sjogren's syndromes)
5. Masseter Muscle	1. Fibrosarcoma 2. Rhabdomyosarcoma 3. Myxoma of the masseter 4. Hypertrophied muscle
6. Ramus of Mandible	1. Osteomyelitis 2. Cysts: Adamantinoma, dental cysts 3. Osteoclastoma 4. Secondaries 5. Winged mandible (Treacher Collins syndrome)
7. Mucosa of Cheek	Squamous Cell Carcinoma
8. Others	1. Branchial cyst 2. Neuroma of the facial nerve 3. Thrombosis of the facial vein 4. Aneurysm of the temporal artery 5. Mastoiditis.

CLINICAL CLASSIFICATION

A swelling in the *parotid region* may be *acute or chronic,* and *cystic or solid.*

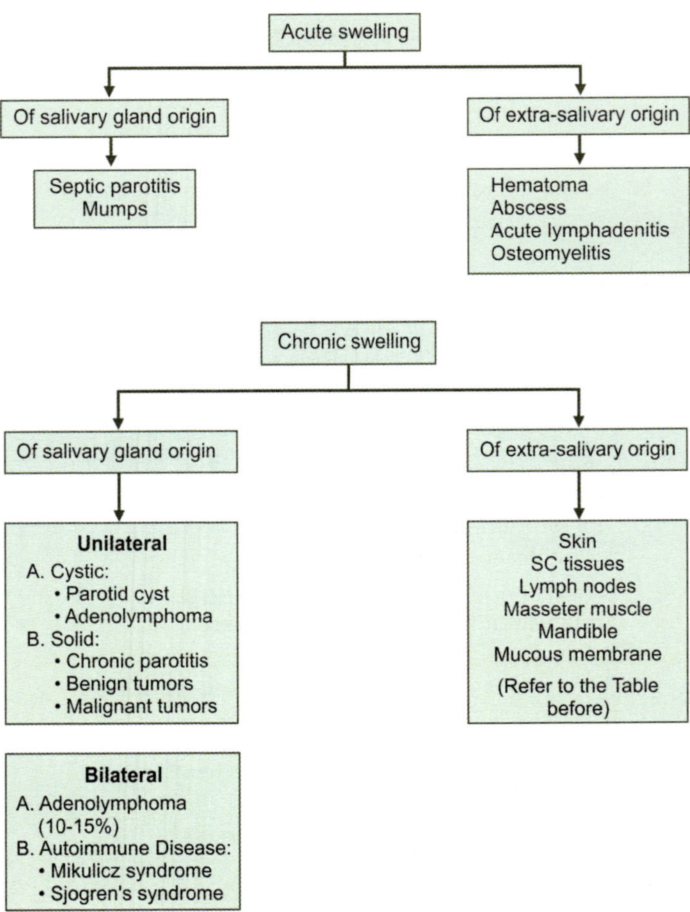

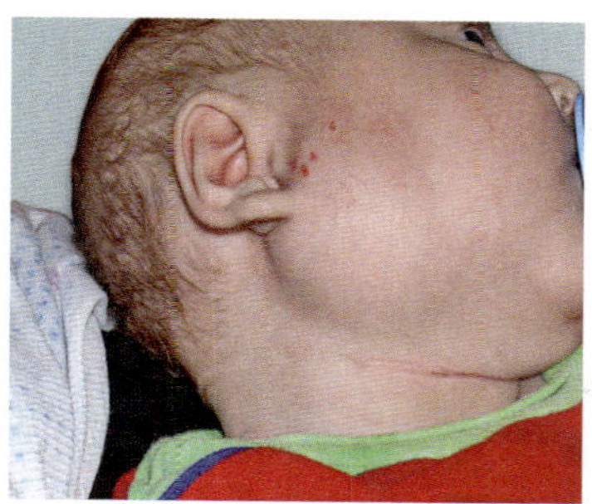

Fig. 1.22: A child with mumps

ACUTE SWELLINGS IN THE PAROTID REGION

Swellings of Salivary Origin

1. *Mumps (Viral infection)*:
   - It affects young children **(Figure 1.22)** and is usually bilateral.
   - It is preceded by a prodromal influenza-like syndrome.
   - The gland is painful, tender, with edema of the face and difficulty of mastication.
   - The temperature is slightly elevated, with mild constitutional symptoms.
   - It may complicate (in adults and in girls) leading to orchitis, oophoritis and pancreatitis.
   - It is self-limited and never suppurates.
2. *Acute Parotitis*:
   - It affects elderly males and infants, and is usually unilateral.
   - It is very painful and tender.
   - Pus can be expressed from the orifice of the duct.
   - Cervical lymph nodes may be enlarged and tender.
   - The temperature is slightly elevated with marked constitutional manifestations.
   - Complications include fistula formation, chronicity, local spread (cellulitis), systemic spread (septicemia).

Pus may rupture into the external auditory meatus, or burrow along the carotid sheath.

CHRONIC SWELLINGS IN THE PAROTID REGION

Swellings of Salivary (Parotid) Gland Origin

Unilateral Cystic Lesions

1. **Parotid Cyst (Figure 1.23):**
   Criteria of diagnosis of a parotid cyst are:
   - Translucency: Parotid cysts are translucent.
   - Duct examination: Presence of inflammatory signs or stone.
   - Aspiration and exam. of the aspirate by:
     - NEA: Clear (cyst) - turbid (infection) - pus (abscess) - hemorrhagic (cancer).
     - Ptyalin Reaction: Positive in the cyst.
     - Cytology: For malignant cells.
   - Radiological examination for detection of stones (PXR, sialography).

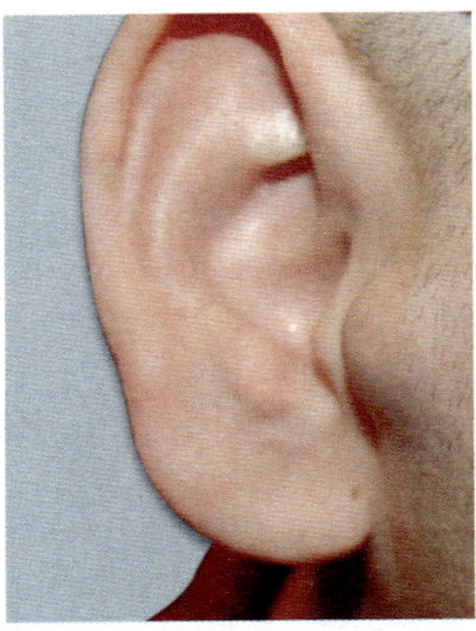

Fig. 1.23: A small right parotid cyst

2. **Adenolymphoma:**
   - It comprises about 5% of all parotid tumors.
   - It characteristically affects men more than women.
   - It is bilateral in 10-15% of cases, which constitutes 70% of bilateral parotid lesions.
   - It should be differentiated from mixed parotid tumors (pleomorphic adenoma) (refer to the Table below).

Unilateral Solid Lesions

1. **Chronic Parotitis:**
   - It is characterized by recurrent attacks of pain and swelling.
   - The gland is diffusely enlarged.
   - It may be bilateral (sialectasia).
   - Saliva may be turbid.
2. **Benign Tumors of the Parotid Gland**

Classification:

1. Pleomorphic Adenoma (Mixed salivary tumor) **(Figure 1.24)**:

   It accounts for 75% of parotid tumors, and may attain a large size without causing facial nerve palsy.

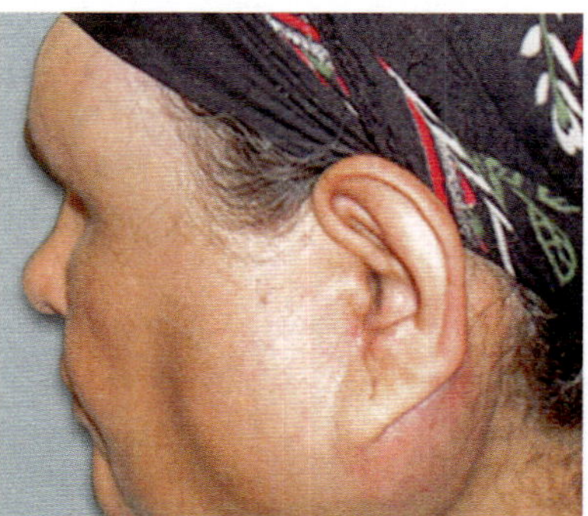

Fig. 1.24: A large pleomorphic adenoma of the left parotid gland in a 39-year-old lady

2. Monomorphic Adenoma:
   a. Adenolymphoma (= Warthin's Tumor = Papillary Cystadenoma Lymphomatosum).
   b. Acidophilic Adenoma (= Oxyphilic Adenoma = Oncocytoma = Mitochondrioma).
   c. Acinar Adenoma (= Serous Cell Adenoma).
3. Benign Mucoepidermoid Tumor.
4. Connective Tissue Tumors:
   a. Lipoma
   b. Fibroma
   c. Hemangioma
   d. Neurofibroma
   e. Others.

Differences between Pleomorphic Adenoma and Adenolymphoma (Warthin's Tumor)

Criteria	Pleomorphic Adenoma	Adenolymphoma
Incidence	75% of parotid tumors	5% of parotid tumors
Gland	Parotid, ± submandibular and minor glands	Almost exclusively in the parotid gland
Age	30–50 years	> 40 years
Sex	Females > Males (or equal)	Males > Females (8:1)
Bilaterality	Unilateral	Bilateral in 5–10% of cases (=70% of all bilateral parotid swellings)
Pathology		
Consistency	Heterogenous (variable)	Soft, may be cystic
Capsule	No true capsule	True capsule
Matrix	Pleomorphic	Full of lymphocytes (mainly B-cells)

Contd...

Contd..

Cut section	Not cystic	Cystic spaces line with columnar cells
C/P		
Site	Mostly begin anterior and superior to angle of jaw (for an unknown reason), but can occur in any part of the gland	Usually develops in lower part of parotid, level with lower border of mandible (lower than pleo. adenoma)
Size	Variable from pea-sized nodules to large masses, 20 cm across !	Small, usually 1-3 cm in diameter
Shape	Spherical when small, lobulated if large	Spherical or hemispherica
Surface	Smooth, sometimes bosselated and occasionally crossed by deep furrows	Smooth, and well-defined
Consistency	Variable	Soft, may be cystic
Relations	Mobile, not attached to overlying skin or deeper structures	Mobile *a little* in all directions, and usually not attached to the skin
Malignant Transform	5-10% (epithelium → duct carcinoma, CT → chondrosarcoma)	Exceptional but documented (epithelium → adeno or epidermoid carcinoma, and lymphoid component → lymphoma)
Treatment	Conservative parotidectomy to avoid recurrence (there is no true capsule)	Resection enucleation, or conservative parotidectomy

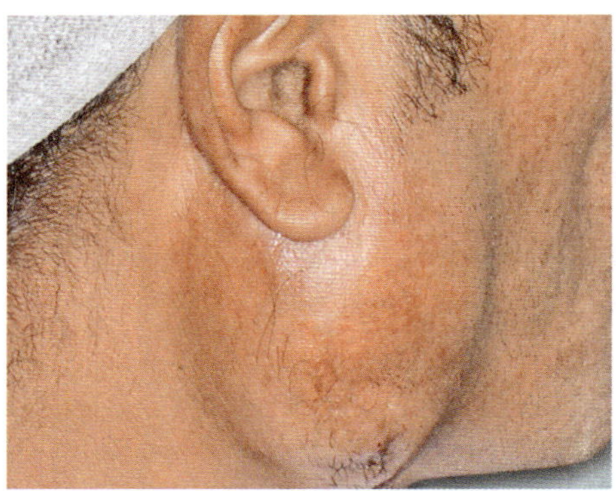

Fig. 1. 25: Large right parotid carcinoma

3. Malignant Tumors of the Parotid Gland

Carcinoma of the Parotid

- *Site*: The swelling lies in the region of the parotid gland **(Figure 1.25).**
- *Skin Over (color)*: If the skin is being infiltrated by the tumor, it may look reddish-blue, and may show dilated veins.
- *Size*: It ↑ inexorably **(Figure 1.25).**
- *Shape*: Basically, a flattened hemisphere, but becomes irregular as it enlarges.
- Surface: Smooth, but irregular.
- *Tenderness and Temp*: The swelling is not tender, but the mass is hyperemic and hot.
- *Edge*: Indistinct.
- Consistency: Firm, dull to percussion, not translucent, and not fluctuant.
- *Relations*: Fixed early to deeper structures (restrict jaw movement) and may be the skin.
- *Lymph Drainage*: Cervical LNs are likely to be enlarged and hard.

- *Local Tissues*: There may be *facial palsy* and so lips deviate to the *normal* side only when the patient is asked to smile or show his teeth. If the mandible is infiltrated, the jaw may be swollen and tender.

Criteria of Malignancy (Signs of Malignant Transformation of Pleomorphic Adenoma)

1. Rapid growth with a short history (1-4 months) ± fungation.
2. Change in consistency → stony hard.
3. Fixation (infiltration of the overlying tissues or deeper structures).
4. Paralysis of the facial nerve (facial palsy—30%): Deviation of the lip towards the normal side **(Figure 1.26)**.
5. Pain (30%), may be referred to the ear (auriculotemporal nerve) ± tenderness.
6. Metastases: Enlarged regional lymph nodes or distant metastases (lungs, bones and abdominal organs).
7. Microscopic evidence of malignancy.
   Only when there is invasion beyond the capsule of the parotid that the tumor will behave clinically malignant.

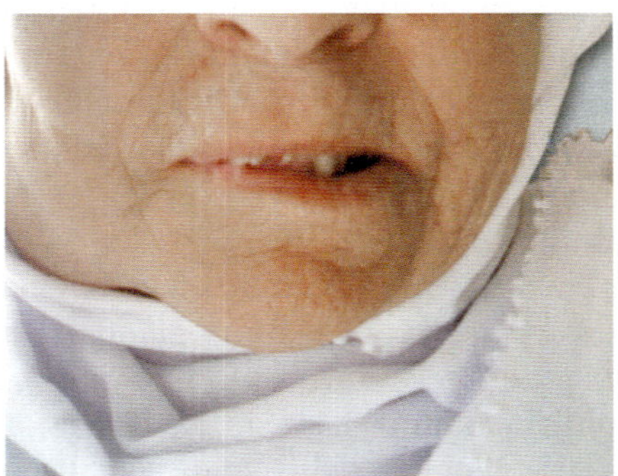

Fig. 1.26: Facial nerve palsy. Note deviation of the mouth (towards the normal side)

Differential Diagnosis between Benign Tumors and Malignant Tumors

Point of Difference	Benign Tumor	Malignant Tumor
Rate of Growth	Slow	Rapid
Sex	Female	Male
Age	Below 40 years	Above 50 years
Pain	Absent	Present (30%)
Mobility	Mobile	Fixed
Consistency	Firm or cystic	Hard
Facial Nerve	Free	Affected (Facial palsy) (30%)
Cervical Lymph Nodes	Not enlarged	May be enlarged
Local or Distant Metastases	Absent	May be present
Sialogram	Regular filling defect	Irregular filling defect
Biopsy	No malignant cells	Malignant cells – invasion

Bilateral Lesions of the Parotid Gland

1. **Adenolymphoma:**
   - About 5-10% of adenolymphomas are bilateral (= 70% of all bilateral parotid swellings).
   - It characteristically affects men more than women.
   - It should be differentiated from mixed parotid tumors (pleomorphic adenoma).
2. **Autoimmune Diseases:**
   - Mikulicz Syndrome: Chronic bilateral enlargement of all salivary glands and lacrimal glands + dryness of the eye and mouth.
   - Sjogren's Syndrome: It is a similar condition associated with keratoconjunctivitis and polyarthritis + other manifestations of SLE.

Swellings of Nonsalivary (Parotid) Gland Origin

1. **Skin:**
   - *Sebaceous Cyst* → It is attached to the skin by a punctum.
   - *Others* → Warts, melanoma, keloid.
2. **Subcutaneous Tissues:**
   - *Dermoid Cyst*
   - *Lipoma* → Mobile, soft, swelling with smooth lobulated surface, slippery edge and skin dimpling.
3. **Lymph Nodes**:
   Swelling of the Preauricular L.N. → The swelling feels superficial (outside the capsule of the parotid) and is characteristically very mobile (to distinguish it from a pleomorphic adenoma). It lies immediately in front of the tragus of the ear. It may be *inflammatory or malignant*; lymphoma or metastatic. A Primary focus (eyelids, forehead, EAM) may be detected.
4. **Facial Nerve:**
   Neuroma of the Facial Nerve → A tender swelling which lies on the course of the facial nerve. It moves in one direction (across the nerve).
5. **Masseter Muscle:**
   - *Idiopathic Hypertrophy of the Masseter Muscle* → Unilateral or bilateral enlargement. It hardens on clenching the teeth and softens on stopping clenching. It does not extend beyond the angle of mandible.
   - *Fibrosarcoma*: Rare.
6. **Ameloblastoma of the Mandible**:
   The swelling is deep to the masseter, fixed to the bone, and hard in consistency. Oral examination reveals expansion of both tables of the mandible. This is the only condition, which leads to expansion of both tables of the mandible.

Cystic Swellings in the Parotid Region Include:

1. Pseudo-cyst:
   - Hematoma
   - Abscess
2. Skin Cyst:
   - Sebaceous cyst
3. Subcutaneous Cyst:
   - Dermoid cyst
4. Parotid Cystic Swellings:
   - Parotid cyst (probably derived from 1st branchial cleft)
   - Adenolymphoma.

II. SUBMANDIBULAR GLAND

Swellings in Submandibular Region

Anatomical Origin

1. Skin.
2. Subcutaneous tissues.
3. Submandibular salivary gland.
4. Submandibular lymph nodes.
5. Mandible.
6. Mucous membrane of the mouth.

Major causes according to origin

A. Salivary Gland Swellings	1. Submandibular Sialadenitis (Acute - Chronic) 2. Salivary Gland Cysts 3. Salivary Tumors (Carcinoma - Mixed salivary tumor)
B. Lymph Node Swellings	1. Inflammatory (Non-specific—TB) 2. Secondaries 3. Lymphoma
C. Oral Lesions with Extension to the Neck	1. Lateral sublingual dermoid 2. Ranula with cervical extension (Plunging Ranula) 3. Tumors of the floor of the mouth
D. Swellings of the Mandible	

Causes According to Clinical Presentation:

Similar to the parotid, the condition may be: Acute or chronic and Solid or cystic:

Acute Swellings	Chronic Swellings	
	A. Of Salivary Gland Origin	*B. Of Extra-salivary Origin*
1. Abscess	1. Chronic Submandibular Sialadenitis	1. Skin
2. Acute Lymphadenitis	2. Cyst	2. SC tissues
3. Acute Submandibular Sialadenitis	3. Tumor: * Benign: e.g. Mixed Salivary Tumor * Malignant: e.g. Carcinoma	3. Submandibular L.Ns
4. Osteomyelitis		4. Mandible
		5. Mucous membrane
		(Similar to Parotid Region)

Clinical Key Points—Swelling in the Submandibular Region

- The submandibular gland is the gland for stone formation, while the parotid gland is the gland of tumors
- Swellings from the submandibular gland are bidigitally felt in the neck as well as in the floor of the mouth. While a L.N. swelling gives only cervical swelling, which can be rolled over the edge of the mandible.
- Swellings originating in the oral cavity are quite evident on examining the mouth (e.g. ranula and lateral sublingual dermoid cyst).
- Swellings of the mandible are hard, fixed to the bone with expansion of one or both tables of the mandible.

Acute Submandibular Sialadenitis

- *Age*:
  Young adults
- *Gender*:
  Males = Females.

- *Complaints:*
  Painful swelling in the submandibular region + salivary colic, i.e. pain and swelling of the gland with meals. Pain may be referred to teeth or tongue.
- *Examination*:
  Tender swelling is felt bimanually. A stone in the duct may also be felt. The orifice of the submandibular duct is congested and edematous. It pours drops of purulent saliva on squeezing the duct.

Chronic Submandibular Sialadenitis (Calcular, Non-calcular):

- *Submandibular Swelling*:
  Firm or hard simulating a tumor that increases in size with meals.
- *Pain* associated with meals (to differentiate it from of dental origin).
- *Lemon Juice Test*:
  Intake of lemon juice causes increase in pain and size of the swelling.
- *Oral Examination of the Orifice of the Duct*:
  It reveals saliva pouring on the unaffected side, whereas little or no secretion is seen ejected from the swollen (affected) side.
- *Bidigital Examination* (finger in the mouth and finger outside):
  A stone may be felt within the duct, or within the gland itself. The swelling may also be felt.
- *Plain X-ray*: May show the stone.
- *Sialogram*: May show filling defect (if stone is translucent).

Tumors of the Submandibular Gland

Types:

- The same as parotid tumors (adenolymphoma occurs almost exclusively in the parotid), the mixed salivary

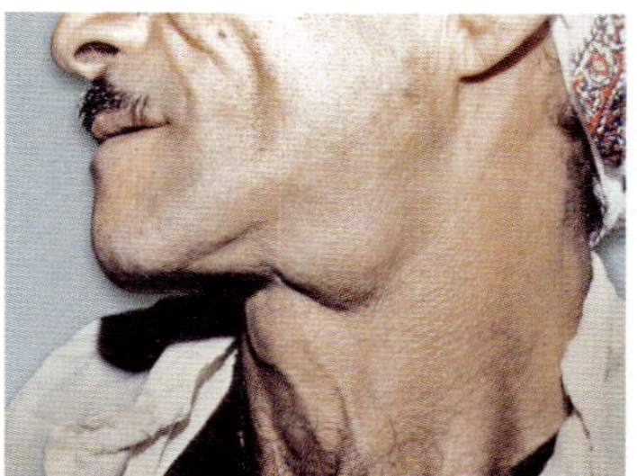

Fig. 1.27: Left mixed salivary tumor. It cannot be rolled over the lower edge of the mandible

tumor being also the commonest, but carcinoma is commoner than in the parotid gland.

1. *Mixed Salivary Gland Tumor* **(Figure 1.27)**:
   - Firm.
   - Smooth.
   - Lobulated.
   - Mobile
   - Of long duration.
   - Cannot be rolled over the lower edge of the mandible.
   - Can be felt by bimanual examination.
2. *Carcinoma*:
   - Hard.
   - Rapidly growing swelling.
   - It may be fixed due to invasion of skin, mandible or floor of mouth.
   - Numbness of the anterior 2/3 of the tongue due to infiltration of the lingual nerve is diagnostic.

Submandibular Lymphadenitis

- TB adenitis: Firm in consistency, and there may be areas of breaking down, mobile, with satellite nodules.

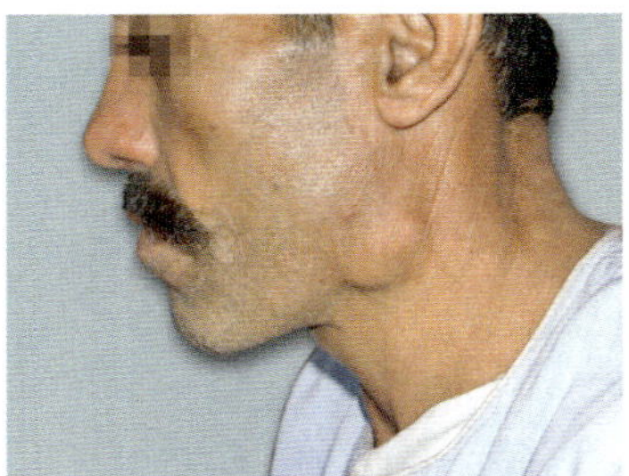

Fig. 1.28: Left submandibular sialadenitis

- If the swelling can be rolled over the lower border of the mandible, it is a L.N, and not a submandibular gland swelling **(Figure 1.28)**.
- Also, a lymph node is not bimanually felt.

Swellings from the Oral Cavity

- *Ranula* is bluish and transparent, and can be seen in the floor of the mouth, to one side.
- *Dermoid cyst* is yellow and opaque.

III. MINOR SALIVARY GLANDS

The Sublingual Salivary Gland

- It is enlarged in Mikulicz's and Sjogrins' Syndromes (+ the major salivary glands and lacrimal glands).
- A *ranula* is a cystic degeneration of this gland.
- About 40% of tumors arising in this gland are benign, and 60% are malignant.

Swellings of Minor Salivary Glands

Tumors arise from the minor salivary glands in the following sites:

1. Inner aspect of the cheek.
2. Floor of the mouth.

3. Base of the tongue.
4. Upper and lower lips.
5. Hard palate (commonest site) ± soft palate.
6. Para-nasal sinuses' openings.

Clinical Picture

- At the beginning, the tumor is symptomless.
- It forms a swelling, firm or hard, mobile or fixed, ulcerating or not.
- If the tumor is neglected, or if it is malignant, it usually invades the underlying bone.

8. CERVICAL LYMPHADENOPATHY

CAUSES OF CERVICAL LYMPHADENOPATHY

Enlargement of the cervical L.Ns is the commonest cause of a swelling in the neck.

Even when only one node is palpable, the adjacent nodes are invariably diseased.

A. Inflammatory	B. Malignant	C. Miscellaneous
1. Nonspecific Lymphadenitis: a. Acute b. Chronic 2. Chronic Specific Lymphadenitis: a. Tuberculosis (T.B) b. Syphilis c. Toxoplasmosis d. Infectious Mononucleosis e. Cat Scratch Fever	1. Lymphoma: a. Hodgkin Disease b. Non-Hodgkin Lymphoma 2. Metastases: From: a. Carcinoma b. Melanoma c. Sarcoma	1. Sarcoidosis 2. Infiltrative disorders: a. Gaucher's Disease b. Niemann-Pick disease c. Histiocytosis-X

A. Inflammatory

1. Nonspecific Lymphadenitis:

a. *Acute Cervical Lymphadenitis*:
   - Short history + presence of a primary focus (oral cavity, nasal cavity, scalp, or face).
   - Affected lymph nodes become enlarged, tender and firm. If untreated, multiple nodes coalesce and central

breakdown occurs and later on suppuration and abscess formation take place.

- Skin overlying may show redness, edema, adhesions, scar, sinus or ulcer.
- Fever and constitutional manifestations are present.

b. *Chronic Nonspecific Lymphadenitis*:

- In association with chronic tonsillitis and pediculosis of the scalp.
- Lymph nodes are enlarged, firm and slightly tender ± abscess formation. They do not become matted nor adherent.

2. Chronic Specific Lymphadenitis

a. T.B. Lymphadenitis:

- It is a common problem in Egypt.
- It is predominantly a disease of children and young adults; however, no age is immune.
- General symptoms of TB toxemia may be present.
- Chronic painless swelling in the neck, of variable size.
- History of fluctuation in size.
- L.Ns are soft to firm, may be matted and slightly tender.
- Caseation (aspiration). If a cold abscess is formed, it becomes cystic (fluctuation). When the abscess has burst through the deep cervical fascia into the SC tissues, it has 2 compartments, one on either side of the D.F., connected by a small central track (= Collar-stud Abscess).
- Sinus or scars of previous sinuses confirms the diagnosis of TB.
- Cord-like structures may be felt between the enlarged L.Ns due to TB lymphangitis.

- Cervical TB lymphadenitis may be:

Criteria	Descending Type	Ascending Type	Generalized
Site	Upper Deep Cervical	Lower Deep Cervical	Anywhere
Age	Children	Adults	Adults
Type	Primary	Secondary to chest disease	Secondary (hematogenous)
Active Pulmonary TB	—	+	±

- Investigations: X-ray chest (If supraclavicular L.Ns are affected), valvular aspiration of a cold abscess (It reveals caseating pus), biopsy.
- *Differential Diagnosis of the different Types of TB Adenitis:*
    1. Lymphadenoid Type: It should be differentiated from lymphoma.
    2. Cold Abscess (Caseating Type): It should be differentiated from other cystic neck swellings.
    3. Fibrous Type (Sinus): It should be differentiated from other sinuses in the neck such as actinomycosis and chronic non-specific lymphadenitis with repeated attacks of suppuration.
    4. Senile (Fibrous) Type: It should be differentiated from metastatic lymph nodes.
    5. Matted Lymph Nodes: It should be differentiated from chronic non-specific lymphadenitis with repeated attacks of suppuration, and lymphoma subjected to irradiation, infection, previous operation, or sarcomatous transformation.

Differential Diagnosis between TB and Chronic Non-Specific Lymphadenitis

Point of Difference	TB Lymphadenitis	Chronic Non-Specific Lymphadenitis
Septic Focus	–	+
Caseation	+	–
Matting	+	–
Sinus	+	–
TB Toxemia	+	–

Differential Diagnosis between TB (Lymphadenoid Type) and Hodgkin's Disease

Point of Difference	TB Lymphadenitis	Hodgkin's Disease
Size of LN	Variable	Variable
Fever	+ (Night fever and sweating)	Pel-Ebstein fever (or other)
Pruritis	–	+
Splenomegaly	–	+ (in 1/3 of patients)
Course	Stationary or regressive	Progressive ↑ in size
Tuberculin Test	+	May be -ve
Cut section (Biopsy)	Tuberculous nodules	Homogenous with destruction
Microscopic Picture	Giant cells with 20 nuclei, surrounded by epithelioid cells	Small DR-cells with 4 superimposed nuclei

Differential Diagnosis between TB (Senile Type) and Metastatic (Secondary) Deposits

Point of Difference	TB Lymphadenitis	Malignant Secondaries
Primary lesion	–	+
History	Long	Short
Course	Stationary of regressive	Progressive
Fixation	–	+ (in advanced cases)
Consistency	Firm or hard	Stony hard
Calcification (PXR)	±	–

b. Syphilitic Lymphadenitis:

- Primary Syphilis: Chancre on the lip or tongue. Local L.Ns are enlarged, painless, discrete and rubbery in consistency. They are not fixed to the skin or deeper structures. They may remain palpable after disappearance of the chancre.
- Secondary Syphilis: Generalized lymphadenopathy. Occipital, mastoid (and epitrochlear) L.Ns are commonly affected. Lymph nodes are painless, shotty, and discrete. WR reaction is +ve.
- Tertiary Syphilis: It is very rare. A true gummatous infiltration does not occur. What occurs is "septic lymphadenitis" which may arise from infection of the 3ry syphilitic lesion. L.Ns are enlarged and elastic in consistency.

c. Viral Lymphadenitis (IMN):

- It is caused by Epstein Barr virus (a herpes virus) that causes irregular fever.
- Lymph nodes are enlarged, particularly the posterior cervical group. They tend to be painful, tender, elastic in consistency, bilateral and symmetrical.

- A sore throat, splenic enlargement and skin rash may occur.

d. Clamydial Lymphadenitis (Cat Scratch Disease):

- Fever, malaise, pustular lesions that subside, and after 2-4 weeks regional lymph nodes (axillary, cervical and inguinal) become enlarged, usually unilateral.
- They are painless.
- Suppuration often occurs, but the pus is sterile.

B. NEOPLASTIC (MALIGNANT) LYMPHADENOPATHY

1. Lymphoma

- Periodic fever and rigors (e.g. Pel-Ebstein fever). Jaundice may be seen due to ↑ hemolysis of RBCs.
- Affection of other L.Ns in the axilla, groin, or mediastinum (causing mediastinal syndrome).
- Enlargement of the spleen and/or liver (diffuse liver infiltration is another cause of jaundice).
- The condition is always progressive, with loss of weight, pallor and jaundice.
- The enlarged lymph nodes have the following characteristics:
  a. Hodgkin Disease:
     L.Ns vary greatly in size. They are smooth, firm or elastic, painless, mobile and discrete. They become matted when they get infected, irradiated or transformed to lymphosarcoma.
  b. Non-Hodgkin Lymphoma:
     Lymph nodes are enlarged, variable in size and consistency, matted and invade the skin early. They are usually painless, but may be painful in children.

2. Metastatic Lymph Nodes:

- The L.Ns are painless (*but later on may become painful*), hard, and often stony hard.
- They start mobile but become fixed later on, and ulcerate and fungate in neglected cases.
- Short history and progressive course.
- The presence of a primary malignant tumor in the field of drainage of the enlarged nodes helps in diagnosis. The primary tumor may be a *carcinoma* (e.g. SCC of the mouth, nose, pharynx and scalp), *malignant melanoma,* or even a *sarcoma* (sarcomas which have a greater tendency to metastasize to regional lymph nodes include synovioma, Ewing's sarcoma, osteogenic sarcoma, Kaposi sarcoma, angiosarcoma, embryonal rhabdomyosarcoma, neurofibrosarcoma, dermatofibrosarcoma protuberance and malignant fibrous histiocytoma).
- Sometimes, metastatic lymph nodes represent the first clinical manifestation of the disease, i.e. occult primary. Sites of occult Primary tumors in the head and neck include:
    a. Nasal sinuses (e.g. maxillary sinus).
    b. Nasopharynx (fossa of Rosenmuller).
    c. Hypopharynx.
    d. Pyriform fossa of the larynx.
    e. Papillary carcinoma of the thyroid gland.

3. Leukemia (Chronic Lymphatic Leukemia)

- Lymph nodes are enlarged, bilateral and symmetrical.
- In addition to lymphadenopathy, there is enlargement of the spleen and liver and may be GIT bleeding.
- Marked increase in the total leukocytic count.

C. Miscellaneous Causes of Cervical Lymphadenopathy

1. Sarcoidosis (Boeck's Sarcoid)

- It is a non-caseating granulomatous disease of unknown etiology that may be entirely asymptomatic and discovered only incidentally at autopsy, or as bilateral hilar adenopathy on chest X-ray obtained for other reasons. Alternatively, it may present with isolated cutaneous or ocular lesions, peripheral lymphadenopathy, or hepatosplenomegaly with insidious onset of respiratory difficulties or constitutional manifestations (fever, night sweats, weight loss), or with an acute onset accompanied by fever, edema, erythema nodosum and polyarthritis.
- Biopsy is essential for diagnosis.

2. Infiltrative and Degenerative Disorders

- Gaucher's Disease:
  It occurs in infants and ends fatally at a young age. It is characterized by marked enlargement of the liver, spleen and lymph nodes, which are infiltrated with Gaucher's cells. There is CNS involvement, skin pigmentation and pigmented scleral thickenings on each side of the cornea. The disease may be associated with pingueculae, dwarfism, and infantilism.
- Niemann-Pick Disease:
  It is characterized by marked enlargement of the liver, spleen and lymph nodes with infiltration of the bone marrow, diffuse neural involvement, pigmentation of the skin, cachexia, anemia, hypercholestrolemia, and visceral involvement affecting the GIT, adrenal glands and lungs.

3. Histiocytosis-X

- It is specific clinico-pathologic entity characterized and defined by proliferation of Langerhan's cells (LC), normally present within the epidermis and related to the mononuclear phagocytic system.
- It includes 3 variants:
  - Acute disseminated LC histiocytosis (Letterer-Siwe syndrome).
  - Unifocal LC histiocytosis (eosinophilic granuloma).
  - Multifocal LC histiocytosis (Hand-Schüller-Christian Disease).

9. SWELLINGS OF THE THYROID GLAND

***Goiter** means "enlarged thyroid gland due to any cause"*
(Normally, the gland is neither visible nor palpable)

Characteristic Clinical Features of a Thyroid Swelling

1. *Anatomical Site:* Lower anterior part of the neck, *deep* to the sternomastoid muscle.
2. *Shape*: Butterfly (2 lobes and isthmus). However, enlargement may be unilateral or asymmetrical.
3. *Mobility with Deglutition*: A goiter moves up and down with deglutition.

Classification of Goiter (Causes of Thyroid Enlargement)

Simple Goiter	Toxic Goiter	Special Goiter
Non-toxic Goiter: 1. Diffuse: a. Physiological b. Colloidal	1. Diffuse (Primary) = *Grave's Disease*	1. Thyroiditis
2. Multinodular	2. Multinodular (Secondary) = Marine-Lenhart Syndrome	2. Neoplastic: a. Benign: Adenoma b. Malignant: Primary or Secondary
3. Solitary Nodule	3. Solitary Nodule=Plummer's Disease	3. Autoimmune
4. Recurrent Nodular	4. Recurrent Nodular	4. Congenital (dyshormonogenesis)

N.B.

Nodules may be seen as *single* lesions (***uninodular***), or several nodules may coalesce and remain segregated *in one lobe* of the thyroid gland (***plurinodular***), or several nodules of different sizes may be scattered irregularly *throughout the thyroid gland* (***multinodular***).

Physiological (Parenchymatous) Goiter

- Enlargement of the thyroid gland as a physiological response to increased demands during stress, e.g. during puberty and adolescence, or during pregnancy and lactation.
- *Complaints:* Fullness or swelling in front of the neck.
- *Clinical Examination:* Enlarged thyroid:
  - Even and uniform enlargement.
  - Smooth surface.
  - Soft or fleshy in consistency.
  - Well-defined.
  - Mobile.

Colloid Goiter

- Return to normal is possible in early stages of parenchymatous goiter if I_2 is given therapeutically, otherwise there will be a slow gradual transition at different rates to the "colloid" condition.
- *Complaints:* Swelling in front of the neck. There may be some pressure effects.
- *Clinical Examination*
  - Enlarged thyroid gland (soft and smooth, more likely to assume a butterfly shape) in an older female than physiological goiter, and with some pressure effects (still unusual).
  - There may be associated evidence of myxedema (hypothyroidism), or rarely, toxicity.

Simple Multinodular Goiter (MNG)

- The gland passes through recurrent cycles of diffuse epithelial hyperplasia followed by involution and the formation of unequal responses in the different portions of the gland. This results in the development of multiple nodular areas, some of which contain abundant colloid, other areas show degenerative changes with cyst formation, recent or old hemorrhage, or calcification.

- *Incidence:* It is the commonest variety. It may be endemic (deficiency of I_2), or sporadic.
- *Age and Sex:* Middle age (usually over 35 years).
- *Sex:* Females > Males.
- *Complaints*:
  - Disfiguring swelling in front of the neck.
  - Dyspnea due to tracheal compression of voice usually do *not* occur, unless there is retrosternal extension, or malignancy.
- *Clinical Examination*:
  - The gland is enlarged and moves with deglutition (under the sternomastoid muscle). It is full of nodules of varying sizes and consistencies present in one or in large goiters, attacks of giddiness and fainting may result from displacement of carotid vessels, but dysphagia and change both lobes; soft, firm or hard when calcification occurs **(Figure 1.29).**

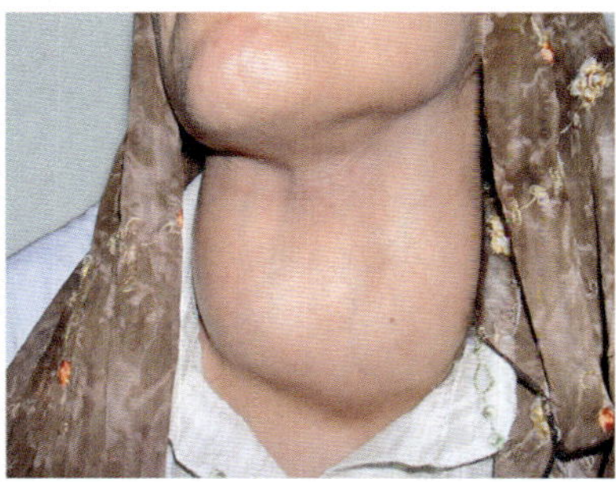

Fig. 1.29: A large multi-nodular goiter involving both lobes and isthmus

- The larynx and trachea are often displaced by the swelling.
- Unlike thyroid cancer, carotids are always palpable and equal on both sides, and lymph nodes are *not* palpable
- *Complications*:
  - *Toxicity:* Simple goiter → Secondary thyrotoxicosis (10–20% of cases, usually in patients >30 years of age).
  - *Retrosternal Extension:* More common in males than in females.
  - *Malignant Transformation:* Criteria of malignant transformation include the following:

Glandular Criteria	Extra-glandular Criteria
Rapid recent growth	Pressure symptoms become more evident
Fixation of the swelling	Vocal cord paralysis (infiltration of recurrent laryngeal nerve)
Consistency becomes harder	Horner's syndrome (infiltration of cervical sympathetic trunk)
Edges become ill-defined	Cervical LN enlargement
Onset of pain	Unequal carotid pulsations
	Evidence of distant metastases

- *Pressure Manifestations:* May result from retrosternal extension, malignancy, or hemorrhage.
  - Pressure on the *trachea* → dyspnea. *How* ??
    - Unilateral goiter causes displacement of the trachea.
    - Bilateral goiter causes compression of the trachea from both sides (*scabbard trachea* - X-ray).

    - Tracheomalacia: softened trachea by absorption of its cartilaginous rings in long-standing cases.
  - Pressure on the *esophagus* → dysphagia (slight).
  - Pressure on the *neck veins* → mediastinal syndrome with congested face.
  - Pressure on the *recurrent laryngeal nerve* → hoarseness of voice (however, it mostly occurs due to malignant infiltration rather than just pressure).
- *Cyst Formation:* Due to rupturing of neighboring acini, hemorrhage, infection, or degeneration of nodules.
- *Hemorrhage:* It causes sudden increase in the size, pain in the neck and sudden compression of the trachea.
- *Calcification* in the capsule or septa. Plain X-ray is diagnostic. It may be mistaken for malignancy (hard).
- *Infection:* It is rare, but more common than in normal thyroid glands.

Solitary Adenoma (Solitary Nodule)

- *Incidence*: Rare in endemic areas, but common elsewhere. It occurs in females > males.
- *Clinical Examination*:
  - Swelling in front of the neck
  - Mobile with deglutition
  - Causing asymmetrical enlargement of the gland
  - Usually situated at the junction of the isthmus with the lateral lobe
  - Smooth
  - Well-defined
  - Soft or firm
  - It is liable to the same complications as multinodular goiter mentioned above.

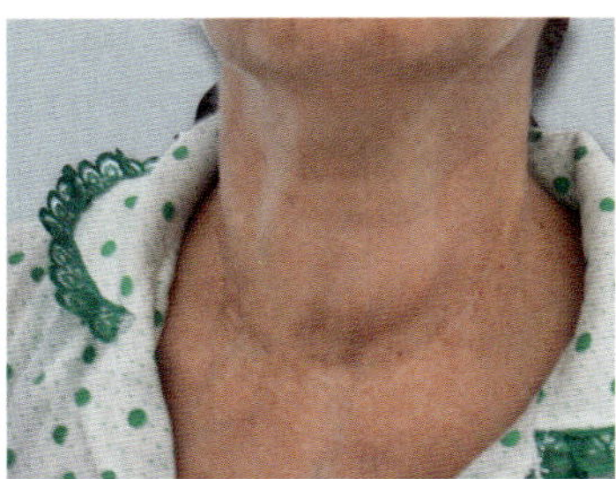

Fig. 1.30: Recurrent goiter. Note previous scar

Recurrent Simple Nodular Goiter

Following a previous thyroidectomy for treatment of simple nodular goiter, a recurrent nodule **(Figure 1.30)** may occur due to:

A. False Recurrence (70%):

1. Foreign body such as a granuloma around a silk ligature, or a small piece of gauge left accidentally.
2. Inadequate excision, e.g. if the isthmus, pyramidal lobe, or postero-medial projections are present, they should be removed completely.

B. True Recurrence (30%)

1. Persistence of the same etiological factors of the primary SNG such as I_2 deficiency, intake of goiterogens, or dyshormogenesis.
2. Inadequate Diagnosis:
   If the operation was designed for SNG (partial or subtotal thyroidectomy), but the pathology proved to be malignant, there may be:
   - Residual malignant tissue.
   - Tumor in the juxtathyroid nodes not treated at the original operation.

   - Spillage of malignant cells from an ill advised incisional biopsy.
3. No postoperative El-troxin (it should be given for life to keep TSH at a low level).

Primary (Diffuse) Thyrotoxicosis (Grave's Disease)

- *Age and Sex*: Third decade (20-30Y) - Female to male ratio is 8:1.
- *Complaints:* Neck swelling + symptoms of toxicity (e.g. dyspnea on effort, tiredness, palpitation, intolerance to heat, ↑ sweating, weight loss despite appetite, diarrhea, nervousness, menstrual disturbances, etc).
- *Local Examination:*
  - The thyroid becomes diffusely enlarged with smooth surface and fleshy consistency.
  - In moderate and severe cases, pulsations due to ↑ vascularity could be seen (inspection). Thrill (palpation) and bruit (auscultation) may be demonstrated.
  - The skin overlying may show dilated veins.
- *General Examination*:
  - *General Appearance*: Exophthalmos, nervous patient, ↓ weight and tendency to falling of hair.
  - *Nails*: The junction of the nail with its bed becomes straight or concave.
  - *Body Metabolism*: ↑ BMR → ↑ sweating, ↓ weight despite good appetite and intolerance to hot weather.
  - *Digestive System*: Diarrhea, nausea and vomiting (thyrotoxic crisis), abdominal distention, ↑ glucose intolerance and glycosuria (polyphagia and polydipsia).
  - *Respiratory System*: Dyspnea on effort.

- *CNS*: Irritability, nervousness and easy excitability, headache and insomnia, fine tremors, and frank psychosis in severe cases.
- *Genitourinary System*: Polyuria, menstrual disturbances (menorrhagia, oligomenorrhea or amenorrhea) and infertility, with impotence in men and frigidity in women
- *Cardiovascular System:* Attacks of palpitation on exertion or on rest. Tachycardia (persists during deep sleep). Cardiac arrhythmias are superimposed on a sinus tachycardia as the disease progresses in the form of:
  - Multiple extrasystoles.
  - Paroxysmal atrial tachycardia.
  - Paroxysmal atrial fibrillation.
  - Persistent atrial flutter not responsive to digoxin.
  - Congestive heart failure (CHF).
- *Musculoskeletal System:*
  - Myopathy: Weakness, most marked in the frontalis muscle, platysma, quadriceps femoris and eye muscles).
  - Osteoporosis.
  - Peritibial myxedema.
- *Eye Manifestations:*
  - Lid retraction (*Dalrymple's sign*).
  - Lid lag (*Von Graefe's sign*).
  - Staring look (*Stellwag's sign*).
  - Absence of wrinkling of the forehead on looking upwards (*Joffroy's sign*).
  - Lack of convergence on looking at a near object (*Moebius sign*).

- Difficulty in passive eversion of the eye (*Giffod's sign*).
- Involuntary spasm of the eyelids when closed (*Rosenbach's sign*).
- Abnormal pulsation of the retinal vessels (*Backer's sign*).
- Abnormal protrusion of the eyeball (*Thyrotoxic exophthalmos*).

- *Differential Diagnosis*:
  - Anxiety neurosis.
  - Organic conditions which cause heart diseases, anemia, or gastrointestinal diseases.
  - Myasthenia gravis, or other muscular disorders.
  - Menopausal syndrome.
  - Pheochromocytoma.
  - Other causes of exophthalmos and primary ophthalmopathy.
  - Thyrotoxic Factitia: Thyrotoxicosis due to increased administration of exogenous thyroxin.

Differences between Thyrotoxicosis and Psychoneurosis

Point of Difference	Toxic Goiter	Anxiety Neurosis
Sleeping pulse	↑	Normal
Appetite	Good appetite	Loss of appetite
Easy fatigability	Relieved by rest	Not relieved
Hands	Warm and sweaty	Cold and sweaty
Lab. tests: T3 and T4	↑	Normal
Drug response	Anti-thyroid drugs	Tranquilizers

Differential Diagnosis of Exophthalmos

Bilateral Causes	Unilateral Causes	
	Pulsating	Non-pulsating
1. Thyrotoxicosis (the commonest cause) 2. Bilateral orbital infiltration as in lymphoma 3. Bilateral nasal sinusitis with spreading infection to both orbital cavities	*Vascular Causes*: 1. A-V fistula (between the ICA and the cavernous sinus) 2. Aneurysm of ICA 3. Aneurysm of ophthalmic artery 4. Thrombosis of the cavernous sinus (usually non-pulsatile) 5. A rapidly growing vascular intraorbital tumor) *Orbitocranial Communications:* 1. Dermoid cyst 2. Neurofibroma 3. Angioma 4. Meningocele	*Acute Causes:* 1. Orbital cellulitis. 2. Cavernous sinus thrombosis 3. Thrombosis of orbital vein 4. Distention of nasal sinus 5. Orbital emphysema 6. Hemorrhage into the orbit *Chronic Causes:* 1. Tumors of the orbit (angioma, osteoma) and optic nerve (glioma) 2. Gumma (syphilis), TB 3. Extension of a space-occupying lesion from the ACF or the MCF 4. Invasion of nasopharyngeal tumor 5. A distended globe due to high myopia, infantile glaucoma, or anterior staphyloma

Secondary Thyrotoxicosis

- It may result as a complication of simple multi-nodular goiter or a simple nodule (→ toxic nodule).

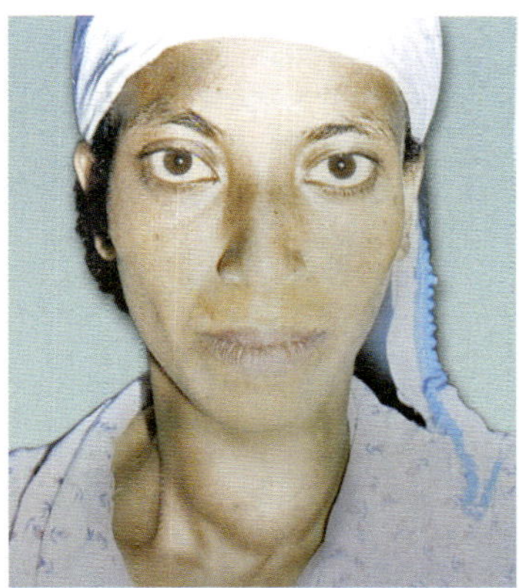

Fig. 1.31: Secondary toxic goiter

- The thyroid gland is characteristically nodular if occurs on top of MNG, and not smooth as in primary thyrotoxicosis.
- There may also be exophthalmos as seen in **Figure 1.31.**
- Secondary thyrotoxicosis has the same manifestations as Primary thyrotoxicosis, but with some differences as shown in the Table below:

Differences between Primary and Secondary Thyrotoxicosis

Point of Difference	Primary Thyrotoxicosis	Secondary Thyrotoxicosis
Age	< 35 years (Young)	> 35 years (Middle age).
Toxic symptoms	Start with gland enlargement	Start after gland enlargement
The gland	Symmetrical, bilateral, fleshy and smooth surface	Asymmetrical, may be unilateral, firm and nodular surface
CVS Manifestations	+	+++

Contd...

Contd...

CNS Manifestations:	+++	+
GIT Manifestations:	++	+
Eye Manifestations:	++++	+
BMR ↑	++	+
Results of I_2 therapy	Often striking improvement	Improvement of a lesser degree

Acute Thyroiditis

- Marked constitutional manifestations.
- *Swelling*: Painful, tender, and indurated with signs of acute inflammation in the skin (red and hot). Fluctuation appears and pus may track subcutaneously low down in the midline of the neck, or into the trachea, pharynx, or mediastinum. Edema of the glottis may occur.
- In few cases, there may be dysphagia or tracheitis that may cause spitting of blood.

Subacute Thyroiditis

Synonyms: Granulomatous Thyroiditis, Giant Cell Thyroiditis, ***De Quervains' Disease***.

- Acute onset, in middle aged females.
- Slightly enlarged thyroid with pain and may be tenderness.
- Pain in the neck, which may refer to the ear and on swallowing.
- Fever, malaise, weakness and palpitation.
- It is self-limited (within 3-6 months); it may undergo remissions and relapses.
- *Investigations:* ↑ ESR, thyroid antibodies are absent, radioactive iodine uptake is usually normal or slightly depressed. Therapeutic test with cortisone.

Chronic Thyroiditis

A. Specific Chronic Thyroiditis

- TB: A hard mass develops in one lobe and gradually softens into a cold abscess, which, if untreated, erupts to the skin surface, or into the trachea or esophagus. Secondary pyogenic infection follows.
- *Syphilis*: It is most commonly seen as a "gumma" (3rd stage), although a more diffuse enlargement has been noted in the 2nd stage of the disease.
- *Actinomycosis*: It occurs as a secondary feature of the disease elsewhere.

B. Non-specific Chronic Thyroiditis:

- Hashimoto's disease.
- Riedle's disease.

Differences between Hashimoto's Disease and Riedle's Disease

Criteria	Hashimoto's Disease	Riedle's Disease
Synonyms	Lymphadenoid goiter	Ligneous thyroiditis, Woody thyroiditis
History	• Sex: Only females (20:1) • Age: Older (menopausal) • Manifestations of hypothyroidism • Little or no pressure symptoms	• Sex: Both males and females • Age: Young adults • Profound hypothyroidism • Profound pressure symptoms
C/E	• Goiter: Uniform enlargement, usually bilateral, firm, mobile with deglutition, smooth surface, and well-defined edges • Signs of hypothyroidism • No palpable lymph nodes	• Goiter: Not uniformly enlarged, uni- or bi-lateral, woody hard, fixed, irregular surface, and ill-defined edges • Profound hypothyroidism • Pressure effects are usual

Contd...

Contd...

Studies	1. Raised titer of thyroid antibodies 2. Serum cholesterol (usually high) 3. RAI uptake (usually low). 4. Needle biopsy (may be necessary)	1. Thyroid function tests show hypothyroidism 2. Plain X-ray chest and neck 3. Needle biopsy

Autoimmune Thyroiditis

- The gland may be partly diffusely affected, small or large, soft or firm. It is at first freely mobile due to confinement of fibrosis within the gland, but later, fibrosis extends outside the gland.
- Initially there is hyperthyroidism due to distention of cells with release of hormones, but hypothyroidism is inevitable due to fibrosis. Cervical lymph nodes are not palpable.
- *Investigations*: High titer of thyroid antibodies: Microsomal, thyroglobulin and second colloid antibody.
- *Complications*: Hypothyroidism, papillary carcinoma or lymphoma.

Differences between Grave's Disease, Colloid Goiter and Thyroiditis

Criteria	Grave's Disease	Colloid Goiter	Thyroiditis
Size	Slight to moderate	Moderate to gross	Small or moderate
Surface	Smooth	Bosselated	Smooth
Consistency	Soft - fleshy	Fleshy	Hard
Tenderness	–	–	+
Bruit	+	–	–

Benign Tumors of the Thyroid Gland

Benign tumors of the thyroid gland include the following:

Epithelial Tumors	Mesenchymal Tumors	Others
• Papillary Adenoma (Fetal Adenoma = Microfollicular Adenoma) • Follicular Adenoma (Cystadenoma = Colloid Adenoma = Macrofollicular Adenoma)	• Lipoma • Leiomyoma • Hemangioma	Teratoma in *children* (not adults)

Characteristic Features of Follicular and Papillary Adenomas

Features	Follicular Adenoma (Macrofollicular)	Papillary (Fetal) Adenoma (Microfollicular)
Incidence	More common	Rare
Age	Older age	Younger (18-20 years, not since birth)
Size	Any size	Usually remains small
Site	Any part of the gland	Usually at junction of isthmus with one lobe
Function	Euthyroid, but may be hot (toxic adenoma)	Euthyroid
DD	1. Nodular hyperplasia 2. Minimally invasive follicular carcinoma 3. Follicular pattern of papillary carcinoma	Other types of adenomata

Malignant Tumors (Cancer Thyroid)

- Sex: Female : Male ratio = 4:1, but in solitary thyroid nodules (males > females).

- *Age*: It is commoner during the 4th and 5th decades. However, the *papillary type* may occur in children.
- *Complaints (History Taking)*:
  - *Swelling in the Neck*: All clinically solitary nodules are "suspect". The swelling is either painful or painless, of recent onset, or on top of simple nodular goiter, and rapidly progressive.
  - *Lateral Cervical Swelling (L.Ns)*: May be the presenting complaint in papillary carcinoma (occult).
  - *Pressure Symptoms*: Dyspnea, dysphagia, hoarseness of voice, Horner's syndrome.
  - *Symptoms of Distant Secondaries*: Bone or lung metastases may be the presenting symptom in follicular, anaplastic or medullary carcinoma.
  - *Watery Diarrhea*: May occur in medullary carcinoma (1/3rd of patients) due to secreted humoral agent.
- *Clinical Examination*:
  - *Thyroid* Gland: Firm or hard, mobile or fixed, tender or not, with or without local invasion.
  - *Cervical Lymph Nodes*: Firm or hard, mobile or fixed.
  - *Carotid Pulse*: May be unfelt or weak at the side of the tumor (Berry's sign)
  - *Distant Secondaries*: Bones and soft tissues may show swelling with palpable thrill and audible murmur.
  - *Endocrine Abnormalities*: In medullary carcinoma of the thyroid: Several endocrine abnormalities may be present e.g. medullary carcinoma + pheochromocytoma + hyperparathyroidism (MEN II). Other abnormalities may be also present due to secretion of certain peptides e.g. ACTH (Cushing syndrome) and calcitonin (hypocalcemia and Secondary hyperparathyroidism).
  - *In Disseminated Lymphoma,* there may be splenomegaly or enlarged lymph nodes at different sites.

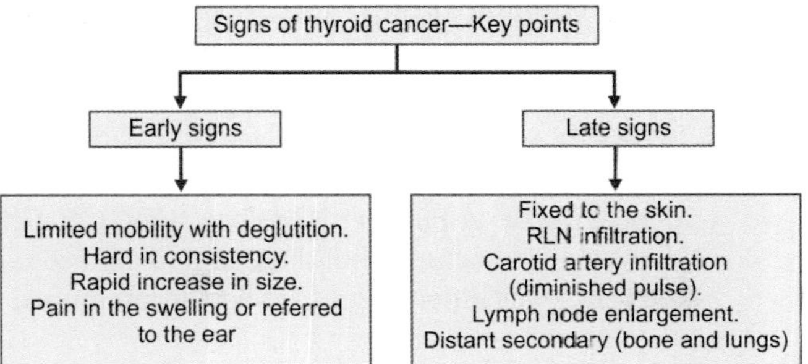

- *Investigations*:

  A. Laboratory:
  - *General Investigations*: Blood, stool and urine analysis.
  - *Serum Calcitonin*: (Normal = 200 picogram/ml). If it reaches > 0.1 mg/ml, it indicates MCT.

  B. Radiological:
  - *Plain X-Ray (Neck and Chest)* may show fine stippling (papillary carcinoma), heavy calcifications (SNG or MCT), tracheal compression or displacement, or pulmonary or skeletal metastases.
  - *Skeletal survey or bone scanning* in order to detect early bone metastases.
  - *CT Scan* to the lungs, liver and bones is useful in detecting metastases.
  - *Ultrasound of the Thyroid*: It can differentiate between solid and cystic swellings.
  - *Isotope Scanning*: Thyroid scan (hot or cold nodule) and *whole body scan* (for functioning secondary).

  C. Endoscopy:

  Indirect laryngoscopy to visualize the vocal cords and assess their condition.

  D. Biopsy:
  - *Frozen Section*: It is essential for R/, but may be difficult to differentiate between nodular

hyperplasia, follicular adenoma, or minimally invasive follicular carcinoma.

- *Core-Needle Biopsy*: Particularly used in diffuse diseases, e.g. Hashimoto's disease. It can confirm the diagnosis of malignancy.
- *Fine Needle Aspiration Cytology (FNAC)*: Gives histological diagnosis, but difficult to diagnose non-invasive (well differentiated) follicular carcinoma.

Characteristic Clinical Features of Individual Types of Thyroid Cancer

Criteria	1. Papillary Carcinoma	2. Follicular Carcinoma
Incidence	60% of thyroid cancer (most common)	20% of thyroid cancer
Age	4th decade, but may affect children and teen-agers (10-20 years)	Older age groups (4th and 5th decades). Does not affect children
Sex	Females > Males	Females > Males
Size	• May be occult • The most slowly growing tumor but may reach a huge size	• Never occult • Usually small in size
Toxic S/S	Rarely gives thyrotoxic effects	May be associated with toxicity
Spread	• Local to soft tissues of the neck • Lymphatics to cervical lymph nodes. May be occult • Blood (late) to the lungs > bone > CNS	• Mainly Blood: to the lungs and bones → painful bony swelling (shoulder girdle, skull, sternum, iliac bones) > to L.Ns • Never occult
Subtypes (Woolner)	A: Occult (< 1.5 cm) B: Intrathyroidal C: Extrathyroidal	A: Non- or minimally invasive B: Invasive (to adjacent tissues, or capsule)
Prognosis	More favorable	Less favorable

3. Undifferentiated Carcinoma (Anaplastic or Sarcomatoid)

- *Incidence*: It is the rarest variety of thyroid carcinoma (10%).
- *Age*: It usually affects elderly people (6th and 7th decades).
- *Sex*: Females > Males.
- *Origin*:
  It may arise on top of:
  - Papillary carcinoma (the most common presentation).
  - Simple nodular goiter.
  - Normal thyroid gland.
- *Spread*:
  - Local spread to the trachea causing compression.
  - Lymphatic and blood spread are rapid.
- *Prognosis*: Survival rate is only approximately 6 months.

4. Medullary Carcinoma of the Thyroid (MCT)

- *Cell of Origin*:
  It arises from "C" *parafollicular cell*, derived from the ultimobranchial body, not from the cells of the thyroid follicles as other primary carcinomas.
- *Age*:
  About 50-70 years, or <30 years or even in childhood.
- *Gender and Race*:
  Any sex or race could be affected.
- *Spread*:
  - Locally to surrounding tissues.
  - Lymphatics 50–60%.
  - Blood spread.
- *Forms of MCT*:
  - Sporadic form (80%).
  - Familial form (20% - autosomal dominant - may be involved in MEN II syndrome).
- It is *not* hormone-dependent and does *not* take up ^{131}I and gives poor response to radiotherapy and chemotherapy.

- *Prognosis*:
  Prognosis is *better* in:
  - Females > males.
  - Children > older patients.
  - Familial > sporadic forms.
  - Tumors confined to the gland.

5. Lymphoma

- The thyroid is a rare site for primary lymphoma.
- It occurs mostly in females over 60 years of age.
- The patient presents with diffuse symmetrical enlargement of the thyroid with or without regional lymph node enlargement.
- Splenomegaly or lymph node enlargement at other sites occurs in patients with disseminated lymphoma.
- Hoarseness of voice is a common feature.

Key Points—Swellings of the Thyroid Gland

Evidence of Retrosternal Extension ??

Males are affected more than females because they have a shorter neck, with strong pretracheal muscles, which direct the swelling into the mediastinum aided by the negative intra-thoracic pressure and the effect of gravity.

- **Reported Symptoms from Retrosternal Goiter (RSG):**
  - Respiratory: Postural dyspnea, stridor, wheezing, cough, hemoptysis not mixed with sputum (due to rupture of enlarged tracheal vein), choking, and death (degeneration hemorrhage).
  - Esophageal: Dysphagia, "lump in the throat".
  - Vascular: SVC syndrome, transient ischemic attacks, cerebral edema, GI bleeding.
  - Neurologic: Vocal cord paresis/paralysis, hoarseness, Horner's syndrome.
  - Metabolic: Thyrotoxicosis, weight loss.
  - Infectious: Abscess in the retro-sternal goiter (reported case).
- **Clinical Examination (Signs of Intrathoracic Swelling):**
  - Enlarged thyroid with impalpable lower border and dullness on percussion over the manubrium.

Contd...

Contd...

- Dilated veins in front of the neck and sternum.
- Flushing of the skin and dilatation of the EJV during raising the arms or hyperextension of the neck (positive **Pemberton's Sign**).

- **Imaging Procedures:** In the diagnostic work up of patients with RSG, imaging procedures include:
  - *PXR* (neck and thoracic inlet) may show a mediastinal, or cervi-mediastinal mass displacing, or compressing the trachea, with or without calcification of the goiter. It is the most cost effective.
  - *CT Scan* demonstrates continuity of the mediastinal mass with a cervical goiter and permits identification of tissue planes of intrathoracic goiterous components.
  - *Radionuclide Scan* (RAI or ^{99c}Tm) to confirm the thyroid origin of the mediastinal lesion. However, it is not always beneficial and sometimes -ve because most retro-sternal goiters do not trap I_2. If scanning with RAI is considered, it should be done prior to evaluation by contrast CT.
  - *Ultrasonography*: In general, it is not necessary, but can be helpful in selected patients.
  - *Magnetic Resonance Imaging (MRI)* can be used. It avoids the use of I2 contrast studies.

A Hard Swelling in the Thyroid ??

- Thyroid cancer.
- Calcified simple nodular goiter.
- Tuberculoma (TB).
- Gumma (tertiary syphilis).
- Hashimoto's disease.
- Reidle's disease.
- Cancer larynx invading the thyroid gland.

A Solitary Thyroid Nodule (STN) ??

- *Metabolic Nodule*:
  - Simple Nodule (about 50% of clinically STNs prove at operation to be multiple).
  - Toxic Nodule.
  - Thyroid Cyst (hemorrhage or necrosis of a hyperplastic nodule).
- *Benign Tumor* (Adenoma).
- *Malignant Nodule*: 10-25%, occurs in males > females, in very young or old patients.
- *Thyroiditis*: Usually Hashimoto's disease, but may be also Reidle's disease.
- *Specific Thyroiditis*: Tuberculoma (TB) or syphilitic gumma.

Contd...

Contd...

Causes of Sudden Enlargement of the Thyroid Gland with Pain ??

- Malignant transformation.
- Hemorrhage or necrosis into a cyst.
- Infection (acute inflammation or abscess formation)

Causes of Hoarseness of Voice in a Patient with Goiter??

- Infiltration of the RLN by thyroid cancer.
- Compression of the RLN by a huge goiter or retrosternal goiter.
- Postoperative (iatrogenic) due to injury of the RLN.
- Myxedematous infiltration of the RLN due to large doses of anti-thyroid drugs.

Causes of Dyspnea in a Thyroid Patient ??

A. Nonoperative Causes

- Simple nodular goiter (retrosternal goiter, large goiter, hemorrhage in a nodule) by displacement of the trachea (in unilateral goiter), compression of the trachea from both sides (Scabbard trachea, in bilateral goiter), softening of the trachea (tracheomalacia).
- Toxic goiter: Thyrotoxic patient, exertional due to increased O_2 consumption.
- Malignant goiter: Due to tracheal compression, infiltration of the RLN, lung secondaries.
- In all goiters: A psychogenic element may play a role.

B. Operative Causes

- Laryngeal edema.
- Tracheal collapse.
- Blood clot or hematoma.
- Foreign body.
- RLN affection.

Cervical Swellings that Move with Deglutition ??

- Thyroid gland (goiter).
- Thyroglossal cyst.
- Median ectopic thyroid tissue.
- Parathyroid swelling (if ever palpable in malignancy!!)
- Prelaryngeal (Delphian) LN and pre-tracheal LNs
- Subhyoid bursa
- Adam's apple bursitis
- Laryngocele
- Laryngeal cold abscess (TB)
- Pharyngeal diverticulum

10. SWELLINGS OF MIDLINE OF THE NECK

Surgical Anatomy

- The midline of the neck extends from the "symphysis menti" above to the "suprasternal notch" below. It, therefore, includes the following regions: submental, hyoid bone, laryngeal/pharyngeal, tracheal regions, and the suprasternal space of Burn.
- Midline neck swellings are classified according to **Anatomical Region** or **Consistency** (Solid or Cystic).

CLASSIFICATION ACCORDING TO ANATOMICAL REGION

I. Swellings Superficial to the Cervical Deep Fascia (DF) Include those Arising from:

1. *Skin*: e.g. sebaceous cyst.
2. *Subcutaneous Tissues*: e.g. Dermoid cyst, lipomata, and neurofibromata.

II. Swellings Deep to the DF are classified according to the anatomic region as follows:

Anatomical Region	Causes
1. Sub-mental Region	1. Abscess related to the mandible (from the central incisors) 2. Submental lymph nodes 3. Sublingual dermoid cyst 4. Ranula (hour-glass ranula)
2. Hyoid Bone Region	1. Thyroglossal cyst 2. Sub-hyoid bursitis 3. Median ectopic thyroid tissue (simulates a thyroglossal cyst) 4. Tumor of the hyoid bone
3. Laryngeal and Pharyngeal Regions	1. Bursa in front of Adam's apple 2. Pre-laryngeal (Delphian) L.Ns - cold abscess (TB lymphadenitis) 3. Retropharyngeal abscess 4. TB chondritis of the thyroid cartilage 5. Laryngocele 6. Tumors of the larynx and pharynx

Contd...

Contd...

4. Tracheal Region	1. Nodule in isthmus of the thyroid gland (adenoma or cystadenoma) 2. Pre-tracheal L.Ns.
5. Suprasternal Space of Burn	1. L.N. enlargement (anterior jugular - superficial vertical group) 2. Thyroid gland (goiter) 3. Teratoma 4. Thymoma 5. Aortic aneurysm, or high aortic arch.

CLASSIFICATION ACCORDING TO CONSISTENCY

A. Solid Swellings	B. Cystic and Pseudocystic Swellings
A. Lymph Nodes: a. Submental b. Prelaryngeal c. Pretracheal d. Suprasternal B. Tumors: a. Hyoid Bone b. Larynx and Pharynx c. Thyroid Gland d. Teratoma e. Thymoma C. Median ectopic thyroid tissue D. Nodule in isthmus of the thyroid gland	1. Mandibular abscess 2. Sublingual dermoid cyst 3. Ranula (Hour-glass) 4. Thyroglossal cyst 5. Subhyoid bursitis 6. Bursa of Adam's Apple 7. Cold abscess (TB) 8. Retro-pharyngeal abscess 9. Laryngocele 10. Thyroid cystadenoma

N.B. Cysts *superficial* to the D.F. include: Sebaceous cyst, dermoid cyst, blood cyst and lymphatic cysts.

Midline Cystic Swellings of the Neck

1. Abscess in Relation to the Mandible:

- It occurs in relation to carious tooth (central incisors) leading to osteomyelitis.
- It forms a "subperiosteal abscess".
- A sinus may be present.

- Plain X-ray appearance is diagnostic: It shows a central area of destruction around the root of the tooth with bone rarefaction surrounded by sclerosis.

2. **Sublingual Dermoid Cyst:**
   - *Age*: Young.
   - *Site*: Submental region. Other dermoid cysts can occur anywhere in the midline of the neck.
   - *Characteristics*: Opaque (Not translucent), rounded, smooth, cystic, mobile.
3. **Ranula:**
   - *Age*: Appears in childhood and adolescence.
   - *Site*: Usually it occurs to one side of the frenulum and when plunging it appears in the submandibular triangle, i.e. on the lateral side of the neck. However, it may be central in the floor of the mouth taking a dumbbell shape (hour-glass ranula) and bulge in the submental region.
   - *Characteristics*: Bluish in color and translucent.
4. **Thyroglossal Cyst:**

- *Age and Sex*: Children or young age (mostly between 15 and 30 years). Women > men.
- *Site*: Suprahyoid, subhyoid, or even pretracheal (**Figures 1.32 and 1.33**).
- *Symptoms*: Painless lump in the midline of the neck, usually present for a long time. Pain, tenderness and an↑ in size occur only if the cyst becomes infected.
- *Color (Skin)*: Normal, but becomes red in presence of infection.
- *Size*: They vary from 0.5-5 cm in diameter.
- *Shape*: Spherical.
- *Surface*: Smooth.
- *Edge*: Well-defined.

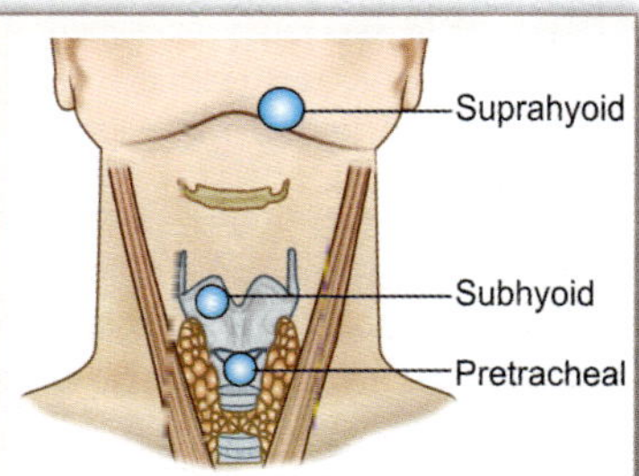

Fig. 1.32: Different sites of thyroglossal cyst

- *Temperature and Tenderness*: Hotness and tenderness are present only if the cyst is infected.
- *Consistency (Composition)*: Cystic or tense cystic (feel firm or hard). Fluctuation may be elicited.
- *Translucency*: It may be translucent.
- *Relations to nearby structures*: Thyroglossal cysts are tethered by the remnant of the thyroglossal duct. *This means that they can be moved sideways, but not up and down.*
- Mobility with protrusion of tongue: The thyroglossal duct is always closely related, usually fixed, to the hyoid cartilage. Since the hyoid bone moves up when the tongue is protruded, the thyroglossal cyst will also move up (characteristic sign); but do not expect to see much movement, it is easier to feel (with the cyst being held between the thumb and the index).

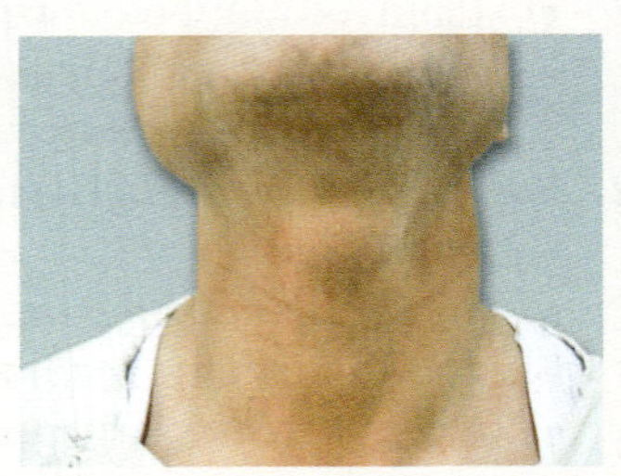

Fig. 1.33: Subhyoid thyroglossal cyst. It characteristically moves upwards with protrusion of the tongue

- *Lymph nodes*: The local LNs should not be enlarged.
- It is not attached to the skin.
- *Local Tissues*: If there is an abnormality of thyroid gland development, examine the base of the tongue for lingual thyroid tissue. It looks like a flattened strawberry sitting on the base of the tongue. A cord may be felt extending from it to the hyoid bone.

5. Subhyoid Bursitis:

- *Age*: Old age.
- *Site*: At the lower border of the hyoid bone.

- *Shape*: Sausage-shaped with its long axis *transverse*.
- *Mobility*: Mobile with protrusion of the tongue.
- *Translucent*.

6. Bursa of Adam's Apple:

- *Site*: In front of Adam's apple (thyroid cartilage).
- It may be inflamed and enlarged.

7. Cold Abscess (TB):

A. *TB Lymphadenitis (Affection of LNs):*
   - Submental - prelaryngeal - pretracheal LNs may be affected.
   - Fixed swelling.
   - Opaque.
   - Multiple sites.
   - Aspiration shows caseous material.
   - Presence of other enlarged LNs in the neck.

B. *TB Chondritis*:
   - The thyroid cartilage is thickened and tender.
   - The abscess is rectangular in shape.
   - TB laryngitis is present.
   - Open pulmonary TB may be present.

8. Retropharyngeal Abscess:

- It is usually due to extension from TB of the cervical spine (Pott's disease).
- Deformity and rigidity of the cervical spine.

9. Laryngocele:

- *Definition*:
  Herniation of the mucus membrane of the pharynx through the gap in the thyrohyoid membrane. It may be central (in the midline of the neck).
- Tense resonant swelling.
- Translucent.
- Compressible (empties on compression).
- Increases in size on straining (coughing).
- It may extend in front of the trachea.
- Associated with dyspnea.

10. Cystadenoma of the Thyroid Gland:

- Mobile with deglutition.
- Other parts of the thyroid gland may be affected.
- Absence of a *cord* between it and the hyoid bone.

11. Other Superficial Cysts:

A. *Sebaceous Cyst*:
   - Site: Can occur anywhere in the midline of the neck.
   - Attached to the skin.
   - Punctum may be seen.
   - Opaque.
   - Cystic or doughy in consistency.

B. *Blood Cyst*:
   - Site: Can occur anywhere in the midline of the neck.
   - History of trauma, or presence of associated blood disease.
   - Bluish in appearance.
   - Aspiration is characteristic.

Key Points—Midline Neck Swelling

Important Causes of Midline Neck Swellings

Cystic Swellings:

1. Sublingual dermoid cyst
2. Subhyoid bursitis
3. Thyroglossal cyst
4. Laryngocele (may occur in front of the neck)

Solid Swellings:

1. Thyroid nodule (goiter)
2. Submental lymph node swellings
3. Median ectopic thyroid tissue
4. Lipoma of the space of Burn's (suprasternal notch).

11. SWELLINGS IN LATERAL SIDE OF THE NECK

A useful way of classifying lateral swellings of the neck to aid in diagnosis is to decide whether the swelling is cystic or solid.

Solid Swellings	Cystic Swellings
1. Parotid Swellings (lower pole of the gland). 2. Jaw Swellings (from the angle of the jaw). 3. Submandibular Gland Swellings. 4. Thyroid Gland Nodule. 5. Carotid Body Tumor. 6. Schwannoma of the Neck. 7. Sternomastoid Tumor. 8. Cervical Rib - Scalene Syndrome. 9. Pan-Coast Tumor (Supra-clavicular). 10. Lipoma. 11. Lymph Node Enlargement: A. Lymphadenitis: a. Acute. b. Chronic: Non-specific - Specific (TB - syphilis). B. Lymphoma: a. Hodgkin's Disease (HD). b. Non-Hodgkin Lymphoma (NHL). C. Secondaries (Metastatic).	1. Ranula. 2. Branchial Cyst. 3. Laryngocele (and Tracheocele). 4. Pharyngeal Diverticulum (Pouch). 5. Retropharyngeal Abscess. 6. Thyroid Cyst. 7. Carotid Artery Aneurysm. 8. Subclavian Aneurysm. 9. Arteriovenous Fistula. 10. Deep Hemangioma. 11. Lymphangioma. 12. Cystic Hygroma. 13 Pneumatocele. 14. Pyogenic Abscess of L.Ns. 15. Cold Abscess (TB). 16. Degenerative Cyst. 17. Cysts Superficial to the Deep Fascia: a. Blood Cyst. b. Lymphatic Cyst. c. Sebaceous Cyst. d. Dermoid Cyst.

I. SOLID SWELLINGS

***Refer back* for:**

- Swellings of the angle of the **jaw**.
- Swellings of the **Submandibular salivary gland**
- Swellings of **the Thyroid gland.**

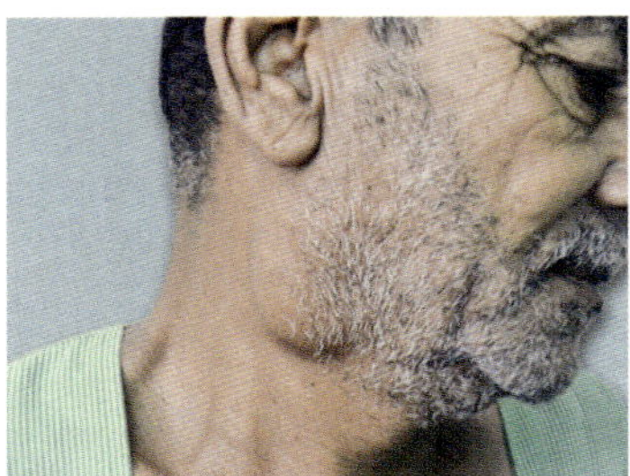

Fig. 1.34: A swelling at the lower pole of the right parotid gland (Atypical site)

Swellings of the Lower Pole of Parotid Gland

- A swelling of the lower pole of the parotid gland may present in the neck behind and below the angle of the mandible **(Figure 1.34)**.
- This situation may give rise to diagnostic difficulty.

Carotid Body Tumor

- *Age:* 40-60 years, may occur in children.
- *Sex:* It occurs more in males.
- *Course:* Long history as it is a slowly growing tumor.
- *Symptoms*: A painless slowly growing lump. Rarely, attacks of transient cerebral ischemia (giddiness, fainting or syncope, transient paralysis or paresis) due to compression of the carotid artery by the tumor.
- *Multiplicity*: Carotid body tumors may be bilateral.

  Site: It is usually solitary at the bifurcation of the CCA. Therefore, it is found in the upper part of the anterior triangle of the neck, level with the hyoid bone, and beneath the anterior edge of the sternomastoid muscle **(Figure 1.35)**.
- *Skin (Color):* Normal.
- *Size:* Variable from 2 or 3 cm in diameter to 10 cm.

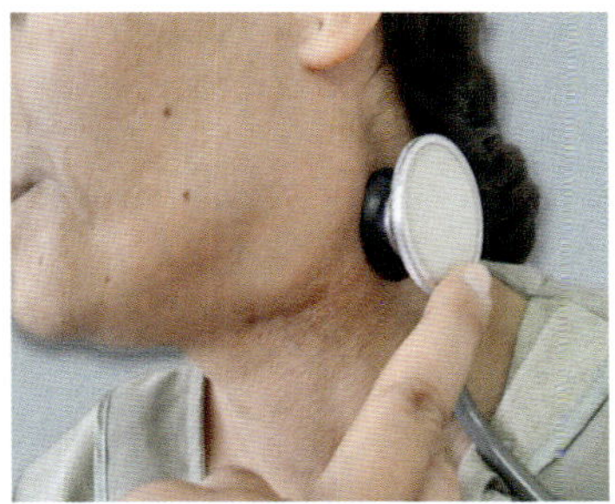

Fig. 1.35: Carotid body tumor in level with the hyoid bone. The ECA may cross the surface of the tumor and its pulsations may be felt

- *Shape:* It is shaped rather like a "potato". ***Hutchinson*** termed it the "*Potato Tumor*".
- *Surface:* Smooth, but sometimes bosselated.
- *Tenderness and Temperature:* Not tender and normal t^o.
- *Edge:* Indistinct.
- *Consistency:* Hard. It is dull to percussion and does not fluctuate. It is fixed to the carotid vessels and shows transmitted pulsations (i.e. not pulsatile by itself).
- *Relations*: It lies deep to the cervical fascia and the anterior edge of the sternomastoid. The CCA can be felt below it. The ECA may pass over its superficial surface (palpable pulsations).
- *Mobility*: It can be moved horizontally with ease, but has very little vertical mobility.
- *Lymph Drainage and Local Tissues*: Local L.Ns are not enlarged and local tissues are normal.
- *Special Investigations*: Angiography (vascular blush + separation of the ECA and ICA by the swelling with narrowing of their lumen) - Biopsy.

Schwannoma

- *Origin:* It may arise from: sympathetic chain vagus or glossopharyngeal nerve, or others.

- *Symptoms:* Painless lump in the neck. There may be pressure effects (on the RLN→ hoarseness of voice, on the esophagus→ dysphagia).
- *Site:* It lies deeply seated, about the middle of the neck.
- *Surface:* Smooth, encapsulated.
- *Consistency:* Firm.
- *Mobility:* It moves from side-to-side and not up and down (not along the course of the nerve).

Sternomastoid Tumor

- *Age*: The lump is noticed at birth or in the first few weeks of life.
- *Symptoms*: The mother may notice the lump or that the child keeps his head turned to one side (torticollis = Wry-Neck). Attempts to turn the head straight may cause pain or distress. As the child grows, the head becomes turned to one side and tilted towards the other side **(Figure 1.36)**.
- *Site*: A swelling in the middle 1/3 of the sternomastoid muscle **(Figure 1.37)**.
- *Size*: Usually 1-2 cm across.
- *Shape*: Fusiform, with its long axis along the line of the sternomastoid muscle.

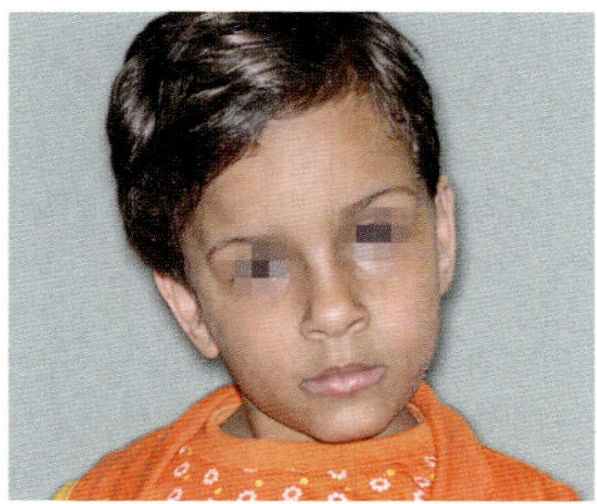

Fig. 1.36: Torticollis, often the sequel of a neglected sternomastoid tumor of infancy

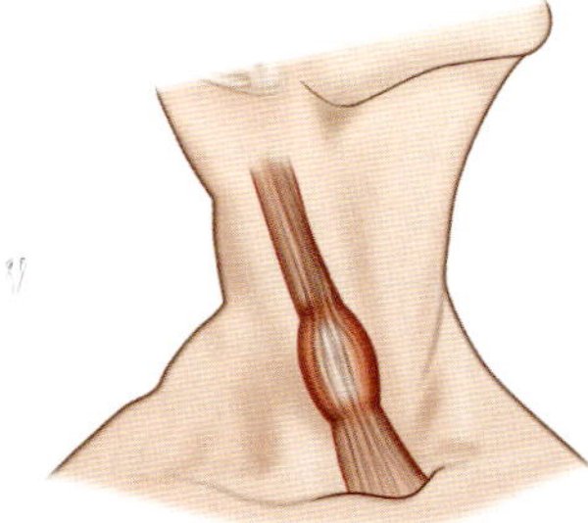

Fig. 1.37: Sternomastoid tumor is at the middle 1/3 of the sternomastoid muscle

- *Surface*: Smooth.
- *Tenderness*: May be tender in the first few weeks of life.
- *Edge*: Anterior and posterior edges are distinct but the superior and inferior edges, where the lump becomes continuous with normal muscle, are indistinct.
- *Consistency*: At first, it is firm and solid and easy to feel, but as it gradually becomes harder it begins to shrink and may become impalpable.
- *Local L.Ns and Surrounding Tissues*: Normal
- *Neck*: Apart from restriction of movement caused by spasm of the muscle, neck movements are normal.
- *Eyes*: Look at the eyes and watch their movements to detect any squint. Torticollis can be a means of correcting a squint. Move the head into a vertical and central position and watch the eyes. If the torticollis is secondary to a squint and not a sternomastoid tumor, the squint will appear as the head is straightened.

Cervical Rib Syndrome

- *Synonyms*: Scalene Syndrome = Superior Thoracic Aperture Syndrome.
- *Symptoms*:
  - Swelling: Sometimes there is fullness at the root of the neck (clinical diagnosis is difficult) **(Figure 1.38)**.

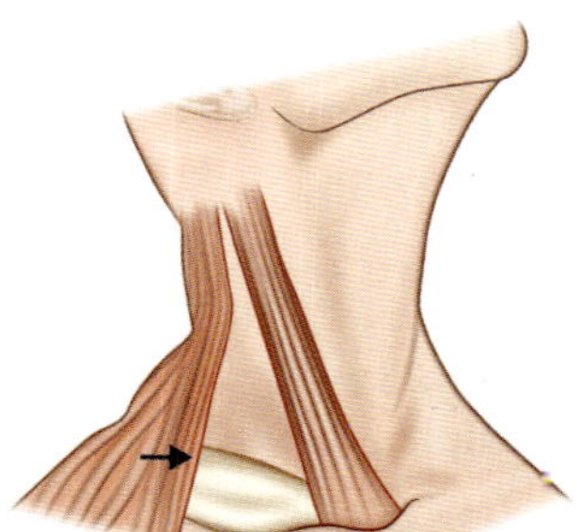

Fig. 1.38: Site of cervical rib: base of the neck

  - Neurological Symptoms (Common): Pain in the C8,T1 dermatomes and wasting and weakness of the small muscles in the hand.
  - Vascular Symptoms: Raynaud's phenomenon, trophic changes, even rest pain and gangrene particularly of tip of index finger. It may cause poststenotic dilatation (subclavian artery aneurysm) → mural thrombus → showers of emboli to the extremities.
- *Age:* Adolescence, and middle age.
- *Sex*: Females > Males (2:1).
- *Site:* A bony swelling may be felt, which is hard and fixed at the base of the neck. It is usually unilateral - right side > left side.
- *Clinical Examination:* Although a cervical rib can cause serious neurological and vascular symptoms in the upper arm, C/E of the neck usually reveals no abnormalities. The abnormal rib is usually detected with an X-ray.
- *Special Test (Adson's Deep-Breathing Test):* Rotation of the head towards the affected side + Taking a deep breath and holding it → diminished radial pulse volume.

Lipoma

- *The edge* is characteristically slippery.
- *The surface* may show dimpling.
- *Soft* in consistency (pseudocystic).

Lymphadenopathy

- *It is the commonest solid swelling of the neck.*
- They are usually multiple, oval and have special anatomical distribution.

II. CYSTIC SWELLINGS

Ranula (Refer Back)

- *Age:* Appears in childhood and adolescence.
- *Site:* When "plunging" it appears in the submandibular triangle.
- *Characteristics*: Bluish and translucent.

Branchial Cyst

Age: Although congenital it usually presents later, usually between the age of 15 and 25 years.
Sex: Males and females are equally affected.
Symptoms: Painless lump in the upper lateral part of the neck (**Figure 1.39**). Pain denotes infection.
Site: Deep to the anterior border of the upper 1/3 of the sternomastoid muscle (a common site for TB cervical abscess) **(Figure 1.40)**. Very rarely, it can bulge backwards *posterior* to the sternomastoid muscle.
Skin: Normal. May be red if the cyst is inflamed.
Size: Most branchial cysts are between 5–10 cm wide.
Shape: Ovoid, with its long axis running forwards and downwards.
Surface: Smooth.

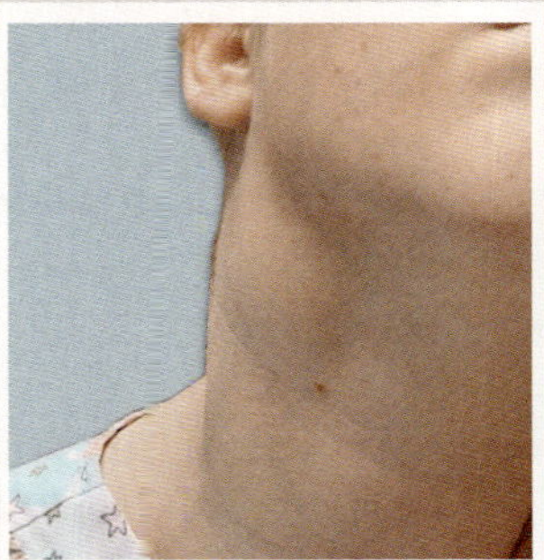

Fig. 1.39: Typical branchial cyst. Note its relation to upper 1/3 of sternomastoid muscle

- *Tenderness:* Absent, unless the cyst is inflamed.
- *Consistency*: It may feel "hard" if tense, or "soft" if lax. It is dull to percussion.
- *Translucency:* It is ***opaque*** as it contains desquamated epithelial cells that make its content thick and white.

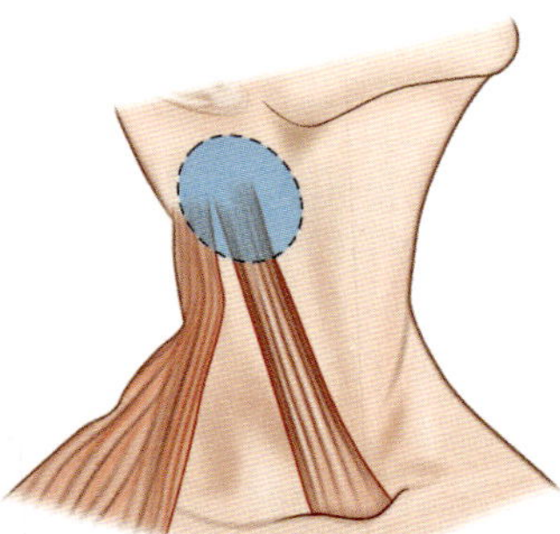

Fig. 1.40: Site of branchial cyst beneath upper 1/3 of sternomastoid

Sometimes, ***aspiration*** reveals fluid which is golden-yellow, rich in fat globules and cholesterol crystals

- *Compressibility:* The cyst *cannot* be reduced or compressed.
- *Relations: Deep* to the sternomastoid and not very mobile as it is closely tethered to surrounding structures.
- *Lymph Drainage:* Local deep cervical L.Ns are *not* enlarged. If they are palpable, you should reconsider your diagnosis in favor of a *tuberculous abscess* rather than a branchial cyst.
- *Local Tissues:* Normal, but if the cyst turns into an abscess, there will be edema + red and hot skin.

Laryngocele

- *Symptoms:* Cervical swelling that appears or ↑ on straining (**Figure 1.41**) and may be associated with dyspnea.
- *Occupation:* It occurs in professional trumpet player, singers and glass-blowers.
- Tense resonant swelling.
- Translucent.
- Compressible (empties on compression).

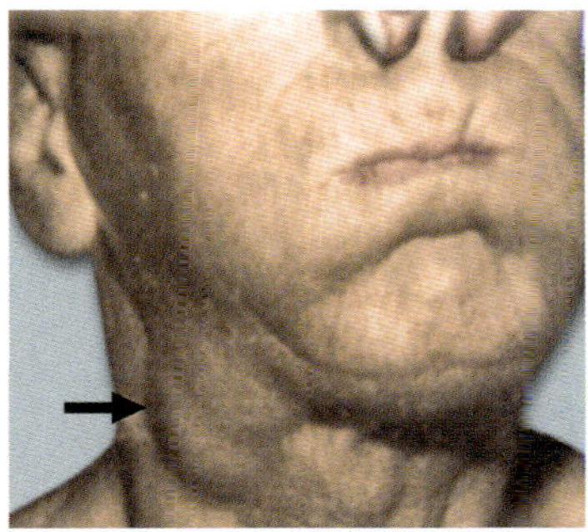

Fig. 1.41: Laryngocele. Swelling appears on blowing the nose

- It ↑ in size on straining (coughing or blowing the nose)
- It may extend in front of the trachea.

Pharyngeal Pouch (Diverticulum)

- *Age and Sex*: Middle and old age - Men > Women.
- *Symptoms*
  - The first symptom is *regurgitation* of undigested food. It may awaken the patient from sleep by a violent fit of *coughing or choking*. If pieces of food are inhaled, a *lung abscess* may develop.
  - As the pouch grows it presses on the esophagus and causes dysphagia.
  - By the time symptoms become severe, the patient notices a neck swelling and discovers that pressure on the swelling causes gurgling sounds and regurgitation. The swelling changes in size and often disappears.
  - If dysphagia continues, the patient becomes *malnourished and loses weight.*
- *Site:* The swelling appears *behind* the sternomastoid muscle at the junction of the upper and middle 1/3 of

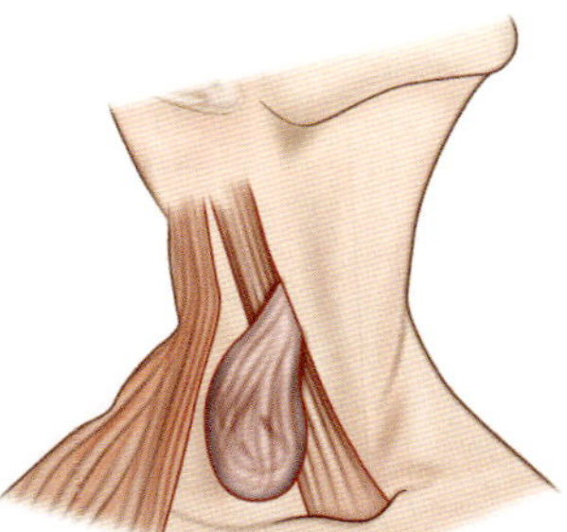

Fig. 1.42: Site of a pharyngeal pouch behind the sternomastoid

the neck (below the level of the thyroid cartilage) (**Figure 1.42**). It is usually on one side, usually the left.

- *Size:* Mostly 5-10 cm, but it ↑ after taking food and straining, and disappears on pressure, with gurgle.
- *Shape* is indistinct because only part of its surface is palpable. *Surface* is smooth and *Edge* is *not* palpable.
- *Consistency (Composition):* Soft, sometimes indentable. It is dull to percussion and does *not* fluctuate or transilluminate. *It can be compressed and sometimes emptied.*
- *Relations:* It lies deep to the deep fascia, behind the sternomastoid muscle, and is fixed deeply.
- *Lymph Nodes and Local Tissues:* Lymph nodes are not enlarged, and local tissues are normal.
- *General Examination:* There may be aspiration pneumonia, collapse of a lobe or a lung abscess.
- *Special Investigation*: Barium swallow will show the diverticulum.

Pyogenic Abscess

- It is painful and tender.
- The skin over it is red and hot.
- There are signs of toxemia.

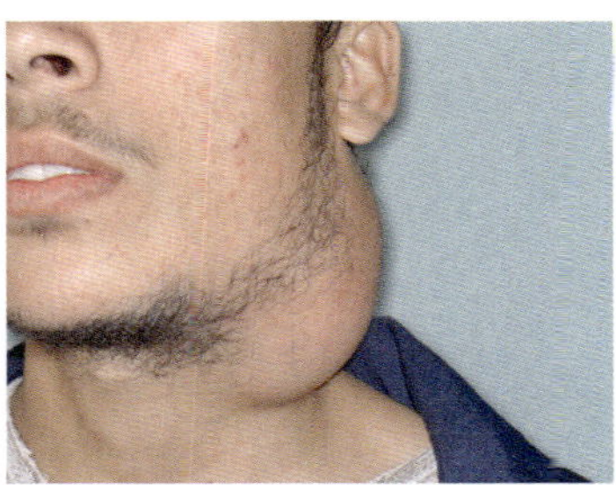

Fig. 1.43: A large cold abscess with no signs of inflammation

Cold Abscess (TB Abscess)

- *It is the commonest cystic swelling in the lateral neck side* (**Figure 1.43**).
- It is common in the upper part, but may occur in any group of lymph nodes.
- Characterized by multiplicity (other L.Ns) (satellites).
- TB toxemia, or other TB lesions may be present.
- It is fixed to surrounding structures (muscle or skin).
- Aspiration reveals caseous material.
- Plain X-ray may show calcification.

Cystic Hygroma (Lymph Cysts, Lymphangioma)

- *Age:* Infancy or childhood.
- *Symptoms*: A disfiguring lump **(Figure 1.44)**.
- *Site*: It usually lies at the base of the neck, filling the whole posterior triangle **(Figure 1.45)**. However, they can be very big occupying the whole of the SC tissue of one side of the neck.
- *Size*: Varies from few cm across to huge lumps filling the side of the neck. Occasionally, as a result of naso-pharyngeal infection, the swelling becomes inflamed and may ↑ in size rapidly.

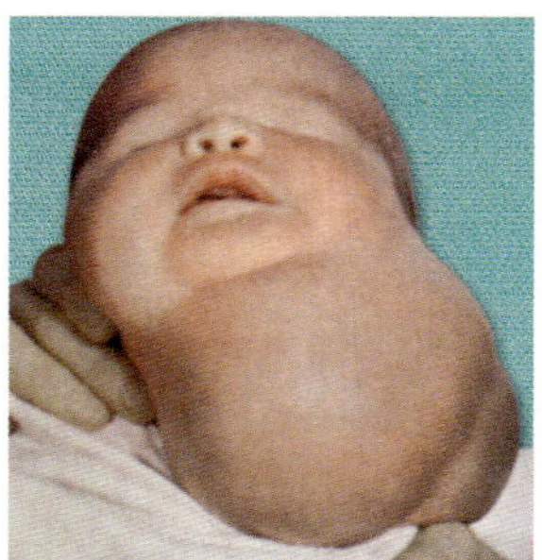

Fig. 1.44: Cystic hygroma

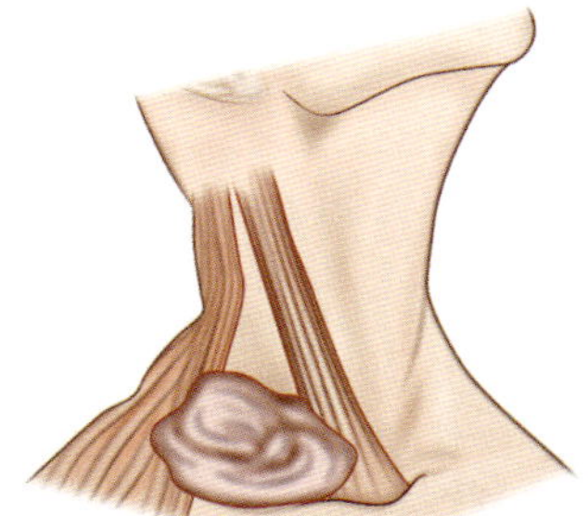

Fig. 1.45: Site of cystic hygroma in the posterior triangle

- *Shape:* It is a mixture of soft uni- and multilocular cysts, so that the whole mass looks lobulated and flattened.
- *Surface:* Deep cysts feel smooth.
- *Temperature and Tenderness:* It is not hot or tender.
- *Consistency:* It is softly cystic and is partially compressible, but *cannot be reduced*. It is dull to percussion and fluctuates easily.
- *Translucency:*
  The swelling is characteristically brilliantly translucent (transilluminable), because it is close to the skin and contains clear fluid.
- *Thrill*: Large cysts will conduct a fluid thrill.
- *Relations*
  They develop in the SC tissues. Thus, they are superficial to the neck muscles and close to the skin but are rarely fixed to the skin.
- *Lymph Nodes and Local Tissues:* Normal.

Carotid and Subclavian Aneurysms

- Swelling in the line of an artery (CCA is vertical, and subclavian is horizontal).
- Mobile across not along the axis of the related artery.

- The swelling may show expansile pulsation.
- Compression of the artery distal to the swelling stops the pulsations.
- A bruit is heard over the swelling.
- Distal pulse is delayed and is weaker than the other side.
- Pressure symptoms on nerves and veins lead to pain and weakness.

Pneumatocele

- Herniation of the apex of the lung through weakness of the supra-pleural membrane.
- It occurs in emphysema.
- It appears on cough and has a typical crepitating feeling.
- Resonant.

Sebaceous Cyst

- You *cannot* pinch the skin from over the swelling.
- It is attached to the skin by a punctum.
- Compression may express the sebaceous material out.
- Doughy in consistency.
- May be multiple.

12. SWELLINGS OF THE CHEST WALL

I. SWELLINGS FROM THE CHEST WALL

A. Cystic Swellings

1. Cutaneous and Subcutaneous Swellings

a. *Hematoma.*
b. *Abscess - Furuncle - Carbuncle - Infected Cyst* (e.g. infected sebaceous cyst or infected hematoma) → pain, tenderness, hotness, pitting edema of the skin over + fluctuation and pus on aspiration.
c. *Sebaceous Cyst:* Attached to the skin by a punctum. Similar to sebaceous cyst elsewhere.
d. *Dermoid Cyst* (in the midline of the sternum). Similar to dermoid cyst elsewhere.
e. *Hemangioma—Degeneration* in a solid tumor.

2. Abscess from Bony Lesions

a. *Pyogenic Abscess*:
   - It usually results from osteitis of ribs or sternum.
   - It used to occur towards the end of a typhoid attack, but may occur years later.
   - At first, there is a firm, tender swelling, which is followed by suppuration.
   - Plain X-ray shows destruction and sequestration.
b. *Cold Abscess*:
   - *From T.B. Osteitis and Periosteitis:* There is a cold abscess which may lie:
     - Outside the ribs.
     - Partly inside and partly outside (hour-glass). It is reducible and gives impulse on cough (resembling empyema necessitans).

- Behind the breast pushing it forwards (Retro-mammary abscess).
- *From TB of the Spine (Pott's Disease)*
  - The cold abscess tracks along the inter-costal nerve to lie at the "lateral border of the sternum".
  - Angular deformity, limited movements of the spine and absent tenderness over the ribs help in diagnosis + absence of tenderness directly over the ribs + plain X-ray + aspiration (reveals caseous material).

B. Solid Swellings

1. Skin and SC Swellings

a. *Benign Tumors*:
- Lipoma: *It is the most common B.T. of the chest wall.*
- Neurofibroma: It may arise from intercostal or superficial nerves.
- Cavernous hemangioma.
- Lymphangioma.

b. *Malignant Tumors*:
- Fibrosarcoma: *It is the commonest primary soft tissue malignant swelling of chest wall.*
- Others: Liposarcoma, neurofibrosarcoma, etc.

2. Bone Swellings (From the Ribs and Sternum)

a. *Benign Tumors*:
- Osteoma: Rare, and present with a very slowly growing, hard mass.
- Chondroma:
  - It is usually single, affecting males and females equally, usually young adults.
  - The swelling is painless and usually grows anteriorly along the costal margin.

b. *Malignant Tumors*:
   - Chondrosarcoma: *The most common primary MT of the skeletal system of chest wall.*
     - Site: It occurs most commonly at the costochondral junction.
     - Age: 20-40 years.
     - It presents as a painless mass (inflammations are painful) that attains a large size. The surface is lobulated and may show areas of cystic degeneration.
     - X-ray picture shows destroyed cortical bone and diffuse mottled calcification.
   - Multiple Myeloma.
   - Metastases:
     - Commoner than primary M.Ts and cause pain and pathological fracture at the site of the swelling.
     - A primary source should be sought in the thyroid, breast, lungs, kidneys, suprarenals and prostate.

II. SWELLINGS FROM WITHIN THE CHEST

These Swellings Have the Following Characteristics:
- Usually cystic.
- Reducible.
- Show impulse on cough.
- The patient may have associated manifestations of the thoracic disease.
- PXR show opacity (soft tissue shadow).

1. **Empyema Necessitans (Pointing Empyema):**
   - Rare nowadays.
   - *Site:* It commonly points at the lateral border of the sternum at the 2nd intercostal space (the widest), but may point anywhere (showing reducibility and impulse on cough).

- The affected side of the chest is stony dull on percussion, with no breath sounds.
- The heart may be shifted to the right
- Aspiration is diagnostic and chest X-ray shows opacity.

2. Pneumatocele (Hernia of the Apex of the Lung):

- *Site:* It appears in the *supra-clavicular region,* in emphysematous patients.
- It shows reducibility with crepitus and impulse on cough.

3. Liver Abscess:

- It may point on the back of the right side of the chest wall.
- Painful swelling in the right hypochondrium, with fever, rigors, and malaise.
- The liver is enlarged, tender, firm and usually smooth.
- There is positive intercostals tenderness with or without rigidity and edema of the overlying skin.
- The chest on the affected side may show signs of diminished air entry.
- *Laboratory tests* show ↑ WBCs anemia, ↑ serum alkaline phosphatase, bilirubin is normal except in multiple abscesses.
- *Plain X-ray chest* shows right basal atelectasis or pleural effusion.
- *Radioactive isotope scanning* shows cold defect(s).
- *US and CT:* Allow determining the site and size of the abscess and also guide therapeutic percutaneous drainage.

4. Pulsating Aneurysm:

- It is rare and results mainly from syphilis.
- The dilated aortic arch erodes the manubrium and presents as a pulsating swelling.

Key Points—Swellings of the Chest Wall

The most common benign tumor of the chest wall is .... **lipoma**.
The most common malignant tumor of the chest wall is ......**secondaries**.
The most common primary soft tissue M.T. of chest wall is .... **fibrosarcoma**.
The most common primary skeletal M.T. is .... **chondrosarcoma**.

13. SWELLINGS OF THE AXILLA

Swellings in the axilla may arise from the **skin** (sebaceous cyst, boil, SCC, melanoma), **subcutaneous tissue** (lipoma, fibroma, neurofibroma, hemangioma - they may turn malignant), **lymph nodes** (acute lymphadenitis, chronic lymphadenitis whether non-specific or specific such as TB, lymphoma or secondaries from the breast or upper limb), **axillary nerves** (neurofibroma), **areolar tissue** (fibrosarcoma, liposarcoma), **blood vessels** (aneurysm), or **bone** (dislocated shoulder, benign tumor such as chondroma, or malignant tumor such as osteoclastoma or osteogenic sarcoma).

I. SWELLINGS FROM THE WALLS OF THE AXILLA

Tumors of the Skin

1. *Sebaceous Cyst*:
   It is cystic or doughy, opaque, and attached to the skin by a punctum. It may present with acute or chronic inflammation.
2. *Acute Abscess*:
   There are well-marked signs of local inflammation and general febrile disturbance.
3. *Chronic or Cold Abscess*:
   It forms a single, fluctuating swelling, which if large, may extend upwards under the pectoralis. Local signs of inflammation are minimal or absent. Aspiration settles diagnosis.

Swellings of the Axillary Wall

a. Anterior Wall:
   - Fibrosarcoma of the pectoralis major.
   - Pectoral lymph nodes.

b. Posterior Wall:
   - Fibrosarcoma of the subscapularis.
   - Lipoma under the subscapularis fascia.
   - Chondrosarcoma of the scapula.

c. Medial Wall:
   - Cold abscess.
   - Chondrosarcoma of the ribs.
   - Metastases in the ribs.

d. Lateral Wall:
   - Aneurysm of the axillary artery.
   - Thrombosis of the axillary vein.
   - Neurofibroma.

Axillary Wall	Type of Swelling	Clinical Presentation
A. Anterior Wall:	1. Fibrosarcoma of pectoralis major:	- Presents in the chest and hardens with contraction of the muscle. It occurs more common in front of the chest wall than in the axilla.
	2. Pectoral L.Ns:	- At the lateral border of the pectoralis major (Primary focus frequently absent).
B. Posterior Wall: From the sub-scapularis or the scapula	1. Fibrosarcoma of the sub-scapularis:	- Firm, slowly growing, taking the shape of the muscle. Bulges only in the axilla not on the dorsal surface of the scapula.
	2. Lipoma under the subscapularis fascia:	- May simulate fibrosarcoma because the dense fascia prevents accurate palpation. It is usually discovered at operation.
	3. Chondrosarcoma of the scapula:	- Hard, lobulated with areas of cystic degeneration. It moves with scapular movements, and bulges both in the axilla and on the dorsal surface of the scapula.

Contd...

Contd...

C. Medial Wall: Fixed to chest wall	1. Cold abscess:	- From TB of ribs or spine (Pott's), cystic, upper thoracic angular kyphosis, FXR is essential for diagnosis.
	2. Chondrosarcoma of ribs.	- Hard, lobulated swelling.
	3. Metastases in the ribs.	- Pain, pathological fractures,etc. A firm, tender swelling may be felt. Common sites of the primary tumor should be searched for.
D. Lateral Wall: Move with the arm	1. Aneurysm of axillary Artery:	- Usually traumatic, after a stab or bullet. Characteristics: Look below **(Figure 1.46)**.
	2 Thrombosis of axillary Vein:	- Thick, tender vein and with swollen painful limb. Usually follows effort.
	3. Neurofibroma:	- Fusiform, tender and mobile across and not along axis of the nerve.

Characteristics of Aneurysm of the Axillary Artery (Figure 1.46)

- Expansile pulsation.
- Systolic thrill.
- May be hot.
- Decrease in size on closure of the subclavian artery.
- The distal pulse is weaker and delayed as compared to the other normal side.

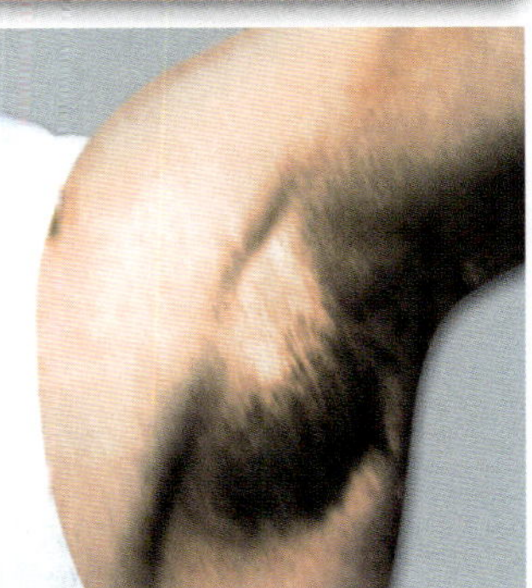

Fig. 1.46: Aneurysm of axillary artery following trauma

- The arm may be swollen due to pressure on veins.
- It may also be painful and weak due pressure on nerves.

II. SWELLINGS FROM CONTENTS OF THE AXILLA

Axillary Lymph Nodes

- These constitute the *most common* causes of axillary swellings.
- Malignant secondaries from the breast are the most important: They are hard, multiple, mobile at the beginning but become fixed later on.
- It may also be inflammatory (e.g. T.B), or neoplastic (e.g. lymphoma).

Axillary Tail of the Breast (Axillary Tail of Spence)

- It lies deep to the deep fascia (passing through the foramen of Langer).
- If carcinoma develops, it resembles enlarged pectoral lymph nodes, but there is one definite mass.

Accessory Breast

- Usually bilateral **(Figure 1.47)**.

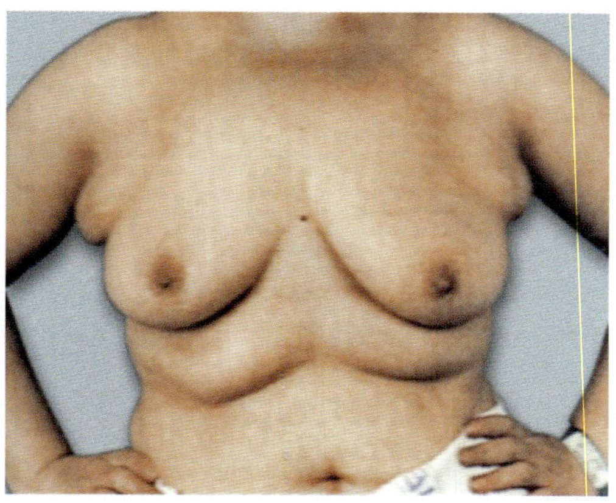

Fig. 1.47: Bilateral accessory breasts

- May manifest only after lactation as a soft lump, attached to the skin, at the lateral edge of the pectoralis major muscle, closely resembling a lipoma.

Lipoma in the Axilla

- It is the *most common* tumor.
- It may attain a large size and extend up under the pectoralis muscles.
- It is a slowly growing (long history), soft, lobulated swelling with a slippery edge and free mobility.
- The skin wrinkles when one attempts to rise away from the tumor. It may show dilated visible veins.

Cystic Hygroma

- Cystic hygroma of the axilla is rare.
- It is usually congenital, but may appear in adult life.
- It either presents in the axilla alone, but more commonly, it burrows from the posterior triangle of the neck through the cervicoaxillary canal along the axillary vessels to present in the axilla, with cross-fluctuation.
- It forms a soft, fluctuating (cystic), quite translucent, and painless swelling, which may grow rapidly (**Figure 1.48**).

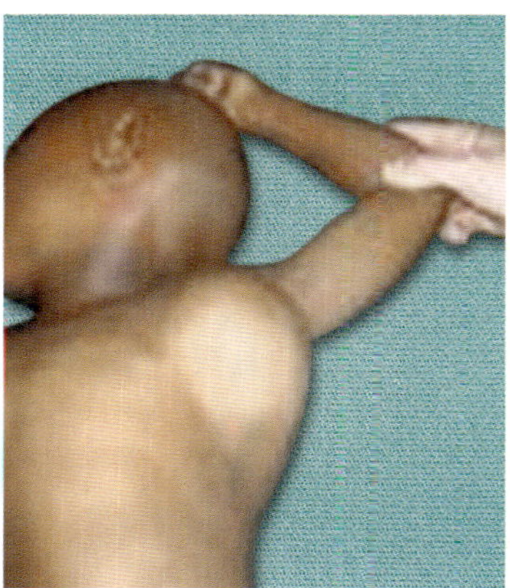

Fig. 1.48: Left cystic hygroma

- It may be mistaken for a lipoma, and diagnosis may not be certain except with excisional biopsy.

Hydradenitis Suppurativa

- It results from chronic infection of the apocrine sweat glands or sebaceous glands.
- It presents with multiple, small, painful abscesses that may open spontaneously resulting in multiple discharging sinuses as shown in **Figure 1.49**.
- It is different to treat as it is liable to recurrence. It may need wide surgical excision and soft tissue coverage.

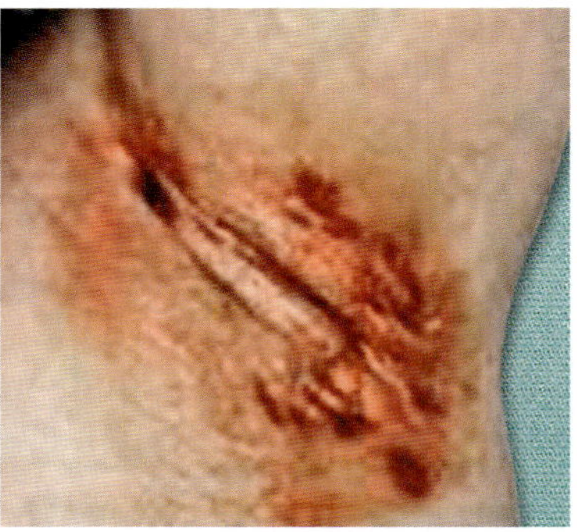

Fig. 1.49: Hydradenitis suppurativa of the left axilla

14. SWELLINGS OF THE BREAST

CLASSIFICATION

Swellings related to the mammary glands could be classified into the following:

1. **Swellings of the *whole* Breast:** *Unilateral or Bilateral.*
2. **Local Swellings *in* the Breast:** *Acute or Chronic - Cystic or Solid.*
3. **Swellings that are *not* in the Breast:** *Swellings that push the breast forward.*

I. SWELLINGS OF THE WHOLE BREAST

Bilateral

1. **Pregnancy and Lactation**:
   This is normal and may cause confusion only if the patient is unaware of her condition. Both breasts are enlarged equally and feel tense and nodular. The superficial veins are usually prominent, and on gentle squeezing a few drops of milk are discharged from the nipple. Montgomery's tubercles will be evident.
2. **Milk Engorgement**:
   The condition follows parturition due to obstruction of the ducts by epithelial debris. When bilateral, both breasts are greatly swollen, dusky, tender, with prominent veins and low-grade fever. Evacuation (manual, by pump, or suckling) causes immediate relief.
3. **Breast Hypertrophy:**
   True hypertrophy is rare. The enlargement is of two types: the commoner where multiple fibroadenomata cause a bilateral enlargement of varying consistency, and the less common consisting of a diffuse lipomatosis of both breasts. The condition is usually bilateral, but may be one-sided, in which case it is very disfiguring.

4. **Gynecomastia in Males:**
Usually there is a history of drug intake (e.g. estrogens, steroids, diuretics, digitalis, or tranquilizers), or chronic disease (e.g. portal hypertension, renal failure, hepatitis, or chronic chest disease). It may be obvious on inspection with a firm, mobile palpable plaque of breast tissue beneath the areola. The mass may involve the whole breast. It is often tender though the overlying skin is normal. *Nipple changes* or *fixation of the mass* suggests malignancy.

Unilateral

Unilateral enlargement of the whole breast is usually found in the undeveloped breast.

1. **Neonatal Breast Enlargement (usually bilateral):**
The enlarged breast is soft and without fixation to the skin or chest wall. The enlargement may be asymmetric and there may be secretion of colostrum. In the absence of stimulation, spontaneous involution occurs over a period of several weeks.
2. **Puberty:**
In girls between 10-13 years, one breast may enlarge several months before the other and may distress the mother. Unless there are obvious signs of inflammation, no notice need to be taken.
3. **Unilateral Hypertrophy:**
It is less common than bilateral hypertrophy.

II. SWELLINGS IN THE BREAST

A. Acute Swellings

1. **Acute Mastitis:**
It usually occurs in a lactating lady. The patient has fever from the start, with a rapid pulse and loss of appetite. The

swelling is painful, tender, hot with a red, edematous and shiny overlying skin. It may take the shape of a sector of the breast. It may occur in infants, puberty and with mumps.

2. **Acute Abscess:**
   - It means localization and pus formation occurring in acute mastitis.
   - It usually occurs within the first few weeks of breast feeding and is characteristically due to *Staphylococcus aureus.*
   - Fever becomes hectic and pain throbbing.
   - Fluctuation may be elicited but is never awaited for.
   - Enlarged tender axillary lymph nodes are felt.
   - All other signs of an acute abscess elsewhere are present **(Figure 1.50)**.
3. **Acute Lactational Carcinoma:**

   It is a rapidly growing type of cancer that occurs in a pregnant or lactating young lady. It resembles an acute abscess but its induration is greater and extends more than that expected for an abscess, it is less tender, and there is no fever. It does not respond to antibiotics.

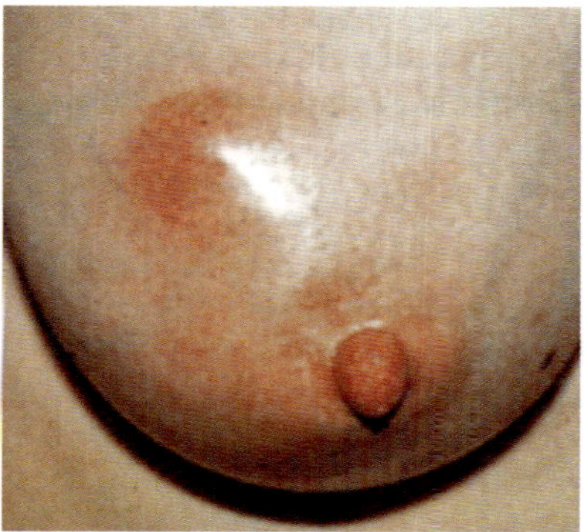

Fig. 1.50: Acute breast abscess. Note signs of acute inflammation

B. Chronic Swellings

1. **Traumatic:**
   - *Traumatic Fat Necrosis (TFN):*
     Hard, irregular, swelling that may be fixed or tethered to the skin simulating cancer. History of trauma and absence of enlarged axillary lymph nodes are suggestive of TFN. However, if there is any doubt about the nature of the swelling, it should be excised with a wide ellipse of surrounding breast tissue, and submitted to histology.
   - *Chronic Hematoma:*
     It results from organization of an acute hematoma and leads to a firm irregular lump that may be confused with carcinoma and therefore should be excised and examined.
2. **Inflammatory:**
   - *Chronic Non-specific Breast Abscess:*
     - Usually there is a history of acute mastitis with abscess that turned into a chronic one.
     - It forms a firm mass due to fibrosis, which may cause nipple retraction and puckering of the skin.
     - The mass is irregular, fixed to the breast substance and may be the pectoral fascia, with enlarged, firm axillary lymph nodes.
     - It simulates carcinoma but may be differentiated from it by history, clinical examination and biopsy.
   - *Chronic Specific Breast Infection: Tuberculous abscess:*
     - It is insidious, starting as a painless irregular swelling, the periphery of which is hard and the center is soft.
     - Later, the skin becomes reddened, and an abscess forms which may burst and leave a sinus.
     - This is the *nodular form,* which differs from an acute abscess in that the duration is much longer, there is little or no pain or fever and the pus, if

examined, reveals no organisms on culture, unless there has been secondary infection.
- Direct examination of stained films of the pus may show tubercle bacilli.
- The sclerosing form of TB forms severe fibrosis resulting in a firm mass and nipple retraction resembling cancer.

- *Gumma of the Breast* (Syphilis):
  - It is rare.
  - It resembles the sclerosing type of tuberculosis.
  - Other stigmata of tertiary syphilis are present.

3. **Fibrocystic Disease (Fibroadenosis)**
   - *The classical triad of presentation is*: Pain in the breast (mastalgia) + lump + nipple discharge.
   - *The lump:*
     - Usually diffuse and bilateral (diffuse type), but may affect only one sector of the breast (sector or nodular type).
     - Felt with the *tips* of the fingers but *not* with the flat of the hand contrary to carcinoma.
     - Firm in consistency.
     - Irregular surface.
     - Mobile within the breast.
     - Not fixed to the overlying skin or underlying structures.
     - May be associated with nipple retraction.
   - *Discharge:* A yellowish, brownish, or even black nipple discharge may be present.
   - *Axillary lymph nodes:* These may be enlarged, but are discrete, slightly tender, and *not* hard in consistency.
4. **Neoplastic:**
   - Benign Tumors:
     - *Duct Papilloma:*

       It arises from one of the *large ducts* near the nipple. It is usually single (may be multiple) and is ***precancerous.***

It usually occurs between 35-50 years (rare before the age of 25 years). Nipple discharge is usually blood stained (bright or dark), rarely serosanguinous. *Cystic swelling* (dilated duct) may be felt under the areola (tumor itself is not felt). The affected duct may be localized by digital pressure along radial lines towards the nipple and the tumor is demonstrated, by *mammography*, as a filling defect in the dilated duct.

- *Fibroadenoma*:
  It is usually single and unilateral (80%) but may be multiple (adenomatosis) and bilateral (20%). Differences between "hard" fibroadenoma and "soft" fibroadenoma are summarized in the Table.

Feature	Hard Fibroadenoma	Soft Fibroadenoma
Incidence:	More common	Much rarer
Age:	14–30 years (peak = 21 years)	Older age (30-50 years)
Pathology:	• Well encapsulated. • Solid • Peri-canalicular fibrosis.	• Not well capsulated. • Partly solid and partly cystic. • Intra-canalicular fibrosis.
C/P:	– Small painless rounded lump – Grows slowly – Firm in consistency – Freely mobile (breast mouse). – Never turns malignant.	– Larger, painless, lobulated lump. – Grows more rapidly – Soft ± cystic (cystadenoma) – Less mobile, may fungate – May turn sarcomatous.

- *Cystosarcoma Phylloides (Giant Soft Fibroadenoma):*
  — *Phylloides* means leaf-like pattern.
  — It is called *sarcoma* because it is a rapidly growing fleshy *hot* tumor with dilated veins and stretched areola and skin, but *without* enlargement of lymph nodes, or fixation to the skin or muscles.

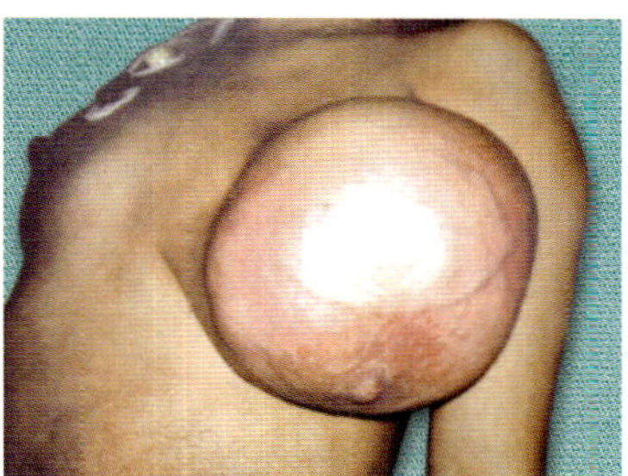

Fig. 1.51: Giant soft fibroadenoma of the left breast

— It usually occurs > 40 years.
— It fills the whole breast in 6-12 months **(Figure 1.51)**.
— The mass is rounded, lobular, well-defined, firm, elastic, very mobile, with stretched skin and dilated veins.
— Hot signs are present (however it is not tender).
— Its characteristic feature is "tear drop appearance" on profile.
— It is a benign condition but may require simple mastectomy, and should be differentiated from cancer of the breast.

- ***Malignant Tumors: Carcinoma of the Breast***

Lump in the Breast:
- Hard in consistency.
- Usually not tender.
- Irregular surface.
- Ill-defined edges.
- Felt with the *flat* of the hand (as opposed to fibroadenosis).
- Fixed within the breast tissue.

- May be fixed also to the skin and/or deeper structures (**Figure 1.52**). It may be *multifocal* (more than one lump in one quadrant) or *multicentric* [other lump(s) in other quadrant(s)].
- The lump is tested for mobility in 2 perpendicular directions before and after muscle contraction.

Nipple and Areola Changes:

- Examine the areola for: Size, surface and the degree of pigmentation.
- Recent retraction (**Figure 1.53**):
  Note that nipple retraction may be congenital (developmental) or due to an inflammatory lesion.
- Erosion: Malignant eczema or Paget's disease.
- Depression.
- Destruction.
- Deviation.
- Discharge:
- Usually there is no discharge, but in duct carcinoma a bloody discharge is present, and in scirrhous carcinoma, a crystal clear discharge is rarely observed.

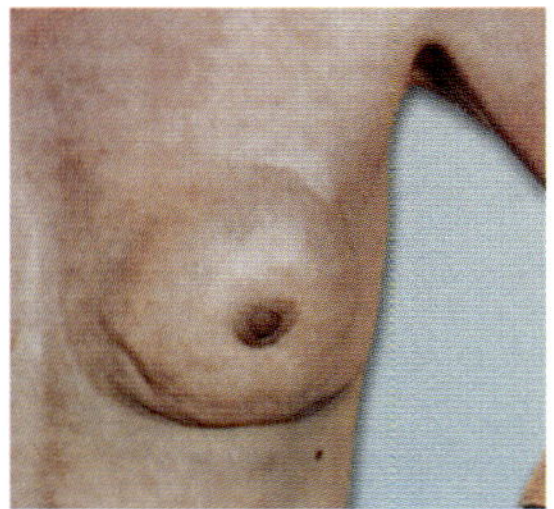

Fig. 1.52: The lump is fixed to the skin and deeper structures. The patient presses her hand firmly into her side to put the pectoralis major into full contraction

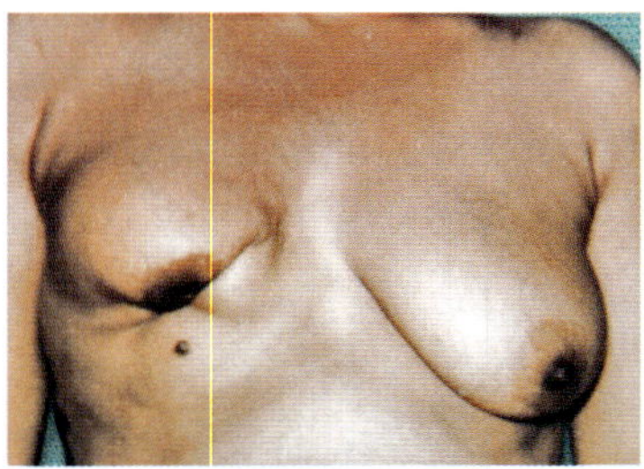

Fig. 1.53: Comparison of nipples. This case of right carcinoma of the breast shows that the nipple is both raised and retracted

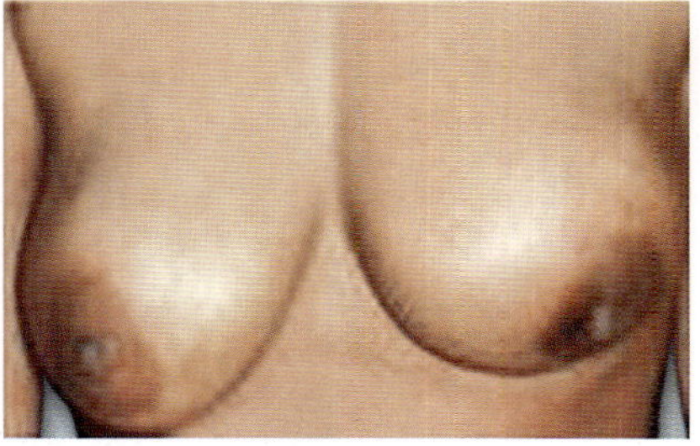

Fig. 1.54: The left breast does not protrude freely being tethered by IDC

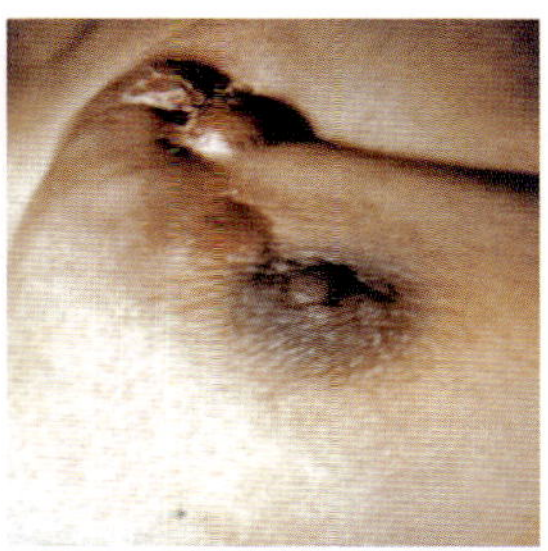

Fig. 1.55: Skin nodules (left breast)

Breast:
- Fibrosis causes the breast to become puckered and displaced. It is pulled upward on raising the arms above the head.
- It does not protrude freely when the patient leans forwards (**Figure 1.54**).

Skin Changes:
- Dimpling and puckering.
- Dilated veins.
- Peau d'orange.
- Skin lymphedema.
- Fixation of the skin to the tumor.
- Cancerous nodules and satellites (**Figure 1.55**).
- Malignant ulceration (**Figure 1.56**).
- Fungation (**Figure 1.57**).
- Cancer-en-cuirasse (late).
- Inflammatory signs (in acute cancer of pregnancy and lactation).
- Nipple and areola changes.

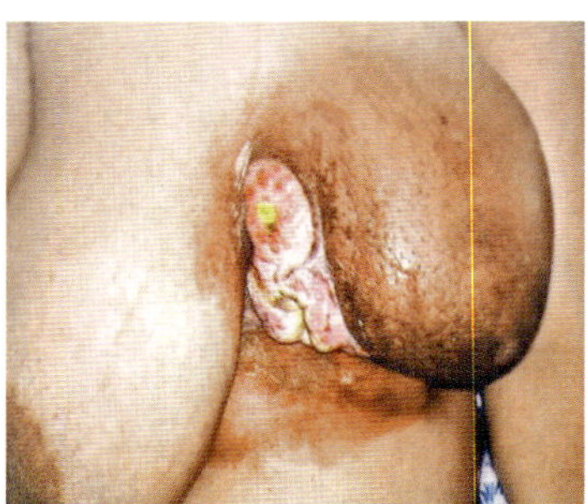

Fig. 1.56: Malignant ulceration of left breast carcinoma

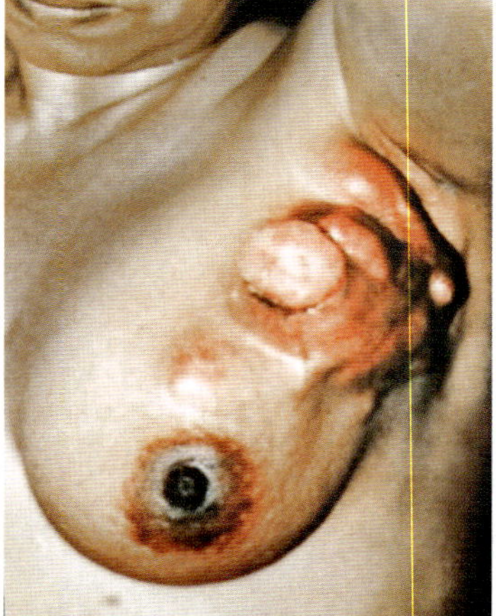

Fig. 1.57: Fungating breast cancer

Opposite Breast:

Metastases may be detected on careful palpation, but when seen early, it seems more probable that it should be regarded as an independent primary growth.

Lymph Nodes: Axillary and supraclavicular LNs, on both sides should be thoroughly examined for:

- Enlargement
- Consistency

- Tenderness
- Mobility.

General Examination:

- *Head and Neck:* For skull metastases and enlarged supraclavicular LNs.
- *Chest:* Pleural effusion, pulmonary deposits and enlarged mediastinal LNs.
- *Abdomen:* Hepatomegaly (tender right hypochondrium), malignant ascites and peritoneal deposits.
- *Pelvis:* PV and PR examination to detect secondaries in the ovaries (Krukenberg's disease).
- *Bones:* Tenderness, weakness, deformity and pathological fractures.
- *Nervous System:* For brain metastases.

Sarcoma of the Breast

It may arise in a soft fibroadenoma. It is characterized by the following:

- A rapidly growing painful lump in the breast.
- A relatively large lump *without* axillary L.N. enlargement (characteristic).
- Warm tender, firm-to-hard (may be cystic due to degeneration).
- Fixed in the breast tissue.
- The skin becomes stretched with marked dilatation of veins.
- No retraction of nipple or other signs of fibrosis.
- The lump is usually not fixed to underlying structures, but fungates through the skin and disseminates to the lungs and viscera.

– The following Table shows the characters of the 4 common breast lumps in the present history and clinical examination:

	Chronic Abscess	Fibroadenoma	Fibroadenosis	Carcinoma
History:				
Onset:	After acute abscess	Accidental	With menstruation	Accidental
Duration:	Short	Long	Long	Short
Course:	May turn to acute abscess	Slow ↑ in size	↑ size + tenderness during menses.	Nipple discharge, metastases.
Associated Symptoms:	Slightly tender axillary LNs.	–	Pain - discharge.	Skin changes, axillary L.Ns
Disappears	–	–	May be	–
Multiplicity:	–	–	+ (usually)	Rarely
Precipitating factor:	Acute abscess	–	Hormonal disturbance	Pre-cancerous lesions
Local C/E:				
Number:	Single	Single	Usually multiple	Single
Site:	Any	Any	Usually whole breast	Usually UOQ
Shape and Surf:	Variable	Oval	Nodular breast	Flat undersurface
Skin Over:	Free or attached	Free	Free	Signs of cancer
Consistency:	Firm or hard	Firm	Firm or rubbery	Hard
Edge:	Ill-defined	Well-defined	Ill-defined	Ill-defined
Tenderness:	±	–	±	–
Mobility:	Fixed in the breast substance	Mobile in the breast substance	Free mobility	Fixed in breast, to skin or deep tissue
Regional L.Ns	± Firm and tender	Free	± Firm and tender	Hard, mobile or fixed

Cystic Swellings of the Breast

A. Duct System (Acinar Cysts):

- *Fibroadenosis*:
  - Complaints: Pain, swelling, discharge.
  - Axillary L.Ns are enlarged and may be tender.
  - The lump is smooth and fluctuant (nodular type); however, fluctuation may be difficult to elicit. Aspiration reveals a clear, green, or yellow fluid. The lump should disappear completely; otherwise, excision biopsy should be done.
- *Galactocele (Milk Cyst):*
  - Occurs in a lactating breast behind an obstructed duct as a single painless swelling deep to the areola, with milky discharge on squeezing the breast.
  - It is mobile in its bed.

B. Stroma (Interacinar Cysts):

- Hydatid cyst
- Blood cyst
- Lymphatic cyst
- Serous cyst
- Inflammatory, e.g. TB

C. Neoplastic:

- *Benign*:
  - Papillary cystadenoma.
  - Duct papilloma (retention cyst).
  - Cystsarcoma phylloides.
- *Malignant*:
  - Degeneration of carcinoma, or sarcoma.
  - Intracystic papillferous carcinoma

D. Cysts of Skin and Subcutaneous Origin:

- Sebaceous cyst.
- Dermoid cyst.

III. SWELLINGS PUSHING THE BREAST FORWARD

These are often mistaken by the patient for breast tumors, and include:

1. **Retromammary Abscess:**
   - It is most commonly *tuberculous*, arising in an underlying rib or in a mediastinal abscess that has tracked along a branch of the internal mammary artery.
   - Sometimes, an *empyema* points beneath the breast, usually in the 5th or 6th intercostal space in the midclavicular line.
2. **Chondroma:**
   - A hard nodular swelling springing from one of the ribs and tilting or pushing the breast aside.
3. **Rib Deformities:**
   - The commonest is a prominence of the costochondral junction of the 3rd rib.
   - It is often bilateral, and may be associated with other abnormalities of the ribs or vertebrae.

MALE BREAST DISEASES

A. Gynecomastia

- Generalized enlargement of the male breast due to increase in the ductal and connective tissue elements.
- Usually there is a history of drug intake (e.g. estrogens, steroids, diuretics, digitalis, or tranquilizers), or chronic disease (e.g. portal hypertension, renal failure, hepatitis, or chronic chest disease).
- It may be obvious on inspection with a firm, mobile palpable plaque of breast tissue beneath the areola. The mass may involve the whole breast (**Figure 1.58**). It is often tender though the overlying skin is normal.
- *Nipple changes* or *fixation of the mass* suggests malignancy.

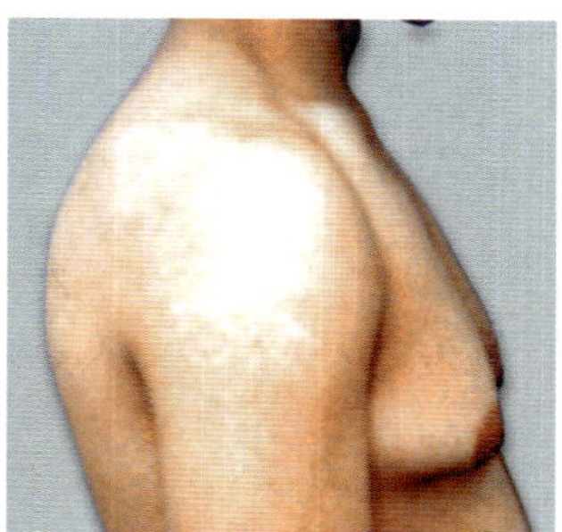

Fig. 1.58: Gynecomastia (profile view), Note enlargement of the breast simulating a female breast (bilateral)

B. Mastitis

1. Mastitis of Infancy
   - It is common in the male as in the female.
   - Clinical signs of acute inflammation are evident.
   - It usually resolves but occasionally suppuration occurs.
2. *Mastitis of Puberty:*
   - It usually occurs in a 14-year-old patient.
   - Complaints include pain and swelling of one breast (80%).
3. *Traumatic Mastitis:*
   - It results from local irritation (manual workers and soldiers).
   - It just requires removal of the cause.

C. Fibroadenosis

Similar to females.

D. Fibroadenoma

Similar to females.

E. Carcinoma

- Male breast cancer accounts for only *1%* of all breast cancers. It is commoner in *UK and USA* than Japan.

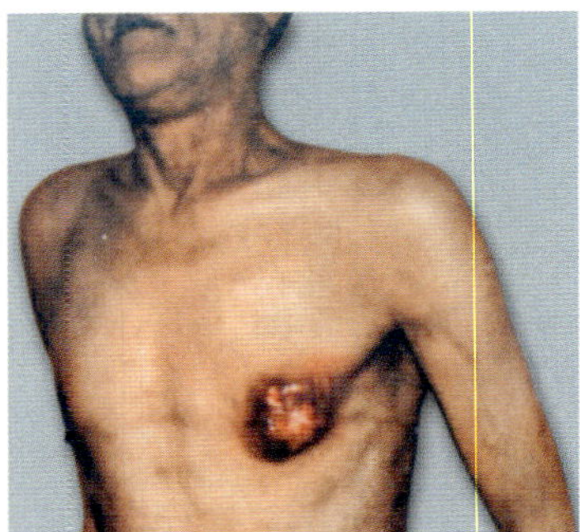

Fig. 1.59: Male left breast cancer with skin invasion and ulceration

- Antecedent *gynecomastia* is present in 10-20% of cases, while *Klinefelter's syndrome* ↑ the risk by 60 times.
- It presents a decade later than in females, with an average age at diagnosis of 60 years.
- It invades extra-mammary tissues early because of scanty subcutaneous tissue.
- Clinical picture:
  - Subareolar mass.
  - Skin ulceration **(Figure 1.59).**
  - Nipple distortion or nipple discharge.
  - Gynecomastia.
  - Enlarged axillary lymph nodes.

BENIGN BREAST CONDITIONS THAT MIMIC BREAST CANCER

Benign Breast Disease in Relation to later Malignancy

To date, microscopic characteristics of pre-malignant conditions, which might indicate their potential for malignant, particularly invasive, transformation are not well defined. The only reliable measure is the extent of in situ changes, which can be determined accurately only by biopsy for histological examination.

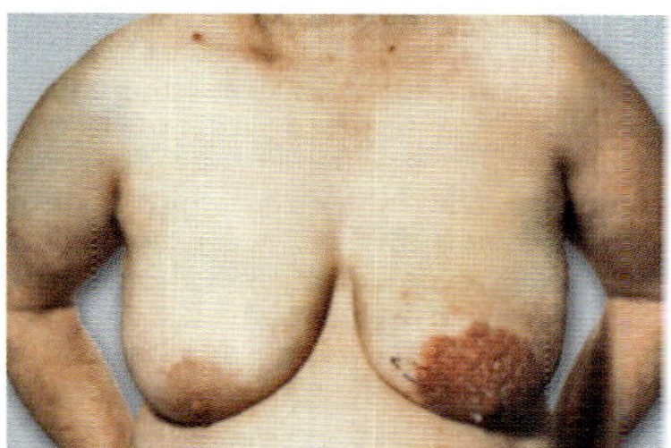

Fig. 1.60: Benign eczema of nipple and areola

No Increased Risk

- Fibroadenomas.
- Ductal ectasia.
- Solitary Papilloma.
- Typical epithelial h yperplasia.

Increased Risk

- Atypical ductal hyperplasia.
- Atypical lobular hyperplasia.
- Cystic disease.
- Papillomatosis.

Benign Lesions that Mimic Breast Cancer with the Signs of Malignancy they cause

Condition ↓	**Signs of malignancy** ↓
Eczema (**Figure 1.60**)	Mimics Paget's disease
MDE	Nipple discharge, retraction and skin changes
Mastitis	Lump, skin tethering
Sclerosing adenosis	Lump, microcalcification on mammography
Solitary papilloma.............. discharge	Discrete mass, bloody or serous discharge.

BREAST LESIONS IN CHILDREN AND ADOLESCENTS

Neonatal Breast Enlargement:

- The enlarged breast is soft and without fixation to the skin or chest wall.

- It may be asymmetric and there may be secretion of colostrum.
- Spontaneous involution occurs in several weeks.

Neonatal Mastitis:

- Uncommon but can lead to severe illness with generalized sepsis.
- The breast area is enlarged, firm and erythematous.
- Fluctuation from abscess formation may be evident.

Premature Development:

- Prepubertal development of the breasts in the absence of other evidence of sexual maturation.
- It may be unilateral or asynchronous.
- Repeated clinical examination and reassurance are all that are necessary.
- Ill-advised excision of the subareolar breast bud in young girls will make normal breast development impossible.

Juvenile Hypertrophy of the Breast:

- It occurs occasionally in adolescent girls and can produce a major cosmetic problem.
- It is usually bilateral, but may be unilateral, and may occur in only one area of a breast.

Breast Abscesses:

- Occur occasionally in adolescent girls and usually respond to antibiotics and drainage.
- Subareolar abscess may be related to mammary dysplasia.

Benign Neoplasms:

- They are most commonly fibroadenomas.
- Other benign conditions include:
  - Fat necrosis.
  - Cysts.
  - Lipomas.
  - Intraductal papillomas.

Malignant Neoplasms:

- Malignancy, whether carcinoma, sarcoma or metastases, is ***rare*** in childhood and adolescence.
- Any unusual appearance of a breast lesion is an indication for biopsy.

Key Points— A Lump in the Breast

Acute Lump
1. Acute lactational carcinoma
2. Acute mastitis
3. Acute breast abscess

Chronic Lump
1. Traumatic: TFN, chronic hematoma
2. Inflammatory: Chronic breast abscess (Non-specific), TB and syphilis (specific)
3. Mammary dysplasia = Mammary duct ectasia (MDE)
4. Neoplastic: BT (fibroadenoma, duct papilloma) - MT (carcinoma, sarcoma)

Painless Lump
1. Carcinoma
2. BT: Duct papilloma, fibroadenoma
3. Breast cysts
4. Fat necrosis

Painful Lump
1. Fat necrosis
2. Abscess
3. Fibroadenosis/cystic hyperplasia
4. Inflammatory carcinomatosa, or advanced carcinoma (fungation, infection....).

Lumpy Axilla
1. Physiological: Obesity (always bilateral).
2. Accessory breast: Presence of a nipple.
3. Lipoma: No nipple, soft, smooth surface and slippery edge
4. Enlarged axillary L.Ns (pectoral L.Ns are deep to the pectoralis major muscle).
5. A tumor in the axillary tail of Spence (superficial to the pectoralis major muscle).

Hard Lump
1. Traumatic
- Traumatic fat necrosis
- Chronic calcified hematoma
2. Inflammatory:
- Non-specific: Chronic abscess
- Specific: TB and syphilis
3. Fibroadenosis
- Interstitial fibroadenosis
4. Neoplastic:
- Benign: Hard fibroadenoma
- Malignant: IDC.

Large (Huge) Lump
1. Giant soft fibroadenoma
2. Encephaloid carcinoma
3. Sarcoma

Large Breast (Massive Breast enlargement)
1. Physiological: Pregnancy and lactation
2. Benign hypertrophy of the breast (Usually bilateral - cause is unknown)
3. Milk engorgement/Acute mastitis
4. Filarial elephantiasis

Bilateral Breast Lesions
1. Fibroadenosis.
2. TB
3. Lobular carcinoma
4. Secondary tumor from a primary in the other breast, or a second primary cancer.

Differences between Mammary Paget's Disease and Eczema

Point of Difference	Paget's Disease	Eczema
Site	Always unilateral	Bilateral
Age	Menopausal	Age of lactation
Nipple Erosion	+	–
Breast Lump	Sub-areolar mass	–
Vesicles	–	+
Itching	–	+
Response to R/	–	+
Biopsy	Paget cells	–

What are the Causes of the Following?

Peau d'orange:

- Breast cancer.
- Fibroadenosis.
- Chronic breast abscess.

Nipple Retraction:

- Breast cancer (IDC).
- Congenital (withdrawn nipple).
- Chronic breast abscess.
- Mammary duct ectasia (MDE).

Nipple Deviation:

- To same side: IDC, chronic breast abscess.
- To opposite side (sarcoma).

Pain in the Breast (Mastalgia/Mastodynia):

- Cyclical mastalgia (the commonest cause), Non-cyclical mastalgia.
- Cracked nipple, post-traumatic.
- Acute inflammatory conditions (e.g. acute mastitis, breast abscess).
- Fibroadenosis (FCD).

- Cancer (e.g. inflammatory breast carcinoma, or advanced cases of other types).
- Non-mammary Causes of Breast Pain:
  - Tietz disease (inflammatory disease of the costo-chondral junction).
  - Cervical rib or cervical root syndrome.
  - Myocardial infarction.
  - Herpes zoster.
  - Pulmonary and GIT causes.

NIPPLE DISCHARGE

Discharge from the nipple may be divided into three classes:

A. Normal Discharges .... *milk*

- *Pregnancy*: Discharge of milk during pregnancy is not uncommon especially in multipara.
- *Lactation*: Usually of a small amount except when the child is put on the breast.

B. Normal Discharges at Abnormal Times

- *Colostrum*:
  A secretion similar to colostrum sometimes occurs in the newly born and again at puberty, due to endocrine stimulation. It predisposes to infective mastitis where secretion becomes purulent.
- *Milk (Galactorrhea):*
  It results from a galactocele, or hyperprolactinemia due to pituitary adenoma, hypothyroidism, or drug-intake, e.g. phenothiazines and methyldopa.

C. Abnormal Discharges

- Serous Fluid:
  - Fibrocystic disease (FCD).

- Duct papillomata.
- May be scirrhous carcinoma or mammary duct ectasia.

- Green Fluid:
  - Pseudomonas infection.
  - Derivatives of hemoglobin (spectroscopy or chemical assay).
- Yellowish Fluid (Pus):
  - Breast abscess.
  - TB lesion (tubercle bacilli in the discharge).
- Grumous or Poultaceous (toothpaste-like) material:
  - Mammary duct ectasia.
    - Lump: Retroareolar, hard and may be difficult to differentiate from carcinoma.
    - Linear nipple retraction associated with MDE is characteristic.
    - Microscopic picture shows ecstatic ducts containing lipid-laden macrophages and surrounded plasma cells, hence the name plasma cell mastitis.
- Serosanguinous discharge:
  - Paget's disease.
  - May be carcinoma.
- Hemorrhagic (blood-stained) or bleeding per nipple:
  The younger the patient the more likely is the cause to be benign; the older the patient the more likely to be malignant.

  Causes from ***within*** *the ducts:*
  - *Benign*:
    - Duct papilloma.
    - Fibrocystic disease.
    - Papillary cystadenoma.
  - *Malignant*:
    - Duct carcinoma.
    - Paget's disease

- *Vascular* (hyperemia or bleeding vessel):
  - Acute mastitis, MDE (not abscess)
  - Pregnancy (engorged breast).
  - Blood diseases (purpura, hemophilia).

*Causes from **without** the ducts:*
- Trauma (abrasions, injury to a duct)
- Chronic Inflammation, TB
- Carcinoma (infiltrating a duct).
- Drugs, e.g. anticoagulants (heparin).

The commonest causes of nipple discharge are:
Duct papilloma.
Fibrocystic disease (FCD)
Mammary duct ectasia (MDE).

15. ABDOMINAL MASSES

Regions of the Abdomen

The abdomen is divided by 2 vertical lines (planes) and 2 transverse lines (planes) into 9 regions:

The 2 vertical planes pass from the mid-inguinal point upwards, on each side.

The 2 transverse planes:

1. The *upper* is roughly midway between the xiphoid and umbilicus, or touching the lower costal margin (*subcostal line*), or at a "trans-pyloric plane", which passes at the lower edge of L1.
2. The *lower* plane is roughly midway between the umbilicus and symphysis pubis, or between the highest points of the iliac crests (*intercostal line*) or between the tubercles of the iliac crest (*intertubercular line*).

*Accordingly, the 9 regions will be (**Figure 1.61**):*

1. Right hypochondrium.
2. Epigastrium
3. Left hypochondrium.
4. Right lumbar region.
5. Umbilical region.
6. Left lumbar region.
7. Right iliac fossa (RIF).
8. Hpogastrium (supra-umbilical region).
9. Left iliac fossa (LIF).

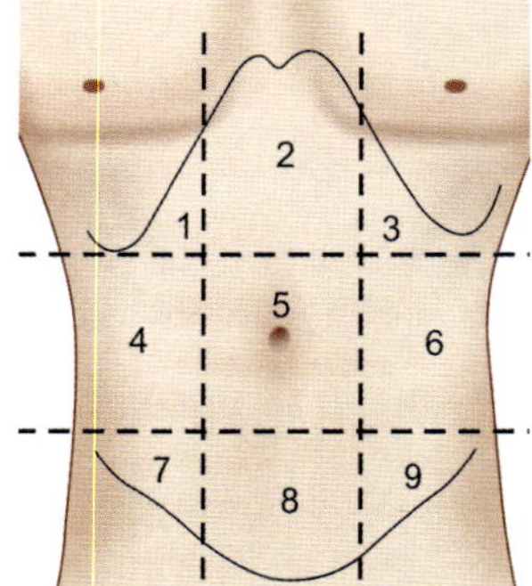

Fig.1.61: Regions of the abdomen

Clinical Approach and Diagnosis

Although recent methods of investigations have facilitated the diagnosis of abdominal swellings, yet the usual scheme of history-taking and physical examination usually lead to a correct clinical diagnosis. The following is a useful approach:

1. **Symptoms:**
   Symptoms of the patient indicate the organ from which the mass originates.
2. **It is parietal or intra-abdominal?**
   A parietal mass bulges more on rising up, while an intra-abdominal mass becomes less prominent or even disappears.
3. **What is the site of the mass?**
   A mass of an abdominal organ occupies the region where it normally lies. However, it may be encroached upon from an organ that lies in another region.
4. **Is it mobile?**
   - Fixed (adherent to the posterior abdominal wall):
     - Retroperitoneal Tumors: lymphoma, secondaries, and benign tumors.
     - Inflammatory Swellings: cold abscess, appendicular mass.
     - Pancreatic Swellings: Tumors, cysts.
     - Advanced Malignant Tumors.
   - Mobile with respiration (related to the diaphragm) → Liver, GB, spleen, kidney.
   - Mobility at a right angle to the root of the mesentery → Mesenteric cyst.
   - Mobility in a transverse direction only → suprapubic mass (UB or uterus), ascending or descending colon.
   - Mobility only vertically → swelling in the epigastrium related to the transverse colon, or omentum
   - Mobility across the sigmoid → cancer sigmoid, bilharzial mass.
   - Mobility in all directions → wandering spleen.

5. **Is it cystic or solid?**
   Cystic intra-abdominal swellings include ovarian, mesenteric and pseudopancreatic cysts, hydronephrosis, encysted TB ascites, cold abscess, and degenerated retro-peritoneal tumor.
6. **Percussion:**
   Most abdominal swellings are dull on percussion. However, the following points are important:
   - Resonance between a mass and the liver or spleen, excludes its relation to such organs.
   - There is a band of resonance (colon) anterior to a kidney swelling, while it is dull posteriorly.
   - There is no band of resonance in front of a splenic swelling while there is a band of resonance posteriorly between the spleen and sacrospinalis.
7. **Investigations:**
   - Laboratory Tests:
     - Complete blood count (CBC).
     - Liver function tests (LFTs).
     - Renal function tests (urea and creatinine).
   - Imaging:
     - Plain X-ray and with contrast such as barium meal, or enema, or IVU.
     - Ultrasonography (US).
     - Computerized tomography (CT scan).
     - Magnetic resonance imaging (MRI).
   - Endoscopy:
     - Upper gastrointestinal endoscopy.
     - Lower gastrointestinal endoscopy.
     - Laparoscopy.
   - Exploration:
     - Undiagnosed intra-abdominal swellings must be subjected to exploration (and biopsy) for diagnosis.

MASS IN THE RIGHT ILIAC FOSSA (RIF)

I. Parietal Swellings

Skin	SC Tissues	Muscles	Abscess
• Papilloma • Sebaceous cyst • Squamous cell carcinoma • Melanoma	• Lipoma • Fibroma • Neurofibroma • Hemangioma • Lymphangioma • Soft tissue sarcoma	• Fibrosarcoma • Rhabdomyoma • Rhabdomyo-sarcoma • Lipoma (inter- or intra-muscular)	Abscess pointing in the parietes (iliac abscess) • Appendicular abscess • Psoas abscess (TB) • Pyogenic abscess

II. Intra-abdominal Swellings

From organs lying *in* the RIF Cecum - Appendix - Terminal ileum - Ascending colon	**From organs encroaching *on* the RIF** Liver - GB - Spleen - Kidney - UB - Fallopian tubes and Ovaries - Uterus - Arrested testis
1. Appendicular mass 2. Cancer cecum 3. Hypertrophic ileocecal TB 4. Ameboma 5. Actinomycosis 6. Intussusception 7. Crohn's disease 8. Mesenteric LNs (Tabes mesenterica, acute NS mesenteric lymphadenitis, lymphoma) or mesenteric cyst	1. Liver: Liver swellings 2. GB: Tumors, mucocele, empyema 3. Spleen: Splenic swelling 4. Kidneys: Renal swelling, unascended, ptosed 5. UB: Huge diverticulum 6. Tubes and Ovaries: Ovarian cyst or tumor, tubo-ovarian abscess 7. Uterus: Fibroid 8. Testis: Tumor in undescended testis

III. Retroperitoneal Swellings

Iliac Lymph Nodes	Iliac Artery	Areolar Tissue	Iliac Bone
• Non-specific lymphadenitis • T.B. - Filariasis • Lymphoma • Secondaries	• Aneurysm	• Sarcoma	• Osteomyelitis • Osteoclastoma • Chondroma • Chondrosarcoma • Osteogenic sarcoma

I. PARIETAL SWELLINGS (ABSCESS POINTING IN THE RIF)

Appendicular Abscess Pointing into the RIF

Features of transformation of a mass into an abscess:
- Increase in the mass size.
- Pain becomes throbbing.
- Temperature becomes hectic.
- Edema and fluctuation.
- Increased leukocytosis.

Iliopsoas Cold Abscess

- *Mass*: Cystic, not tender, not painful, lying in the RIF and below the inguinal ligament with cross fluctuation, and associated with psoas spasm (hip flexion).
- *Signs of primary cause*: Limited lumbar spine movement (losing its normal lordosis).
- *Diagnosis*: Aspiration + plain X-ray of the spine and sacroiliac joints.

Iliac Abscess of Pyogenic Origin

- Fever.
- Pain is not shifted as in acute appendicitis.
- Severe tenderness and erythema.
- A clear space may be formed out between the abscess and the iliac crest in appendicular abscess, but not in an iliac abscess.

II. INTRA-ABDOMINAL SWELLINGS

Appendicular Mass

- History of neglected acute appendicitis for 2-3 days.
- There may be nausea and vomiting (usually with constipation), and psoas spasm.
- Elevated temperature.

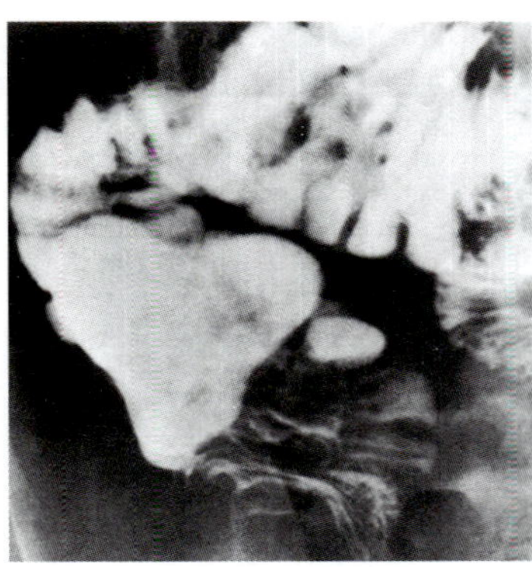

Fig. 1.62: Peri-appendiceal abscess. There is fixation and a mass effect at the base of the cecum with no filling of the appendix

- Appendicular mass: painful, tender, oblong in shape, firm in consistency and dull to percussion, fixed at the beginning, but later on it becomes movable. Borders are ill defined and the surface is irregular. It is usually tympanic on percussion.
- In case of an ***appendicular abscess*** fluctuation is difficult to detect unless the abscess is big and superficial, or the patient is very thin. If neglected, it approaches the surface and shows signs of acute inflammation (redness, edema and fixation to skin). Barium (**Figure 1.62**) helps diagnosis.
- *Investigations:* Leukocytosis, US, CT.

Cancer Cecum

- Age: Usually > 40 years of age
- Sex: Men > Women.
- The mass may be the first indication of the disease, but usually it indicates a late disease; the mass is firm or hard, with irregular surface, ill-defined edge, and is fixed or mobile.

- Unexplained weakness or anemia.
- Dyspepsia, diarrhea alternating with constipation and persistent right abdominal discomfort.
- Intestinal obstruction (occurs late).
- Occult blood with stools.
- *Investigations:*
  - Barium studies (filling defect).
  - CT scan.
  - Lower GI Endoscopy and biopsy.

Hypertrophic Ileocecal TB

- Age and Sex: Usually a female - young age.
- Gradual onset of pain in the RIF.
- Diarrhea alternating with constipation.
- Anemia.
- Abdominal mass: firm, tender, fixed or mobile.
- In case of obstruction: there is colicky pain, abdominal distention and visible peristalsis.
- TB manifestations of lung or L.Ns may be present.
- *Investigations*: Barium studies may reveal
  - Filling defect.
  - Iliac stasis with obstruction.
  - Obtuse ileocecal angle.
  - Sterling's sign (barium as if jumping from the ileum to the hepatic flexure).

Ameboma

- History of dysentery.
- Pain in the right lower quadrant.
- Two localized zones of tenderness: over the McBurney's point, and over the sigmoid.
- Enlarged, tender cecum and ascending colon. The mass simulates cancer.

- There may be intestinal obstruction due to adhesions resulting from pericolitis.
- It responds to antibiotics and anti-amebic drugs.
- *Investigations*:
  - Demonstration of Entameba histolytica in stools.
  - Barium enema demonstrating concentric narrowing.

Actinomycosis

- Young adult male with a *mass* in the RIF: very hard, fixed, irregular and tender.
- Multiple sinuses, discharging sulfur-like granules (colonies of the organism).
- Sometimes, the condition follows as operation on the appendix.
- Loss of weight and anemia.

Intussusception

- *Infantile Type*:
  It begins in the right iliac fossa, but only at a very early stage a lump may be formed here (usually higher up in position and with red current jelly passing per rectum).
- *Adult Type*:
  - Intestinal obstruction: abdominal pain, vomiting, and constipation.
  - Mass: firm, sausage-shaped (convex backwards and concave towards the umbilicus).
  - Bleeding and passage of mucus per rectum.
- *Investigations*:
  Barium enema shows a cup-shaped filling defect at the apex of the intussusceptum (**Figure 1.63**).

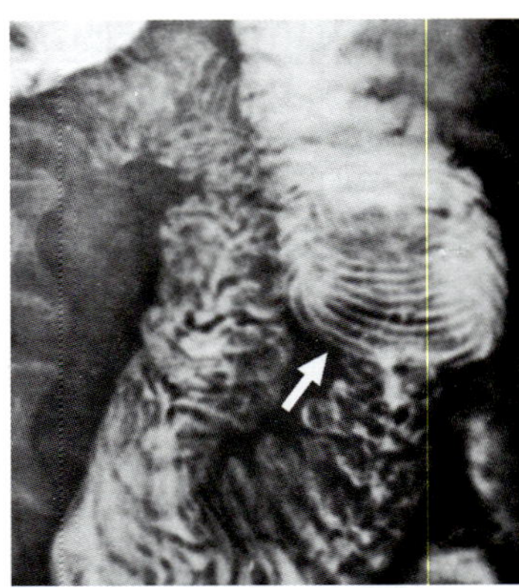

Fig. 1.63: Jejunojejunal intussusception coiled spring appearance

Crohn's Disease (Regional Ileitis)

- *Acute Stage*: It simulates acute appendicitis, however, diarrhea is always present.
- *Subacute Stage*: Diarrhea, colicky pain, blood and mucus with stools + Abdominal mass (matted loops of intestine): slightly tender, firm, mobile + Anemia and loss of weight.
- *Chronic Stage*: Intermittent intestinal obstruction.
- *Complicated Stage*: Abscess formation - fistula (external or internal).
- *Investigations*: Barium studies → String sign of Kantor, i.e. purse-string appearance of the terminal ileum due to narrowing of the affected part.

Mesenteric Lymph Nodes

- *Acute Non-Specific Mesenteric Lymphadenitis:*
  - The patient is usually a child with a history of upper RTI and he is usually free between attacks.
  - Fever reaches 40° C.

  - Diarrhea is common and shifting tenderness is characteristic (i.e. shifting on lying on the left side due to mobility of the mesentery).
- *Tabes Mesenterica (TB Mesenteric Lymphadenitis)*:
  - It commonly occurs in young children who present with alternating attacks of diarrhea and constipation, TB toxemia and a mass (Tender, firm and nodular).
  - Plain X-ray may show mottled calcification of the L.Ns.
- *Lymphoma*
  - A Non-Hodgkin lymphoma (NHL) that commonly affects children.
  - The mass moves in one direction (across the root of the mesentery), but may be fixed. It is usually hard, irregular and nodular and the intestine itself may be involved in the mass.

Other Causes

- *Misplaced Kidney*
  An ectopic or mobile kidney may be felt in the RIF. It is reniform in shape, firm in consistency and slightly tender. It can be pushed back into the renal angle, if it is a mobile kidney.
- *Ovarian Cyst*
  There is a smooth, cystic swelling, which occupies the supra-pubic region as well as the RIF. It is usually mobile and is dull to percussion.
- *Tumor in Undescended Testis*
  The mass is usually hard, irregular and fixed + empty scrotum.

III. RETROPERITONEAL SWELLINGS

Iliac Lymph Nodes

- *Acute Non-specific Lymphadenitis:*
  A child or young adult with very high temperature, severe toxemia and an abdominal mass (just above the inguinal

ligament, painful and tender, firm and fixed, suppuration leads to abscess formation, flexion and spasm of the hip joint (psoas spasm).

- *Filarial Nodes:*
  Periodic attacks of fever with simultaneous enlarged and tender nodes. Eosinophilia + Demonstration of microfilaria in blood drawn at night.
- *Lymphoma:*
  Young subject with rapid LN enlargement, variable in size and consistency. Usually not tender.
- *Secondaries:*
  Lymph nodes are hard, nodular, fixed, not tender. Finding the primary settles the diagnosis.

Aneurysm of the External Iliac Artery

- Swelling with expansile pulsations, palpated thrill and audible bruit.
- Lies along the line of the artery and mobile across it (i.e perpendicular to it).
- History of chronic ischemia of the right lower limb.

Retroperitoneal Sarcoma

- Young patient, with a lump that grows rapidly into a huge, firm, nodular mass with no early symptoms.
- It is fixed to the PAW and therefore does not move with respiration.
- Later on, pressure on the IVC causes edema of the lower limbs.

Iliac Bone Swellings

- *Chondrosarcoma*: It presents with a huge mass, lobulated, hard with cystic areas. The outer table of the iliac bone may be swollen also in the gluteal region.

- *Osteomyelitis*: Usually subacute and may end in an abscess and sinus. The bone is thickened and tender.
- *Bone Secondaries*: Should also be considered particularly in patients over 40 years of age.

THE MOST COMMON CAUSES OF A SWELLING IN THE RIF (FIGURE 1.64)

1. Appendicular mass (50%).
2. Cancer cecum (25%).
3. Non-specific acute lymphadenitis.
4. Hypertrophic ileocecal TB.
5. Ameboma.
6. Actinomycosis.

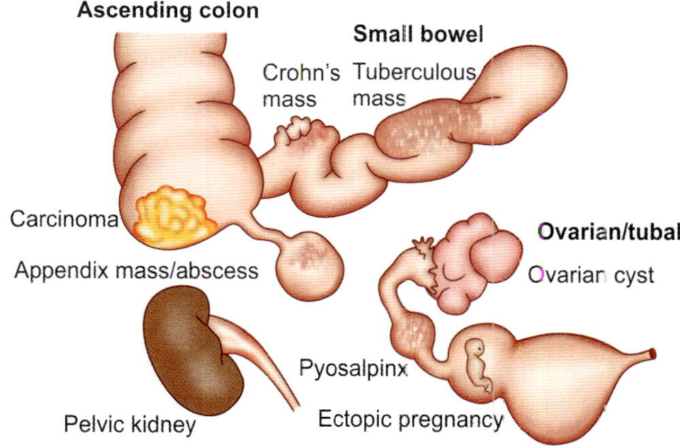

Fig. 1.64: Mass in the right iliac fossa

Investigations

CBC: Anemia (tumors) - Leukocytosis (Crohn's, appendicitis, diverticulitis).

US: Ovarian lesion, appendix/diverticular mass or abscess, Crohn's mass, pelvic kidney. Allows guided drainage of abscesses.

CT: Appendix/diverticular mass or abscess, Crohn's mass. Allows guided drainage of abscesses and biopsy of some tumors.
Colonoscopy: Colonic tumors, diverticular disease. Allows biopsy.
Barium Enema: Diverticular disease, colonic tumors.
Small Bowel Enema: Terminal ileal Crohn's disease.

MASS IN THE RIGHT HYPOCHONDRIUM

A swelling in the right hypochondrium may arise from the liver, GB, or right kidney. Being related to the diaphragm, it moves up and down with respiration. It may also arise from the hepatic flexure of the colon, or from the pylorus.

Classification

Classification of mass in the right hypochondrium table is given on the next page.

I. PARIETAL SWELLINGS

Hematoma:

- History of injury.
- Ecchymosis of the skin.
- It is at first cystic and then turns solid.

Cold Abscess:

- Cystic swelling in the right hypochondrium.
- It may arise in the transverse process, ribs or dorsal spine.
- Spread is usually along the lymphatics.
- Other evidence of TB may be present.

II. INTRA-ABDOMINAL SWELLINGS

A. Liver Swellings

Criteria of a Liver Swelling

- It is an intra-abdominal swelling that lies just beneath the anterior abdominal wall and moves with respiration.

Classification of Mass in the Right Hypochondrium

	Congenital	Traumatic	Inflammatory	Neoplastic	Others
Parietal		Hematoma	Cold abscess	Lipoma Neurofibroma	
Liver	Riedle's lobe Polycystic liver Hepatoptosis	Subcapsular hematoma	Liver abscess Amebic abscess Hydatid cyst	BT: Adenoma Hemangioma Hamartoma MT: Primary Secondaries	
G.B.	Choledochal cysts		Empyema Cancer head of pancreas	Adenocarcinoma	
Kidney	Polycystic kidney Fused kidney Congenital hydronephrosis		Hydronephrosis Stones	Wilm's tumor Hypernephroma Suprarenal tumors	
Hepatic flexure			TB (right side)	Cancer	Intussusception
Pylorus				Cancer	Perforated peptic ulcer

- It lies in the right hypochondrium, but may extend to the epigastrium or downwards to the right iliac fossa.
- It is dull to percussion, which is continuous with the normal dullness of the liver.
- The characteristics of the swelling (tenderness, surface, edge, consistency, etc.) depend on the cause.

Riedle's Lobe

- It is a normal anatomical variation in which a tongue-like lobe projects from the lower border of the right lobe along the anterior axillary line.
- Its dullness is continuous with that of the liver and can be mistaken for an enlarged GB.
- It does not extend to the loin.

Polycystic Liver

- It is rare and may be associated with polycystic kidney.
- The liver is occupied by cysts of variable sizes.
- It becomes irregularly enlarged.

Subcapsular Hematoma

- It usually results from a direct blow or road accidents.
- If the pressure inside increases, it ruptures spontaneously giving signs and symptoms of internal hemorrhage.
- Investigations that may reveal diagnosis include US and CT scan.

Pyogenic Liver Abscess

- It may be single (**Figure 1.65**) or multiple (or multiloculated usually resulting from portal pyemia, **Figure 1.66**).
- There is a painful swelling in the right hypochondrium, with fever, rigors and malaise.

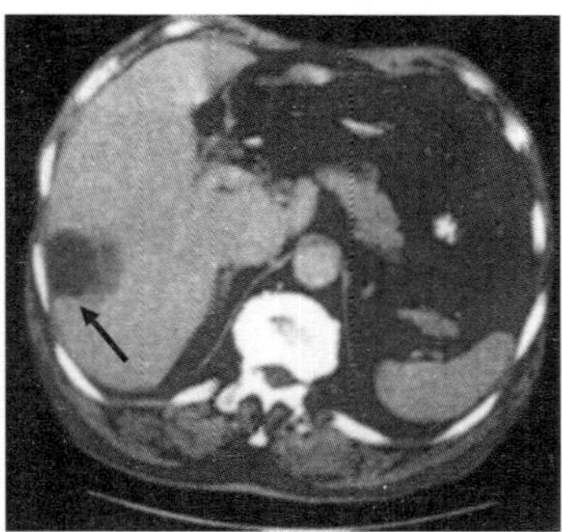

Fig. 1.65: CT with contrast (defines abscess more clearly) showing a solitary right lobe liver abscess

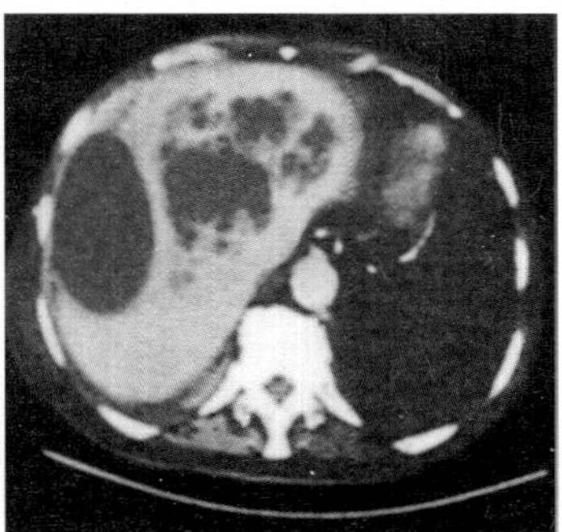

Fig. 1.66: CT showing a multiloculated right lobe liver abscess following portal pyemia

- The liver is enlarged, tender, firm and usually smooth.
- There is positive intercostal tenderness ± rigidity and edema of the overlying skin.
- The chest on the affected side may shows signs of ↓ air entry.
- *Laboratory tests* show WBCs ↑, anemia, bilirubin is normal except with multiple abscesses, serum AP ↑.
- *Plain X-ray* may show air-fluid level in the region of the liver.

- *Chest X-ray* shows right basal atelectasis or pleural effusion.
- *US and CT* can establish the site and size of the abscess and guide percutaneous drainage.

Amebic Abscess

- *History* of amebic dysentery before (usually a mild attack).
- *Age*: It usually affects middle-age adults (3rd–5th decades).
- *Sex*: Males > Females (9:1).
- *Symptoms*: pallor, ↓ of weight, earthy complexion, ± diarrhea. Fever, rigors, sweating, anorexia and malaise. Pain in the liver area and often referred to the right shoulder. Dry cough due to irritation of the diaphragm.
- *Clinical Examination*:
  - General Examination: Fever (38°C or more); Anemia and loss of weight; Jaundice (uncommon).
  - Abdominal Examination: Tenderness and rigidity in the right hypochondrium. Liver enlargement (50–70%) (smooth, firm and displaced downward). In the left lobe, the abscess may point in the epigastrium.
  - Chest Examination: Basal lung signs: crepitations + dullness on the right side due to pleural effusion. Intercostal spaces may show bulging, skin edema and deep tenderness.
- *Investigations*:
  - Laboratory:
    - Leukocytosis (but < pyogenic abscess), eosinophilia and anemia.
    - Stool analysis may reveal E. histolytica (if -ve do not exclude it).
    - Serological tests for detection of antibodies in the serum.
  - Imaging:
    - Plain X-ray → Elevation and fixation of the right copula of the diaphragm, obliteration of the

costophrenic angle, and collapse of the lower lobe of right lung.
  — Scanning of the liver using Rose Bengal or ^{99m}Tc (filling defect).
  — US, CT, MRI can help in localizing the abscess.
- Sigmoidoscopy: Flask-shaped ulcers, scrapings from the ulcer may reveal E. histolytica.
- Exploratory aspiration: Performed in the "OR" → anchovy pus (confirms diagnosis).
- Therapeutic test: Marked improvement with Emetine HCl (if still in the hepatitis stage).

Hydatid Cyst

- *Age*: Infestation occurs at a very young age, but takes many years to produce symptoms.
- *Number*: In its early stages, the cyst is univesicular and fertile, but later on, hundreds of cysts develop.
- *Distribution*: The disease is relatively common in sheep-rearing countries, e.g. Australia, Turkey, Iran, Iraq.
- *Site*: The commonest site is the upper posterior part of the right lobe of the liver.
- *Symptoms*:
  - It may be completely symptomless and discovered accidentally.
  - A smooth painless mass in the right hypochondrium.
  - Epigastric discomfort and sensation of pressure. Pain is rare and usually denotes complications.
  - It may present with one of its complications, e.g. jaundice, rupture or infection.
- *Clinical Examination*:
  - A smooth cystic swelling, mobile with respiration, may be palpable with downward displacement of the liver.
  - A hydatid thrill is rarely elicited on examination.

- *Investigations*:
  - Laboratory studies: Blood picture (eosinophilia) - LFTs.
  - Immunologic studies: The use of these studies ↓ in the present time because of imaging techniques.
  - Imaging studies:
    - Plain X-ray may show elevation, fixation, or distortion of the diaphragm. There may be a calcified intrahepatic shadow (water-lily appearance). Dense calcification denotes a dead cyst.
    - Radioisotope scanning gives information about location and number of the cysts.
    - CT and US help in localization and diagnosis of liver cysts. CT is the best in showing the number of cysts, location, daughter cysts and the density of the contents, which denotes if the cysts are dead or alive.
  - Endoscopic: ERCP delineates the biliary anatomy in obstructive jaundice due to hydatid disease.

Liver Tumors

Benign Tumors

Hemangioma: It occurs at all ages and is of equal sex distribution. It is usually symptomless. It may reach a huge size and cause pain in the right upper quadrant, or palpable mass (if it reaches > 4 cm in diameter).

Hepatic adenoma: Right upper quadrant pain occurring in women on birth control pills. There may be nausea and vomiting. Right upper quadrant mass. Spontaneous hemorrhage into the tumor or peritoneal cavity, due to rupture→ pain and shock.

Focal nodular hyperplasia (FNH): The right lobe is affected > the left. It occurs at any age, mostly 20–45 years. Women > men (no relation to oral contraceptives use). Only 20% of cases are symptomatizing causing right upper quadrant discomfort or pain. Occasional mass, bleeding or portal hypertension may occur.

Primary Malignant Tumors (Hepatocellular Carcinoma, Cholangiocarcinoma, Mixed type)

- It usually affects persons > 50 years; but may affect children mainly under 2 years of age.
- *Symptoms*:
  - Pain in the right hypochondrium that may be severe due to tumor necrosis.
  - Anorexia with rapid loss of weight.
  - Intermittent fever is usually present.
  - Abdominal swelling.
- *Signs*:
  - Mass (hepatomegaly): hard, nodular liver, which is usually tender. A bruit may be heard over it.
  - Ascites in late cases and splenomegaly.
  - Compression of PV → portal hypertension.
  - Fever is common (due to tumor necrosis).
  - There may be jaundice (it indicates cirrhosis or extensive unresectable tumor, or duct obstruction due to seedling into the biliary tract).
  - Generally, there is anemia. Rarely, they may present by massive hemorrhage. Evidence of spread or liver failure, which is the main cause of death.
- *Systemic Effects (Paraneoplastic Manifestations)*:
  - Hypoglycemia.
  - Erythrocytosis.
  - Hypercalcemia.

- Others (dysfibrinogenemia, carcinoid syndrome, ↑ production of ACTH and HCG).
- *Systemic Effects due to Spread:*
  - Lymphatics → Lymph nodes in the porta hepatis → thoracic duct → mediastinal lymph nodes (by retrograde spread) → Virchow's lymph nodes.
  - *Blood Spread* → Hepatic vein and IVC → Lungs and bones rapidly.

Secondary Malignant Tumors

These are more common than the primary. The Liver is the 2nd most common site of spread from tumors after lymph nodes.

- The liver is enlarged (hard, tender, irregular or nodular).
- Pain in the right hypochondrium, anorexia, loss of weight and fatigue.
- There may be obstructive jaundice, ascites or peritoneal deposits, and cachexia (late cases).
- Evidence of the primary tumor, e.g. cancer colon.

Differential Diagnosis: Differences between Hepatoma and Secondary Tumors

Criteria	Hepatoma (HCC)	Secondary tumor
History	—	Previous operation for Primary MT (±)
Age	Young and old	Usually old
Cirrhosis	+	—
Growth Rate	More rapid	Less rapid
Serum AP	↑	↑↑
Serum AFP	↑	—
CT Scan	Area(s) of ↓ attenuation with variable enhancement	Multiple areas of ↑ attenuation with variable enhancement

B. Gallbladder Swellings

Criteria of a Gallbladder Swelling

- Site: In the right hypochondrium immediately beneath the AAW, at the tip of the 9th rib.
- Shape: Pyriform with a smooth rounded lower boundary (fundus), but no upper boundary (i.e. continuous with liver dullness).
- Mobility: It moves with respiration and liver movement, and can be moved from side by side but not vertically.

Choledochal Cyst

- It presents after 8-10 years, although it is congenital. Females are more affected than males.
- It presents with a triad of jaundice, cholangitis and abdominal mass.

Inflammatory Conditions

The GB cannot be felt unless hugely distended which can result from two causes:

1. Stone in the cystic duct: The secretions of the GB will accumulate to cause hydrops or *mucocele* of the GB if the wall is healthy, or *empyema* in cases there is infection. In both conditions the patient is *not* jaundiced. In *mucocele,* the swelling is cystic and not tender. In *empyema,* the patient suffers from fever, rigors and malaise. The GB is tender, and may be difficult to feel due to rigidity of the overlying muscles.
2. Carcinoma of the head of the pancreas: It will cause back-pressure causing dilatation of the biliary tree, distention of the GB and hydrohepatosis. According to *Couvoisier's law,* "jaundice with palpable GB indicates carcinoma of the head of the pancreas, but without palpable GB indicates stone in the CBD".

Tumors of the GB

- Benign tumors: Adenoma, villous papilloma, polyp. They may cause GB neck obstruction causing cholecystitis.
- Malignant tumors: Carcinoma of the GB per se does *not* cause jaundice. *The mass is hard and irregular.* Symptoms are usually late and vague (continuous pain if present, nausea, loss of appetite and weight) causing late diagnosis. It may simulate chronic cholecystitis or even acute cholecystitis. Some cases are discovered during exploration.

C. Kidney (Renal Swelling) and Suprarenal Gland

Criteria of a Renal Swelling

- Site: Loin - full renal angle - ballotable.
- Reniform in shape.
- Slightly mobile with respiration.
- Percussion is dull posteriorly, but has a band of resonance anteriorly (gas in the colon).
- You can insinuate your hand between it and the costal margin.

Congenital Causes

- *Polycystic kidney*: Age: Intrauterine, early infancy or adult life. It is always bilateral, and consistency is firm (not cystic) because the fluid in the small cysts is under high tension.
- *Fused kidneys*: Both kidneys are on the right side, being fused together.
- Congenital hydronephrosis.

Renal Trauma

Trauma → disruption of the parenchyma → collection of blood and fluid inside the intact capsule resulting in "hematonephrosis" which presents with a large swelling that is liable to infection.

Inflammatory Causes

It is the commonest cause of kidney enlargement and result from *stones, ureteral stricture or retroperitoneal fibrosis.* These cause **hydronephrosis** or **pyonephrosis** (if there is infection) due to gradual obstruction, while acute renal obstruction results in atrophy of that kidney. The lower the ureteric obstruction, the gradual ↑ in pressure and more ↑ in kidney size.

Hydronephrosis	Pyonephrosis
• Painless, but there may be dull back ache	• Severe pain.
• Not tender and no fever (unless infected).	• Tender, with hectic fever and rigors.
• Mobile.	• Fixed or ↓ mobility due to peri-nephritis.
• May reach a large size.	• Usually does not reach a big size.

Renal Tumors

- *In children*: Wilm's Tumor → grows rapidly in size to fill the whole abdominal cavity causing rapid emaciation of the child. It may cause painless hematuria.
- *In adults*: Hypernephroma → a renal swelling and total painless, intermittent hematuria which is present in 60% of cases. Sometimes, the tumor in the kidney is so small causing osteolytic secondaries in the bone before the Primary tumor is evident.

Suprarenal Tumors

- Neuroblastoma: It appears in childhood and grows rapidly to attain a big size (crosses the midline). It is fixed (early). Metastases are common and occur early.

- Pheochromocytoma: It is usually not felt but presents with systemic effect (hypertension).

D. Colonic Causes

1. Cancer of the Hepatic Flexure or Right 1/3 of Transverse Colon:

- The tumor is irregular, firm or hard but may be hidden by the liver.
- The patient, usually an adult male over 40 years, presents with anemia, dyspepsia, alteration of bowel habits, and ↓ weight.
- Sometimes the patient presents with secondaries in the liver or skeleton.

2. TB Colon:

- Young male, with TB toxemia, and vague abdominal signs.
- Later on, the patient presents with signs of intestinal obstruction.

3. Intussusception:

- Recurrent attacks of obstruction.
- During the attack a firm sausage-shaped mass is felt.

E. Gastric Causes

Tumors of the Pyloric End of the Stomach, and the Duodenum:

- The patient usually presents with vomiting, dyspepsia, rapid emaciation, and rarely a mass.

III. RETROPERITONEAL SWELLINGS

1. Malignant (80%) - Retroperitoneal Sarcoma:

- Large mass, irregular, hard, fixed, with resonance (intestinal loops) in front it.
- It does not move with respiration.

- Later compression on the IVC causes edema of the lower limbs.

2. **Benign (20%):**
   - Most of these are "cysts"

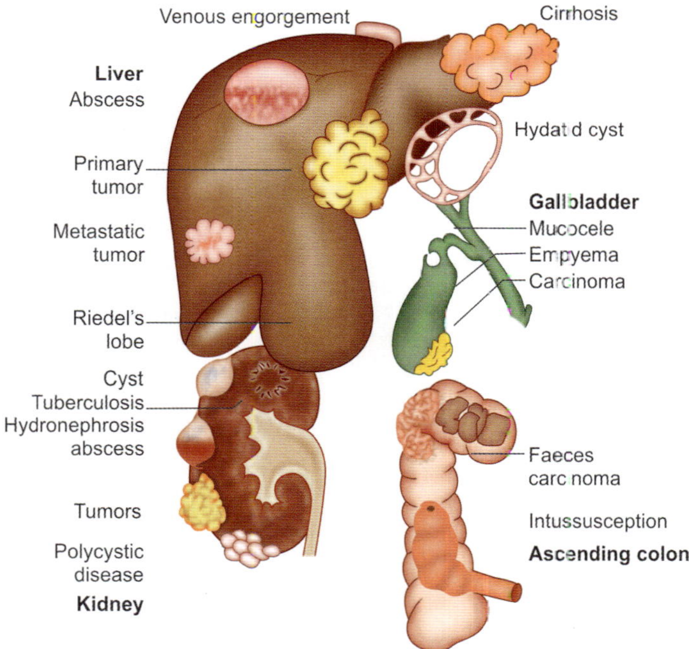

Fig. 1.67: Mass in the right hypochondrium

Investigations

- **CBC**
- **LFTs**
- **US**
- **CT scan**
- **Colonoscopy**
- **Barium enema**

MASS IN THE EPIGASTRIC REGION (FIGURE 1.68)

A swelling from another region, mainly the umbilical region, may encroach on the epigastrium

I. Parietal Swellings

1. Skin swellings.
2. SC tissue swellings.
3. Fatty hernia of the linea alba, epigastric hernia.
4. Abscess: Liver abscess, epigastric abscess, subphrenic abscess.

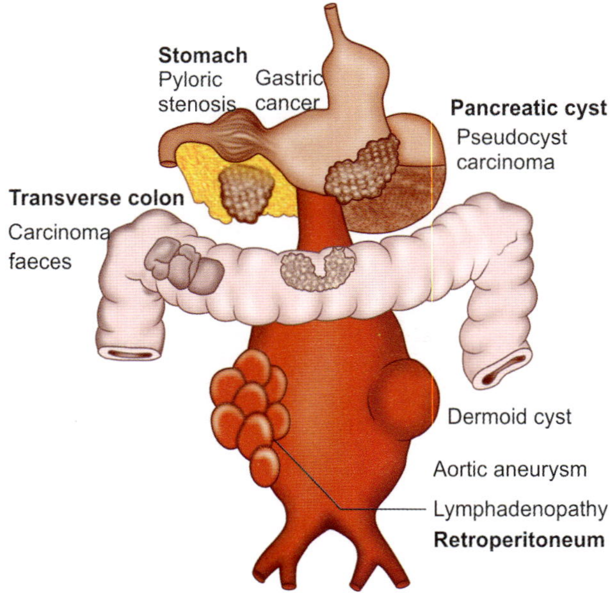

Fig. 1.68: Mass in the epigastric region

Investigations

- **CBC:** Anemia (Tumors) – WBC count (Lymphoma)
- **LFTs:** Hepatic lesions.

- **US:** Pancreatic (Pseudo) cysts – Aortic aneurysm.
- **CT scan:** Lymphadenopathy – Pancreatic tumors – Retroperitoneal cysts – Aortic aneurysm – Omental deposits.
- **Gastroscopy:** Gastric tumors.
- **Colonoscopy:** Colonic tumors.
- **Barium (Meal/Enema):** Gastric tumors and colonic tumors.

II. Intra-abdominal Swellings

Liver (Left Lobe)

1. Acute causes: Hepatitis, abscess, congestion.
2. Chronic causes: Hydatid cyst, tumor (primary - secondary).

Stomach and Duodenum

1. Pyloric stenosis:
    - Causes: Congenital hypertrophic pyloric stenosis, or stenosis following peptic ulcer.
    - The dilated stomach is resonant, with succussion splash and visible peristalsis from left to right
2. Subacute perforation of peptic ulcer → a tender mass.
3. Carcinoma of the stomach:
    - It may present with a hard mass in the epigastrium.
    - Laboratory tests: Anemia.
    - Imaging: Barium meal shows an irregular filling defect (**Figure 1.69**).
    - Endoscopy: UGI endoscopy allows also biopsy for confirmation of diagnosis.

Pancreas

1. *Tumors*:
    - These are rarely felt as abdominal lumps.

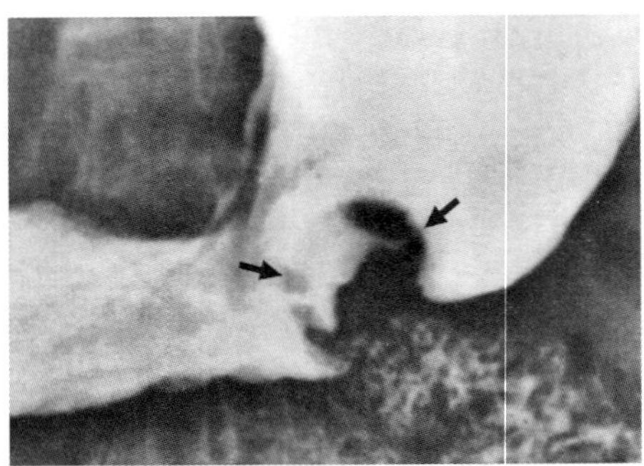

Fig. 1.69: A huge malignant ulcer in the pyloric region (arrows)

- If felt clinically, the mass is:
  - Hard.
  - Irregular.
  - Fixed.
  - Ill-defined.
  - Covered by a band of resonance (colon).

2. *Pseudopancreatic cyst.*

- It results from trauma or a mild grade of infection resulting in a swelling which is:
  - Smooth.
  - Rounded with indistinct lower border.
  - It is fixed and you cannot get above it.
  - Fluctuation may be difficult to illicit if the cyst is tense.
  - It shows "transmitted" pulsations that are lost when the patient acquires the knee-elbow position.
  - A barium meal (lateral view) shows the swelling to lie behind the stomach (**Figure 1.70**).

Transverse Colon

1. Diverticulitis: Tender, irregular mass - less common than the left colon.

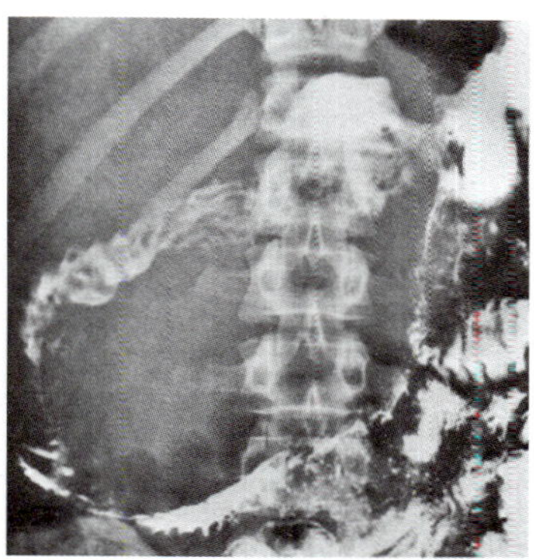

Fig. 1.70: Pancreatic pseudocyst

2. Bilharzial mass: Less common than the left colon.
3. Hyperplastic TB.
4. Tumors (Carcinoma): Hard, irregular mass, which is mobile vertically and is not tender. It may present with intestinal obstruction. Barium enema and endoscopy are diagnostic.
5. Intussusception.

Omentum

TB peritonitis: The omentum is rolled up to form a transverse ridge in the epigastrium, usually in children or young adults with poor health.

III. Retroperiotneal Swellings

Sarcoma

The mass is hard, irregular and fixed.

Aneurysm of the Upper Abdominal Aorta

- There is a tense cystic epigastric swelling with expansile pulsations which are *not* lost in the knee-elbow position and systolic thrill.
- Aortography is diagnostic.

Lymphadenopathy

Lymph nodes in the lesser omentum or para-aortic lymph nodes may be enlarged due to secondaries or lymphoma.

MASS IN THE UMBILICAL REGION (FIGURE 1.71)

Parietal Swellings

1. Skin swellings.
2. SC tissue swellings.
3. Umbilicus: Hernia, polyp, secondaries.
4. Rectus sheath: Hematoma, abscess, desmoid tumor.

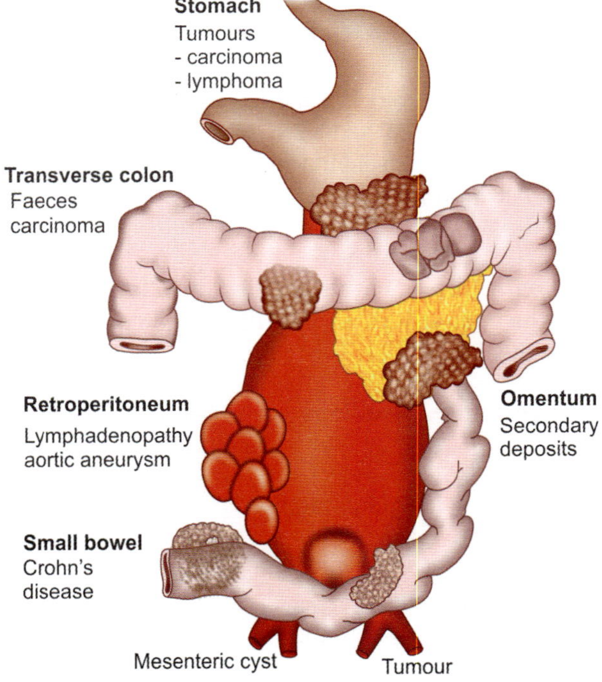

Fig. 1.71: Mass in the umbilical region

Investigations

- **CBC:** Anemia (Tumors).
- **WBC Count**: Lymphoma – Crohn's disease.
- **US**: Lymphadenopathy – Aortic Aneurysm.
- **CT Scan**: Lymphadenopathy – Retroperitoneal cysts – Mesenteric cysts - Aortic aneurysm – Omental deposits.
- **Gastroscopy**: Gastric tumors.
- **Colonoscopy**: Colonic tumors.
- **Small Bowel Enema**: Small intestinal tumors.

Intra-abdominal Swellings

Small Bowel	Mesentery	From Above	From the Side	From Below
Tumors (rare) • Benign: 1. Lipoma 2. Myoma • Malignant: Non-Hodgkin lymphoma	A.Lymph Nodes: • Tabes mesenterica • Lymphoma B.Cysts: • Dermoid cyst • Lymphatic cyst • Hydatid cyst • Degenerated tumor (pseudocyst)	Stomach Pancreas Colon Spleen	Kidneys	Urinary bladder Uterus and ovaries

Retroperitoneal Swellings

1. Sarcoma: Fixed swelling.
2. Retroperitoneal lymphadenitis:
   - Tuberculosis
   - Filariasis.

MASS IN THE SUPRAPUBIC REGION

Parietal Swellings

1. Skin and SC swellings.
2. Parietal abscess.
3. Urachal cyst:
   - The swelling is cystic, fixed to the posterior surface of the anterior abdominal wall
   - Unlike other parietal swellings, it becomes less prominent on contraction of the recti.

Intra-abdominal Swellings

Urinary Bladder (UB)	Uterus and Ovary	Sigmoid Colon and Small Bowel
1. Urine retention 2. Cancer bladder 3. Huge diverticulum 4. A big stone in the UB may be felt	1. Pregnant uterus 2. Sub-involuted uterus 3. Fibroid uterus 4. Ovarian cyst 5. Hematocolpus 6. Metropathia hemorrhagica	1. Bilharzial mass 2. Diverticulitis 3. Cancer colon 4. Intussusception

Differences between Full Bladder and Bladder Carcinoma

	Distended (Full) UB	Carcinoma of the UB
Symptoms	Cessation of passage of urine (acute or chronic retention)	Hematuria, pneumaturia, nocturia, dysuria, interrupted stream
Signs (Swelling)	You can't get below the swelling which lies above the pubis, may reach the umbilicus	You can not get below the swelling

Contd...

Contd...

	Cystic and dull to percussion Well-defined borders Bimanually felt Pressure induces the desire for micturition Disappears after passage of urine	Hard and nodular Ill-defined borders Can be felt bimanually and rectally

Differences between Pregnant Uterus, Fibroid and Ovarian Cyst

	Pregnant Uterus	Fibroid	Ovarian Cyst
History	Amenorrhea	• Lump • Menorrhagia	• Lump • Menstrual troubles
Signs *Mass*	• Smooth • Dull • Firm (firmer than full UB) • Cannot be moved independently from the cervix	• Bosselated • Dull • Firm • Well-defined edges • Slightly mobile in a transverse direction	• Smooth • Dull • Soft (cystic) and mobile • Well-defined edges • Moves independently on bimanual palpation
Cervix	• Cervix: soft and patulous	• The mass moves with the cervix, on bimanual palpation	• It may be felt per vagina or rectum

Pelvic Abscess

- It results from pelvic appendicitis, salpingo-oophoritis, etc.

- It is best felt by PR examination as a swelling which is:
  - Tense
  - Tender
  - Pushing the anterior rectal wall backwards or the vaginal wall forwards.
- History of symptoms of rectal irritation (tenesmus) is evident.
- History of urinary bladder irritation (frequency of micturition) is present.

Retroperitoneal Swellings

Pelvic Bone Tumors

- Hard in consistency.
- Fixed.
- Plain X-ray.

MASS IN THE LEFT ILIAC FOSSA (LIF)

Parietal Swellings

- Skin swellings
- SC tissue swelling
- Muscle swellings
- Iliac abscess: Pericolic, psoas abscess, ilioadenitis.

Intra-abdominal Swellings

Sigmoid and Descending Colon	From Above	From Below
Bilharzial mass	Splenic swelling	Left ovary (ovarian cyst)
Diverticulitis	Left renal swelling	Left fallopian tube
Cancer colon		Tumor in undescended testis
Intussusception		
Crohn's disease		

The main three causes of mass in the LIF

Criteria	Carcinoma	Bilharzial Mass	Diverticulitis
History:	*Short (old patient)*	*Long*	*Long*
Clinically:			
Pain	Colicky, lower abdomen	±	Recurrent, ± severe
Mass	Not tender, hard, irregular (can be indented).	Firm, oblong, tender, irregular, mobile or fixed.	Firm, tender, mobile or fixed.
Bleeding PR	Small and persistent	Blood + Diarrhea + Mucus	Profuse and periodic.
Bowel habits	Constipation (obstruction)	Dysentery (diarrhea)	Chronic constipation
Liver	± secondaries	Cirrhotic (fibrosis)	–
PR Exam	Ballooned	Polyps	Painful
Investigations			
Barium enema:	Localized, fixed, irregular filling defect	Honey-comb appearance (multiple filling defects)	Diffuse change, sawtooth appearance
Sigmoidoscopy:	Annular or tubular carcinoma. The rest of the mucosa is normal	Various Bilharzial changes: Congestion, polyp, ulcer	Long segment of inflammatory changes. Mouth of diverticulum may be seen

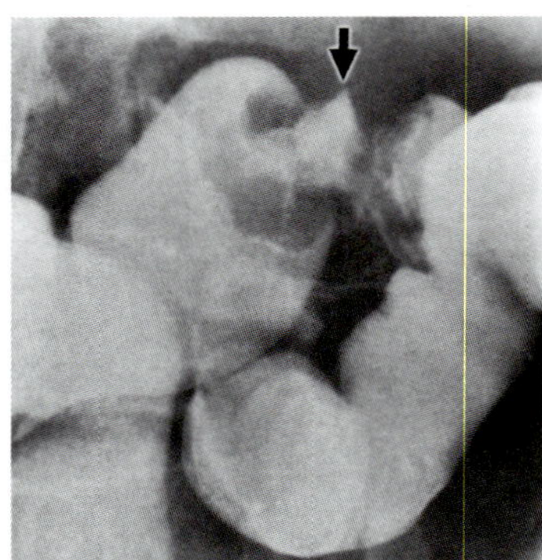

Fig. 1.72: Carcinoma of the sigmoid colon

A Carcinoma in the Left Colon

It is usually constrictive (stenotic) in nature (**Figure 1.72**), and may not be felt as a mass in the left iliac fossa except when it causes:

1. Fecal impaction above the tumor where an indentable mass could be felt.
2. Perforation, forming a peri-colic mass or abscess, which has the following characteristics:
   - Tender
   - May show pitting edema
   - Fluctuation may be demonstrated
   - Resonance on percussion due to the presence of gas.

Different causes of a mass in the left iliac fossa are depicted in **Figure 1.73**.

RETROPERITONEAL SWELLINGS

Similar to those of the RIF.

Investigations

Similar to those of the RIF.

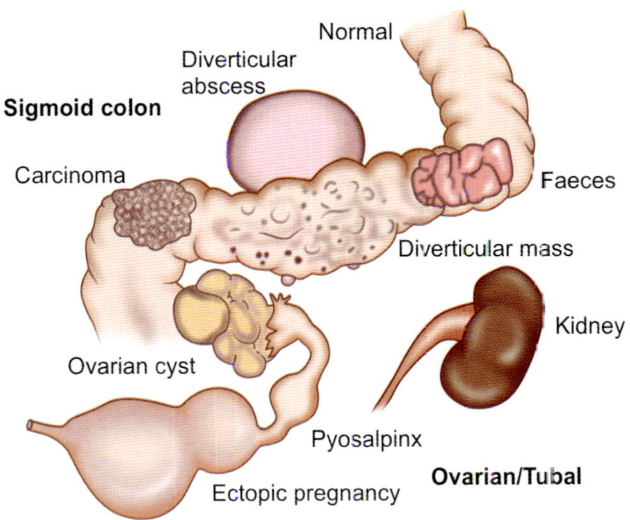

Fig. 1.73: Mass in the left iliac fossa

MASS IN THE LEFT HYPOCHONDRIUM (FIGURE 1.74)

I. Parietal Swellings

1. Skin swellings.
2. SC tissue swellings.
3. Muscle swellings.
4. Abscess:
   - Liver abscess (left lobe).
   - Left subphrenic abscess.

II. Intra-abdominal Swellings

1. **Splenic swelling (splenomegaly)**
   It is the most common swelling encountered in the left hypochondrium encountered in Egypt due to schistosomal portal hypertension causing fibro-congestive splenomegaly.

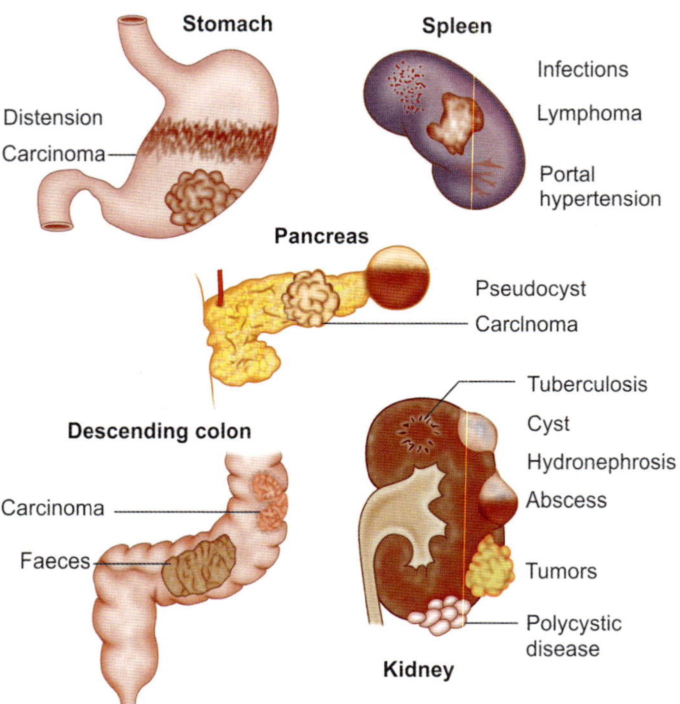

Fig. 1. 74: Mass in the left hypochondrium

Investigations

- **CBC**
- **LFTs**
- **US**
- **CT scan**
- **Colonoscopy**
- **Barium enema**

Criteria of a splenic swelling:

- Intra-abdominal lying immediately beneath the anterior abdominal wall in the left hypochondrium.

- You cannot insinuate your hand between it and the costal margin, i.e. you cannot get above it.
- Borders are rounded, and it has a definite notch on its anterior border.
- Moves with respiration.
- Grows downwards and medially, towards the umbilicus and RIF.
- Does not fill the renal angle.
- Dull on percussion. Its dullness is continuous with that of the normal splenic dullness.

2. **Splenic flexure of the colon.**
3. **Left lobe of the liver.**
4. **Left kidney.**
5. **Left suprarenal gland.**
6. **Stomach.**
7. **Pancreas.**

III. Retroperitoneal Swellings

Retroperitoneal Sarcoma

- Hard or variable in consistency (due to degeneration)
- Fixed

MASS IN THE LUMBAR REGION

I. Parietal Swellings

1. Skin swellings.
2. SC tissue swelling.
3. Lumbar hernia.
4. Abscess: Cold abscess - perinephric abscess.

II. Intra-abdominal Swellings

1. Renal swellings (Right or left).
2. Right side:
   a. Ascending colon:
      - Cancer colon
      - Tuberculosis
      - Intussusception.
   b. From above:
      - Swellings of the liver
      - Swellings of the gallbladder
3. Left side:
   - Descending colon: Cancer, diverticulitis, intussusception.
   - From above: Splenomegaly.

III. Retroperitoneal Swellings

Retroperitoneal Sarcoma

Refer back.

Abdominal Masses - Important Clinical Notes

Commonest abdominal swellings according to region:
- Right hypochondrium .... Gallbladder swellings.
- Left hypochondrium .... Splenomegaly.
- Right iliac fossa .... Appendicular mass.
- Left iliac fossa .... Bilharzial mass.
- Hypogastrium .... UB (Retention).

Causes of Huge Cysts of the Abdomen

1. **Hydronephrosis:**
   It may be bilateral if the obstructing lesion is in or distal to the neck of the urinary bladder.
2. **Ovarian Cyst:**
   - A painless lump associated with menstrual troubles of long duration.

- There may be attacks of acute abdominal pain (due to twisting).
- The umbilicus is displaced upwards, while in ascites it is displaced downwards.
- The swelling is freely mobile, and felt by vaginal (or rectal) examination to move independently of the uterus.

3. **Mesenteric Cyst:**

   Movement in the plane from the right hypochondrium to the left iliac fossa but not in the opposite direction is pathognomonic.

4. **Pseudopancreatic Cyst:**
   - A rare condition, which follows an attack of pancreatitis or trauma.
   - Its site depends on which part of the pancreas is involved.
   - It is situated above the umbilicus, tense cystic, smooth and immobile.

5. **Degeneration Cyst:**
   - A degenerated retroperitoneal tumor may be cystic in areas.
   - It is characterized by being fixed and rapidly growing.
   - There may be ascites.

6. **True Pancreatic Cyst.**
7. **Hydatid Cyst.**
8. **Choledochal Cyst.**
9. **Mucocele of the GB.**
10. **Encysted TB Peritonitis and Cold Abscess:**

- Encysted TB ascites is a rare condition that affects adults, usually females.
- The patient complains of a painful mass in the lower abdomen, which is:
  - Ill-defined.
  - Tender.
  - Fixed.
- It is associated with anorexia, fever and night sweats.

Causes of Huge Abdominal Distention (5F)

Never forget that pregnancy is the commonest cause of enlargement of the uterus, and of abdominal distention.

Fetus

Diagnosis is usually given by the patient. However, a woman may conceal her pregnancy. Never squeeze an enlarged uterus during a bimanual examination - you might cause an abortion!!

Diagnosis

- The uterus enlarges to the xiphisternum by the 36th week of pregnancy. At this stage, the fetus is palpable and jumping about. Diagnosis of pregnancy in the first 20 weeks, when the uterus is smaller and there are no fetal movements.
- A pregnant uterus is a smooth, firm, dull swelling, arising out of the pelvis.
- Bimanual examination reveals that the mass cannot be moved independently of the cervix, which is soft and patulous.

Flatus = (Tympanites)

Causes

1. Aerophagy.
2. Acute dilatation of the stomach.
3. Mechanical intestinal obstruction.
4. Paralytic ileus.

Diagnosis:

- Distended bowel has no palpable surface or edge.
- There is hyper-resonance.
- Increased peristalsis (visible/audible), and +ve succussion splash (shaking the patient → a splashing sound as the thin layer of fluid in the distended bowel splashes about. This is particularly common in gastric distention secondary to pyloric stenosis).

Fat

- Fat rarely causes distention, but frequently makes the patient "pot-bellied".
- A large fat abdomen may be caused by a thick layer of SC fat, or by excess fat in the omentum and mesentery.

Feces

Causes: The colon can become grossly distended with feces. The common causes are:

1. Hirschsprung's disease or acquired megacolon.
2. Chronic intestinal obstruction and chronic constipation.

Diagnosis (Physical characteristics of feces are):

- The masses (may be multiple and separate) lie in a part occupied by the colon, i.e. flanks and lower epigastrium.
- Feces feel firm or hard but are indentable.
- If there is no mechanical obstruction, PR → full rectum with rock-hard feces, but if there is obstruction → empty rectum.

Fluid

A. Free Fluid (Ascites):

Diagnosis: Fluid thrill + shifting dullness.
Etiology:

1. Causes of ↑ Portal Venous Pressure:
   - Prehepatic: Portal vein (PV) thrombosis - compression of the PV by L.Ns.
   - Hepatic: Cirrhosis - multiple hepatic metastases.
   - Posthepatic: Budd-Chiari syndrome.
   - Cardiac: Constrictive pericarditis - right HF - mitral stenosis.
   - Pulmonary: Pulmonary hypertension.
2. Causes of Hypoproteinemia:
   - Renal disease associated with albuminuria.

- Liver cirrhosis.
- Cachexia of wasting disease, malignancy and starvation.
- Protein-losing enteropathy.

3. Causes of Chronic Peritonitis:
   - Physical: Post-irradiation - Talc granuloma.
   - Infection: TB peritonitis.
   - Neoplasms: Secondary peritoneal deposits of carcinoma - mucus-forming tumors (pseudomyxoma peritonei).
4. Causes of Chylous Ascites:
   - Direct leakage of lymph from the lacteals or cisterna chyli into the peritoneal cavity as a result of congenital abnormalities, trauma, and primary and secondary gland disease.

B. Encysted Fluid:

Etiology:

- Ovarian cysts: These are differentiated from ascites by percussion and PXR of the abdomen and US. In case of huge cyst, the small bowel is displaced in the upper abdomen.
- Hydronephrosis, polycystic kidneys, urine retention.
- Pancreatic cysts.
- Mesenteric cysts.
- A large aortic aneurysm (it has no thrill being subjected to repeated intrinsic percussion - the pulse. It is diagnosed by the presence of expansile pulsations.

Diagnosis: Dullness, fluid thrill, no shifting dullness (differentiates it from ascites).

Solid Tumors

A. Organomegaly: E.g. Hugely enlarged spleen or kidney.
B. Large Tumors:
   - Fibroid uterus.

- Large cancer of the colon.
- Carcinoma of the pancreas.
- Retroperitoneal sarcoma or lymphadenopathy.
- Ganglioneuroma and neuroblastoma in children.
- Renal swellings: Polycystic kidneys - Carcinoma of the kidney.

16. SWELLING IN THE GROIN

INGUINAL SWELLINGS

Inguinal swellings are properly those in the *region of the inguinal canal,* i.e. related to the medial half of the inguinal (Poupart's) ligament and the part immediately above it. The following are some of the most important:

Groin Hernia

- A "Groin Hernia" may be inguinal (direct or indirect), or femoral.
    1. *Direct inguinal hernia* (DIH) protrudes through the posterior wall of the inguinal canal *medial* to the inferior epigastric vessels (Hesselbach's Triangle).
    2. *Indirect inguinal hernia* (IIH) passes through the deep inguinal ring (DIR) *lateral* to the inferior epigastric vessels and traverses the whole canal in front of the cord.
    3. *Femoral hernia* passes through the femoral canal, but may be large enough to extend upwards over the medial end of inguinal ligament and thus, become an inguinal swelling.
- A hernia, unless obstructed, gives an impulse on cough and is reducible. Psoas abscess and saphena varix give these signs, but they are *below* Poupart's ligament.

To Differentiate Between Inguinal and Femoral Hernia

1. *Pubic tubercle test:* Inguinal hernia may be direct (above and lateral to the tubercle) or indirect (above and medial). Femoral hernia lies below and lateral to it.
2. *Relation to inguinal ligament: Inguinal hernia* lies above it. *Femoral hernia* lies below it, but if large it may ascend over the ligament and lies above it.
3. *Direction of reduction: Femoral* (downward and medial, then backward, then upward), *IIH* (upward, backward and laterally), *DIH* (backwards).

4. *Ring test:* Close femoral opening after reduction of hernia, it does not descend on coughing.

Point of Difference	Femoral Hernia	Inguinal Hernia
1. Sex	Commoner in females > males	Commoner in males > females
2. Site	Lateral to the pubic tubercle and below the inguinal ligament.	Medial to the pubic tubercle and above the inguinal ligament.
3. Inguinal Canal	Obviously empty	Felt occupied by the inguinal hernia
4. Femoral Ring Test	The hernia does not come down	The hernia comes down
5. DIR Test	The hernia comes down	An "IIH" does come down
6. Irreducibility	More likely	Less likely

To Differentiate Between Direct and Indirect Inguinal Hernia (Figure 1.75)

Point of Difference	DIH	IIH
Age	Old (common after 40 years)	Any age (young and middle age)
Site	More likely to be bilateral	Usually unilateral
Clinical Picture		
Shape	Hemispherical	Oblong
Descend to scrotum	Negative or very rare	Common
Reduction	Backwards	Upward, backward and laterally
Descent	Forwards	Downward, forward and medially
SIR size	Normal	Wide
SIR test	Impulse felt on finger pulp	Impulse felt on fingertip
DIR test	Negative	Positive
Complications	Less common due to wide neck	More common (narrow neck)

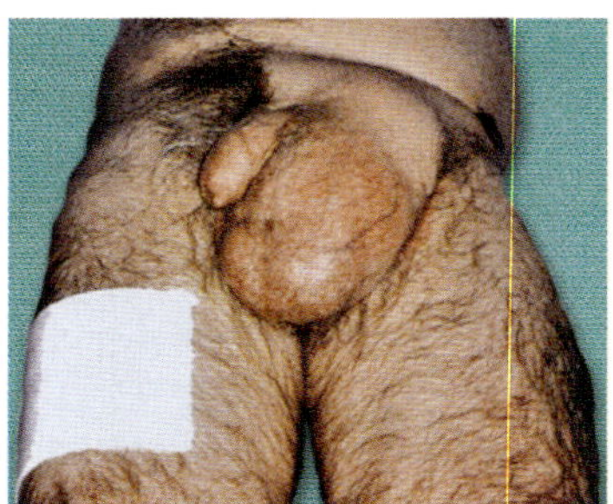

Fig. 1.75: Left indirect inguinal hernia. An oblong swelling reaching down to the scrotum

Enlarged Lymph Nodes

- Enlarged inguinal lymph nodes are:
  - Nearly always multiple.
  - Usually subcutaneous, so that they are easy to recognize as lymph nodes.
- Clinical findings depend on the cause of enlargement.
- The primary source should be always searched for.
- The following are some causes for enlargement of inguinal lymph nodes:
  - Irritation:
    - Mechanical irritation.
    - Chemical irritation.
  - Non-specific infection: Septic lymphadenitis.
  - Specific infection: TB, syphilis, filariasis, lymphogranuloma inguinale.
  - Neoplastic: Lymphoma
    - Lymphoma: Hodgkin disease/Non-Hodgkin lymphoma.
    - Lymphatic leukemia
    - Metastases (secondaries).

Cause	Presentation and Diagnosis
1. Mechanical or Chemical Irritation	Nodes become slightly enlarged and tender in young men, particularly in athletes, often due to epidermophytosis of the feet or mechanical irritation of a truss
2. Septic Infection	It may follow bites of parasites such as pediculus pubis. Lymph nodes become firm and tender, but if suppuration occurs, a fluctuant center appears. The areas drained by the nodes should be searched for a septic focus
3. Tuberculosis	Lymph nodes do not separate for months, and then but with little inflammatory reaction. The source of infection may be from neighboring tuberculous nodes, but more likely from a sore or ulcer in the foot or leg
4. Syphilis	A true syphilitic lymph node is hard, movable, painless and only moderately enlarged. The presence of indurated chancre makes diagnosis easy. Spirochaeta pallida may be detected, WR may be +ve. Instances of mixed infection by sepsis and syphilis are common
5. Lymphogranuloma Inguinale (LGI)	Nodes are swollen and the intervening fibrosis gives to the mass a lobulated, firm feeling. The condition persists for many months with slight tenderness and eventually the mass may break down and discharging sinuses or ulcers appear on the groin skin. Frei's serological test is +ve
6. Filariasis	• Blood examination is pathognomonic • Other evidence of filariasis
7. Hodgkin's Disease	• Groin lymph nodes are rarely affected alone, and the smooth, soft enlargement without signs of inflammation, associated with anemia and intermittent fever, and possibly enlargement of the spleen suggest the diagnosis. • Biopsy may be necessary.

Contd...

Contd...

8. Non-Hodgkin Lymphoma	• Usually they are not the only lymph nodes affected • They grow rapidly and remain smooth and fairly soft to firm until they attain a great size. • Biopsy is necessary
9. Lymphatic Leukemia	• Blood examination is pathognomonic • Other signs of leukemia
10. Secondaries	• Nearly always secondary to a primary epithelioma of the skin or mucous membrane drained by the nodes such as the anus, scrotum, penis. • Nodes are hard with progressive growth and no signs of inflammation. They become adherent to the deep fascia and skin. • Melanotic growths of the skin (in a toe) may give rise to rapidly growing smooth lymph nodes, often cystic; the pigment may be visible through the skin.

Abscess: Acute or Chronic

Acute Abscess

- An acute abscess in the groin has only one common cause, namely, suppuration of the lymph nodes, and a search for the primary source of infection must be made.
- An appendicular abscess may point just above the inguinal ligament; but there is then a history of the characteristic symptoms of acute appendicitis.

Chronic Abscess

- It may due to a disease of the hip, sacroiliac joint, or lumbar spine, although these usually point below the inguinal ligament.
- It is usually due to a cold abscess of ***tuberculous*** lymph nodes.

- ***Actinomycosis*** of the appendix is another possible causative condition.

Hydrocele of the Cord or of the Hernial Sac

Encysted Hydrocele of the Cord

- It occupies part of the inguinal canal, and is a rounded oval tense irreducible swelling, transilluminated with difficulty.
- It may be mistaken for an inguinal hernia, but being cut off from communication with the abdominal cavity, does *not* give an expansile impulse on coughing, but rather is pushed forwards by the thrust of the abdominal wall.
- It moves down with traction of the cord, but its side-to-side movement is restricted.

Hydrocele of the Hernial Sac

- The neck of an inguinal hernia may become obstructed, usually by omentum, and a hydrocele may develop in the sac.
- Such a hydrocele extends up to the internal ring forming a cystic swelling distinguished from a bilocular vaginal hydrocele by the history of previous hernia, and by palpating the swelling up to the inguinal ring.

Retained Testis: Undescended or Ectopic

Undescended Testis

- It is one, which is retained at any point along its normal line of descent.
- The scrotum is therefore empty and not well developed, and the groin swelling (testis) may give the characteristic testicular sensation, or the condition may be associated with attacks of pain which may be mistaken as acute appendicitis or intestinal colic.
- It is associated with actual or potential inguinal hernia.

Ectopic Testis

- After descending out of the SIR, the testis deviates from its normal path (to scrotum).
- The testicle may, therefore, lie superficial to the external oblique aponeurosis and felt as a groin swelling. The testicle is usually more developed than the undescended testis.

Tumors of the Cord or Round Ligament

Lipoma

- It is so soft and displaceable that it gives an impulse on coughing and is often mistaken for an omental hernia, especially in stout patients.
- It is irreducible and difficult to diagnose except at operation.
- A hernia and a lipoma of the cord may co-exist.

Fibromyoma

- It is hard and smooth.
- It somewhat simulates the ovary or a thick-walled hydrocele of the canal of Nuck, a possible diagnosis being possible only at exploration.

Endometrioma of the Round Ligament

- A history of a swelling that becomes painful and more swollen at the time of menstruation will suggest the diagnosis.

Aneurysm of the External Iliac Artery (and Other Vascular Swellings)

- ***Aneurysm of the external iliac artery*** may be mistaken for a ***vascular sarcoma*** arising from the pelvis.

- It can generally be recognized by the classic signs of an aneurysm, such as expansile pulsation, bruit, weakening and delay of the corresponding femoral pulse, and marked reduction of the size of the swelling as a result of pressure on the common iliac artery.

FEMORAL SWELLINGS

Femoral swellings are properly those, which lie in the *region of the femoral (Scarpa's) triangle*. The following are some of the most important:

Femoral Hernia (Reducible)

- It is more common in women than men, but this is not sufficient for diagnosis.
- The swelling lies below the inguinal ligament, below and lateral to the pubic tubercle as opposed to IIH which lies above and medial to the tubercle (**Figure 1.76**).
- If large enough, it may extend above the inguinal ligament, thus simulating an inguinal hernia. More rarely, it extends downwards along the femoral vessels.

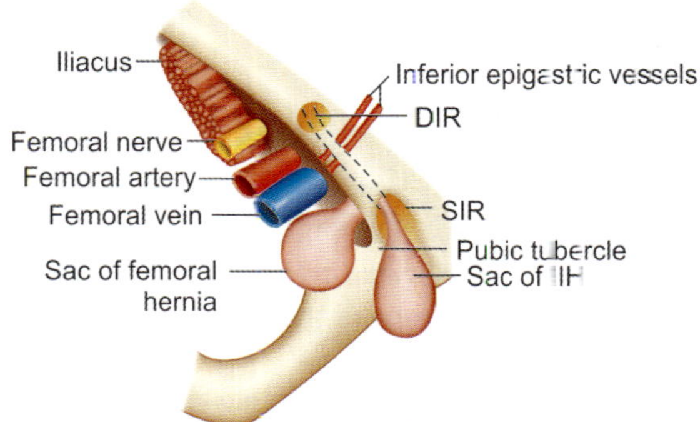

Fig. 1.76: Site of appearance of femoral hernia and IIH in relation to the pubic tubercle

- If it is large and contains intestine, it will be resonant, and a gurgling may be heard or felt on reduction, distinguishing at once from all other femoral swellings.
- If it is reduced and the finger held over the femoral ring, the hernia will be felt projecting forcible against the finger when the patient is asked to cough.
- Invagination test: The little finger is invaginated in the inguinal canal, which is empty (*H. Bailey*).

Femoral Hernia (Irreducible)

- It presents as a rounded elastic swelling in the femoral triangle.
- Irreducibility may be accounted for in four ways:
  1. Strangulation.
  2. A piece of omentum, adherent and plugging the neck.
  3. An empty sac but with a mass of extra-peritoneal fat around it.
  4. A hydrocele of the hernial sac.
- If strangulation has occurred, there will be signs of bowel obstruction and the hernia will be tense and tender.
- It is quite impossible to say, without dissection, whether the swelling is due to a plug of omentum inside the sac or to a collection of fat outside it.

Hydrocele of the Femoral Hernial Sac

- The neck of the femoral hernial sac is plugged with omentum, and thus communication with the general peritoneal cavity is closed.
- The sac may then become cystic and filled with fluid, i.e. a hydrocele is formed.
- It may be mistaken for an irreducible femoral hernia, but a hydrocele is "translucent".

Saphena Varix

- A localized dilatation of the saphenous vein at the saphenous opening, just before joining the femoral vein.
- *Compressible* swelling below the inguinal ligament (may be mistaken for femoral hernia).
- It appears on standing and ↓ (disappears) on elevating the lower limb.
- It has a blue tinge.
- Associated with varicose veins of the limb, though none may show between the knee and Scarpa's triangle.
- A thrill is felt when the patient coughs (*Cruveilhier's sign*), or if the vein is tapped with the finger.

Psoas Abscess (Cold Abscess)

- A cold abscess arising from TB of the body of one of the lumbar vertebrae and tracking along the psoas sheath to the insertion of the psoas major gives rise to a cystic swelling (may be reducible).
- It is painless unless infected (suppurative).
- It usually points in the femoral triangle, below the inguinal ligament, with +ve cross fluctuation.
- If pulsation of the femoral artery is felt, the swelling will be found to lie lateral to the femoral artery.
- Examination of the back (Pott's disease, e.g. kyphosis, caseous aspiration, wedging on plain X-ray) and the iliac fossa shows the primary lesion and clarifies the diagnosis.

Femoral Artery Aneurysm

- History of trauma or atherosclerosis.
- Expansile *pulsations* and a *bruit* may be heard.
- Emptying on compression and refilling on release of pressure.
- Reduced when the external iliac artery is compressed.
- Mobile in one direction - perpendicular to the artery line.

Arteriovenous Fistula

- History of trauma.
- Dilated veins around (Secondary varicose veins) and audible to-and-fro murmur.

Enlarged Lymph Nodes (Cloquet)

- Chronic inflammatory or neoplastic lymph nodes may be difficult to differentiate from ***irreducible femoral hernia.***
- The primary source is searched for by examination of the feet, legs, buttocks, perineum, anus and genitals (glans penis) for a new growth, boil, blister or an abrasion.
- A lymph node has some degree of mobility. Multiplicity is in favor of diagnosis of enlarged lymph nodes.

Ectopic Testis

- One of the places into which a testis may be drawn abnormally is Scarpa's triangle, which it reaches by passing over Poupart's ligament.
- The fact that the swelling has the shape of a testis, though generally smaller than normal, and that the corresponding half of the scrotum is empty, make the diagnosis easy.

Femoral Neuroma (Very Rare)

- Hard, smooth, moves laterally but not vertically, pressure may cause pain in the distribution of the femoral nerve.

Primary Tumors

Lipoma

- It is relatively common in the subcutaneous tissues over Scarpa's triangle.
- It has the characteristic soft texture and lobulated outline.
- It is felt lying outside the fascial envelope of the thigh with no deep connections.

Fibroma and Sarcoma

- These are rare in these situations.

INGUINAL-FEMORAL SWELLINGS

Certain swellings are neither truly inguinal nor truly femoral, but betwixt and between, bulging the Poupart's ligament forwards. They are generally deep, and on that account obscure:

1. **Psoas bursa (Bursitis):**
    - It may be mistaken for a femoral hernia, and is often difficult to distinguish from a psoas abscess.
    - The bursa becomes distended between the tendon of the ilio-psoas muscle and the capsule of the hip joint, and diminishes in size when the hip is flexed.
    - The hip shows signs of osteoarthritis.
2. **Effusion of the hip joint** as in TB of the hip.
3. **Osteophytic outgrowths** from the acetabulum in osteoarthritis of the hip joint.

Clinical Key Points — Groin Swellings

Groin swellings **(Figure 1.77)** can be categorized into four groups according to consistency as follows:

Reducible	Pulsating	Cystic	Solid
1. Reducible inguinal hernia. 2. Reducible femoral hernia. 3. Saphena varix.	1. Femoral (or external iliac) artery aneurysm. 2. A-V fistula.	1. Psoas abscess. 2. Psoas bursa. 3. Encysted hydrocele of the cord. 4. Hydrocele of hernial sac. 5. Abscess (acute/chronic).	1. Enlarged lymph nodes 2. Tumors (lipoma) of the cord and round ligament. 3. Retained testis. 4. Femoral neuroma. 5. Primary tumors (lipoma).

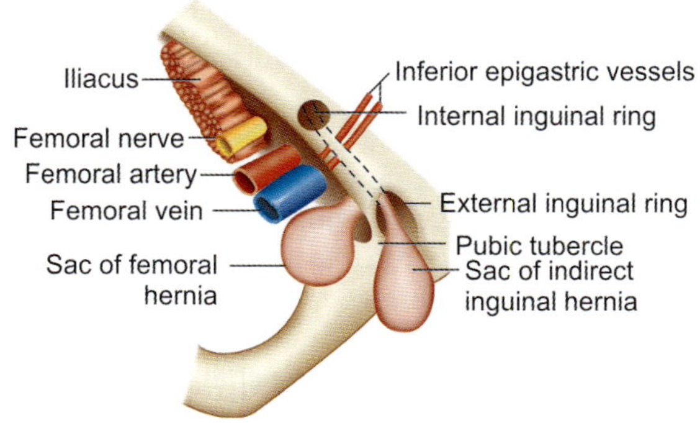

Fig. 1.77: Groin swelling

Investigations

CBC: For causes of lymphadenopathy.
US: For femoral aneurysm, saphena varix, psoas abscess, ectopic testis.
CT: For causes of psoas abscess.

17. INGUINOSCROTAL SWELLINGS

CAUSES

- Inguinoscrotal swellings almost necessarily arise in the constituents of the spermatic cord or in a persistent funicular process.
- The following must be considered:
  1. Hernia (Reducible, irreducible, strangulated).
  2. Hydrocele (Congenital, hydrocele of the cord, hydrocele of the hernial sac).
  3. Varicocele.
  4. Other spermatic cord lesions (causing thickening of the cord):
     a. Traumatic (Hematocele of the cord).
     b. Inflammatory.
     c. Malignant thickening of cord.
  5. Testicular causes.

Hernia

Indirect Inguinal Hernia (Reducible)

- It is by far the most common inguinoscrotal swelling and has two cardinal features:
  1. It gives an impulse on cough.
  2. It shows reducibility (can be reduced into the abdomen).
- If it contains bowel, it is elastic, resonant and reduces with a gurgle.
- If it contains omentum, it will feel soft, doughy or granular, dull on percussion and reduces without a gurgle.

Irreducible Hernia

- It presents as a tubular swelling along but *in front of the cord,* going up to the internal ring and extending downwards for a variable distance, but ending below in a rounded fundus **(Figure 1.78)**.

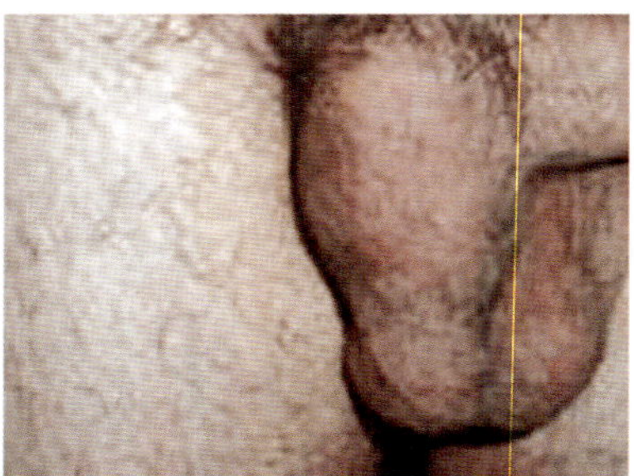

Fig. 1.78: Right IIH (inguinoscrotal)

- History of a previously reducible swelling settles the diagnosis without confusion.

Strangulated Hernia

- A strangulated hernia is irreducible, but also tense, tender and loses it cough impulses.
- There is evidence of intestinal obstruction (which is incomplete in strangulated Richter's hernia).
- Strangulated *omentum* resembles inflamed hydrocele of the cord, but the latter is very rare, and both demand operation.

Hydrocele

Congenital Hydrocele

- It is a persistence of the processus funicularis throughout its length, and differs from a congenital hernia in that its communication with the abdomen is shut off, or so nearly shut off that bowel or omentum *cannot* enter it.
- The swelling fills the tunica vaginalis and obscures the testis, and continues as a tubular prolongation up the inguinal canal. It is elastic or fluctuant, and transilluminates easily.
- It is differentiated from a hernia by its translucency, and absence of both impulse on cough and reducibility.

- Though irreducible many congenital hydroceles have a small communication with the abdomen indicated by its reduction in size during the hours of sleep.
- The appearance of bilateral congenital hydrocele in a baby is often an index of peritoneal mischief, such as tuberculous peritonitis.

Bilocular Hydrocele

- It occurs when a completely patent processus funicularis remains unobserved in infancy and becomes distended during adult life.
- It has the same physical characters mentioned above except that it does not vary in size.

Encysted Hydrocele of the Cord

- It occurs if the processus funicularis is shut off from both, the tunica vaginalis and peritoneum, leaving a patent portion in between, which becomes distended with fluid. It may give an inguinal, scrotal or inguinoscrotal swelling depending on the patent part of the funicular process.
- The swelling is oval, cystic and translucent.
- Traction test is positive.

Hydrocele of the Hernial Sac

- There is collection of fluid in the hernial sac, the opening of which at the internal ring being closed by a plug of omentum.
- There is a history of hernia, and the testis is felt separate.

Varicocele

It is an inguinoscrotal swelling that is chiefly scrotal.

- It is nearly always on the left side, the patient being usually a young adult with dragging pain particularly after prolonged standing (**Figure 1.79**).

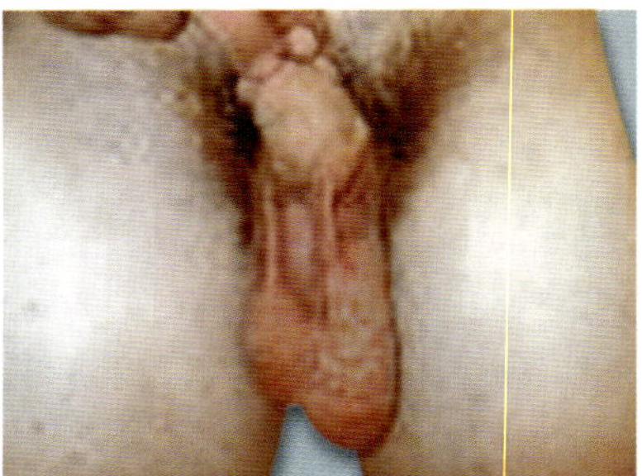

Fig. 1.79: Left varicocele

- The distended veins of the pampiniform plexus resemble a "bag of worms". With a lax scrotum, the blue color of veins can be seen.
- A varicocele is said to have an impulse on coughing, but the sensation is that of a fluid thrill or a small tap on the examining finger rather than an impulse.
- Squeezing empties the swelling, which refills immediately. Recumbency with the scrotum raised also causes it to disappear.

Differences Between Primary and Secondary Varicocele

Criteria	Primary varicocele	Secondary varicocele
Incidence	More common	Less common
Etiology	• Genetic factor (familial tendency) • Wall weakness • Venous hypertension (congestion)	• Abdominal mass or retroperitoneal fibrosis • Hypernephroma invading the renal vein, or causing compression from outside
Age	Young adults	Older age (40-50 Y)
Side	Left side (96%), right side (2%), bilateral (2%)	According to cause and site of obstruction
Onset	Gradual	Rapid and sudden

Contd...

Contd...

C/P	1. Dragging pain 2. Impulse and thrill on cough 3. Bowing test +ve 4. Softer and smaller testicle 5. No evidence of primary cause	1. Painless 2. No impulse and no thrill 3. Bowing test -ve 4. Larger and firmer testicle 5. Evidence of primary cause

Other Spermatic Cord Lesions

Trauma (Hematocele of the Cord)

- It presents as an ill-defined opaque swelling which is tender and irreducible.
- It occurs soon after trauma such as a kick in the groin.

Inflammation

- Inflammatory thickening of the cord may be an extension of inflammation of the epididymis and testis.
- *Tuberculous funiculitis:*
  - There is generalized fullness of the cord.
  - More typically the "beaded" vas may be felt.
- *Filarial funiculitis:*
  - It is usually acute with high fever swelling and redness of the skin.
  - The cord becomes thickened, tender and matted.
  - There is always a well-pronounced hydrocele.
  - The prostate and seminal vesicles are normal.
  - The patient usually comes from an endemic area.
  - Blood shows leukocytosis and eosinophilia and may show microfilaria.
  - Sometimes a residual mass is felt in the cord after the acute attack resolves.

– It resembles a *bilharzial mass*, but differentiation can be made by the following:

Filarial Mass	Bilharzial Mass
• Cord is matted	• Cord not matted
• Mass diffusely affect the cord	• Mass selects the lower 2 inches of the cord
• Normal prostate	• Enlarged, firm, irregular prostate
• Patient comes from an endemic area	• History of bilharziasis
• No bilharzial ova in urine	• Ova in urine

Lymph Varix (Lymphangiectasis, Diffuse Hydrocele of the Cord)

- There is dilatation and tortuosity of the lymphatic vessels of the cord, caused by obstruction due to *filaria*.
- It gives an impulse (thrill-like) on coughing and reduces spontaneously on lying down.
- It may feel soft, cystic or doughy.
- It is diagnosed by the history of periodic attacks of fever with development of swelling and tenderness of the cord, eosinophilia and living microfilaria in blood.

Neoplastic

- *Diffuse lipoma of the cord* is rare.
- The cord feels soft and lobulated.
- The swelling is irreducible and has no impulse on cough.
- *Malignant extension from the testis* may occur along its lymphatics.
- The inguinal condition is, however, overshadowed and explained by the scrotal one (i.e. the testicular tumor).

Testicular Causes

Undescended Testis Associated with Hernia

- It gives either an inguinal or inguinoscrotal swelling.

- Absence of the testis from the scrotum and its presence in the inguinal canal is evident.
- There is expansile impulse on cough and reducibility.

Torsion of the Testis

- It usually occurs with the undescended testis, but may occur with a completely descended one (**Figure 1.80**), so it should be differentiated from a strangulated hernia.
- The swelling is tense and tender, dull on percussion, and without an impulse on coughing.
- Elevation of the testis causes more pain.
- There is slight fever, and constipation (not absolute).
- Doppler US can settle the diagnosis by showing absence of blood flow.

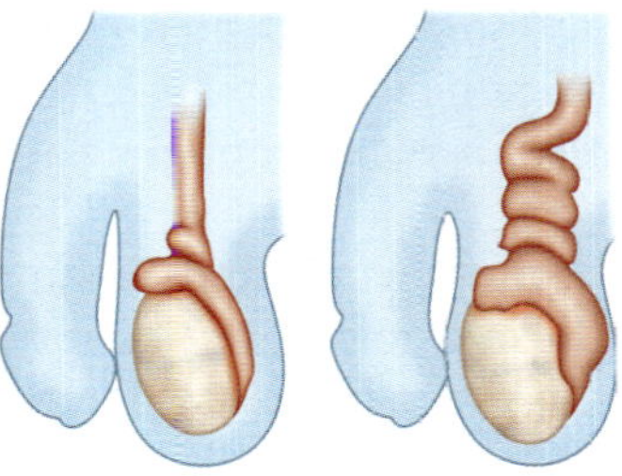

Fig. 1.80: Normal anatomy and torsion of testis (cord)

18. SCROTAL SWELLINGS

It is first essential to prove that the swelling is *purely scrotal.* This is done by grasping the root of the scrotum between the thumb and index finger to determine whether any of the swelling extends along the cord into the inguinal region.

True scrotal swellings may arise in: (1) the skin, (2) connective tissue coverings of the testicle, (3) tunica vaginalis, (4) testicle, (5) epididymis, (6) lower end of the spermatic cord, (7) urethra and (8) bones of the pubic arch. Of these swellings in the cord, testicle, epididymis, and tunica vaginalis are the most important.

SWELLINGS AFFECTING THE SKIN

- The nature of these is usually obvious. The only common ones are boils, soft sores and chancre (syphilis), sebaceous cysts, warts and epithelioma.
- A scrotal *sebaceous cyst* may suppurate and leave an open sore.
- *Epithelioma* ulcerates early and commonly occurs in sweeps or in those who work in tar, or petroleum. The groin lymph nodes soon become enlarged.

SWELLINGS OF THE CONNECTIVE TISSUE COVERINGS

Scrotal Edema

- It may result from *generalized* edema of acute or chronic renal disease.
- Diagnosis is confirmed by renal function tests, and by albumin and tube-casts in urine.
- Gross edematous scrotum also occurs with ascites or IVC thrombosis, and may accompany the abdominal swelling of pellagra and infantile Kwashiorkor.

Scrotal Swellings					
Scrotal Origin				**Extra-Scrotal**	
Coverings	**Contents**			**Urethra**	**Pubic Bones**
	Testis/Epididymis		**Spermatic Cord**		
	Cystic	*Solid*			
Scrotal Skin • Boil • Erysipelas • Soft sore • Hard chancre • Sebac. cyst • Wart • Papilloma • Epithelioma **SC Tissue** • Cellulitis • Edema • Lipoma • Neurofibroma • Elephantiasis **Tunica Vaginalis:** • Hydrocele • Hematocele • Chylocele • Pyocele	• Spermatocele • Epididymal cysts • Hydatid cyst of Morgagni	*Acute* • Torsion • Acute epididymo-orchitis • Hernia testis *Chronic* • TB • Syphilis • Tumors	• Varicocele • Hydrocele • Cord lipoma • Inflammatory (TB, $) • Parasitic: (filariasis, bilharziasis)	• Periurethral abscess • Primary urethral epithelioma • Rupture urethra (extravasation of urine) • Urethral stone	• Osteomyelitis • Acute necrosis • Osteosarcoma • Chondro-sarcoma

- Neurodermatitis affecting the scrotum may also cause scrotal edema, as does moniliasis.

Elephantiasis Scroti

- It results from infection with *Filaria sanguinis hominis*.
- It is limited to the Tropics and causes symmetrical enlargement.

Tumors

- These are rare, but occasionally a fibrosarcoma may occur.
- These swellings are movable upon the testicle.

SWELLINGS OF THE TUNICA VAGINALIS

The tunica vaginalis may become distended with serous fluid, blood, or pus. Distention with fluid may be primary (the ordinary vaginal hydrocele), or secondary to disease of the testis or epididymis. You can get above the swelling (**Figure 1.81**), i.e. it is purely scrotal.

Primary Vaginal Hydrocele

- It usually arises slowly.
- The patient is well complaining of a lump or the drag it causes.

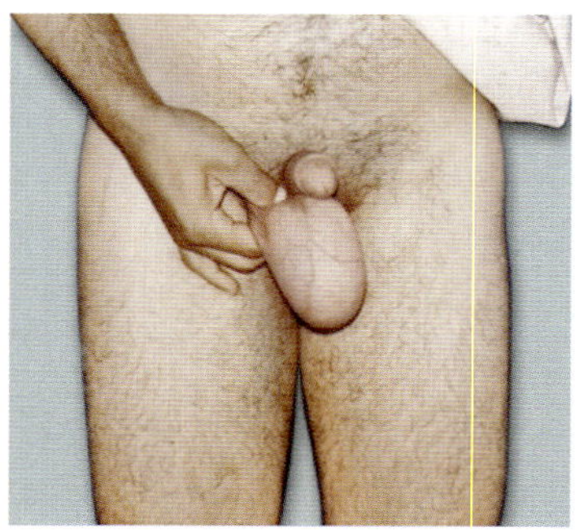

Fig. 1.81: Hydrocele: purely scrotal swelling

- The swelling is usually large, heavy, ovoid, tense and elastic rather than fluctuating, though fluctuation can be proved if the swelling is fixed by an assistant or the patient.
- Neither the testis nor the epididymis can be felt apart from the swelling.
- It can be transilluminated (**Figure 1.82**). The testicular shadow will be felt at one edge of the swelling, usually behind.

Secondary Hydrocele

- It follows disease of the testis or epididymis such as:
  - Acute epididymo-orchitis.
  - Syphilitic orchitis.
  - TB epididymitis.
  - Newgrowths of the testis.
- The amount of fluid is usually small, and the swelling lax, so that the finger can touch the testis.
- The complaint is of the causative disease rather than of the hydrocele.
- Transillumination confirms the presence of fluid (**Figure 1.82**).

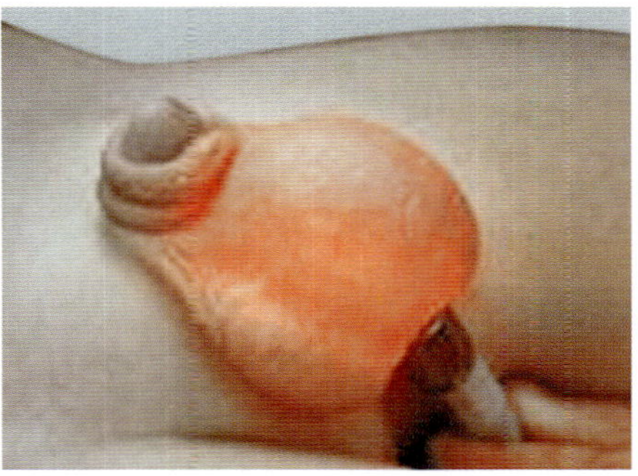

Fig. 1.82: Hydrocele: Transillumination shows the fluid

Hematocele

- It has the physical characters of a hydrocele except that it is not translucent (i.e. opaque).
- Hematocele is due to **t**apping of hydrocele, **t**rauma, **t**orsion, or **t**umor of the testis, and its discovery is therefore the indication for exploration unless the history of trauma is recent and definite.
- *Tapping* may be required for diagnosis.
- If it becomes *chronic*, the blood clots and hardens simulating tumor or gumma.

Pyocele

- It is merely part of a suppurative process arising in the testis or the epididymis such as epididymo-orchitis.
- In addition to the enlarged, tender epididymis and testis, a cystic, tender swelling exists in front of and on the testis.
- It is hot, red, tender, and the overlying skin is edematous.

Chylocele

- It is rare.
- It is only diagnosed on aspiration of a milky fluid (due to fat droplets floating on the surface).
- The specific gravity is low.

SWELLINGS OF THE TESTICLE/EPIDIDYMIS

- Swellings of the testicle affect either the ***body of the testis***, or the ***epididymis***, rarely, the two together (epididymo-orchitis).
- The first group includes *torsion, mumps, gumma, and new growth.*
- The second group includes T*B, gonorrhea, Bacillus coli infection and cysts.*

- Swellings of the testis and epididymis are either cystic or solid, the latter is either acute or chronic.

Cystic Swellings

Spermatocele

It is a large, single, translucent swelling that should be differentiated from hydrocele.

1. A spermatocele is placed above and behind the testicle, from which it is distinct.
2. Though attached to the epididymis, it is rounded. Being thin-walled it does not feel as tense as a hydrocele.
3. It tends to have several rounded projections rather than a simple surface.
4. The fluid withdrawn is milky or opalescent (not golden yellow), of low specific gravity (not as high as 1030), containing little albumin but showing numerous cells under the microscope, some of which may be spermatozoa.

Multiple Cysts

- These occur in men past middle age, and probably analogous to cystic degeneration of the breast.
- They are painless, lobulated, fluctuating swellings that are strikingly translucent and increase in size very slowly.

Hydatid Cyst of Morgagni

- It is rare.
- It is typically situated on the upper aspect of the testis **(Figure 1.83)**.

Acute Solid Swellings

*Torsion of the Testis (Cord) (**Figure 1.84**)*

- The patient, usually a boy around the age of puberty, complaining of sudden, agonizing pain in the scrotum

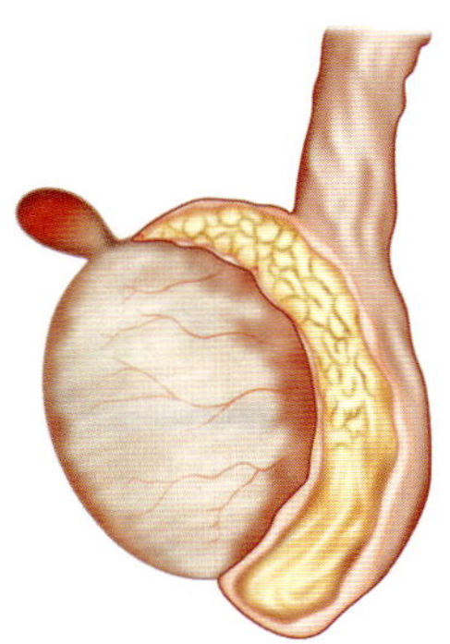

Fig. 1.83: Hydatid cyst of Morgagni

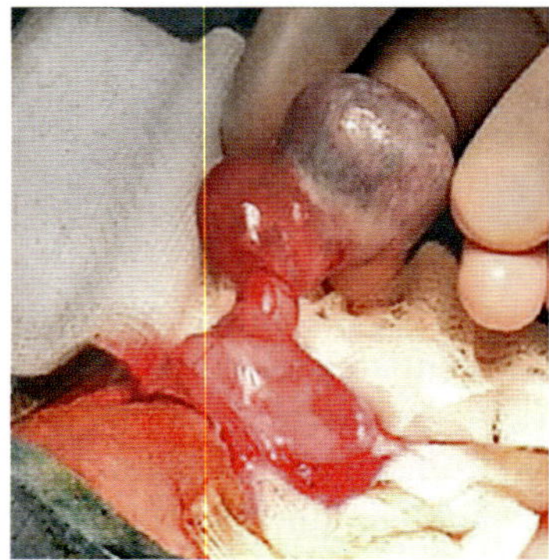

Fig. 1.84: Torsion of the testis

that may be referred to the groin and abdomen, together with nausea and vomiting.

- *Local signs* include moderate enlargement of the testicle, tenderness, the presence of a small hematocele, and the appearance after a few hours of edema of the scrotal wall on the affected side. The testis is higher in position than its counterpart and is transversely situated (**Figure 1.85**). If neglected, necrosis of the testis takes place (**Figure 1.86**) and pain subsides.
- It should be differentiated from acute epididymo-orchitis (Table below) and strangulated hernia.
- *Recurrent, subacute* torsion of the testicle is not uncommon, and in these cases the signs and symptoms are less pronounced than in the acute variety into which they eventually pass.
- *Chronic torsion,* which is occasionally seen in adults, is the result of a blow or an injury in the saddle.

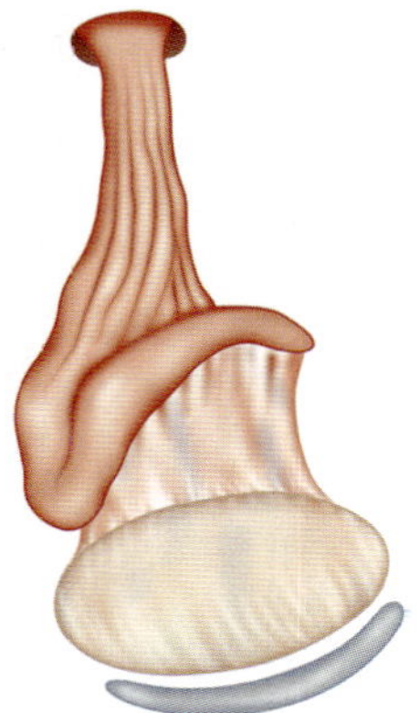

Fig. 1.85: The affected testis is found to lie horizontally (and higher in position than its counter-part)

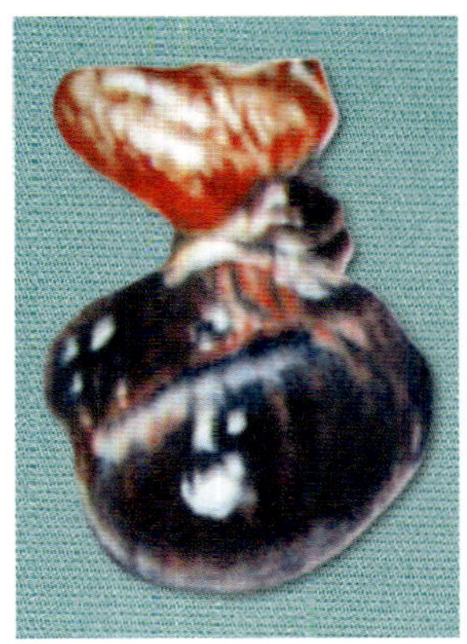

Fig. 1.86: Torsion of the left testis of 24-h duration in a 15-year old boy simulating acute epididymo-orchitis. Note gangrene of the testis

Acute Epididymo-orchitis

- It is usually due to *E. coli* or gonorrheal infection of the urethra, and starts when the urethral discharge ceases.
- The patient, usually > 25 old, complains of severe pain and swelling associated with erythema of the scrotum, fever and pyuria, dysuria, frequency ± urethral discharge. Pain is relieved by elevating and supporting the testis. The testis and epididymis become swollen, and acutely tender. There may be a small secondary hydrocele.
- Diagnosis is confirmed by the history and finding the gonococci in the discharge collected after prostatic massage. The prostate is firm and tender. Pressure on it may bring turbid prostatic fluid from the external urethral meatus.
- In *subacute epididymo-orchitis, filariasis* (besides pyogenic infection) may give rise to ill-defined enlargement of the testis and epididymis.

Point of Difference	Acute Epididymo-Orchitis	Torsion of the Testis
1. Age	Unusual below the age of 25 years	Young age (15-25 years)
2. History of fever or UTI	+ve	-ve
3. Urethral discharge	±	-ve
4. Site of testis	Normal site	Higher up
5. Elevate and support testis	Relieves pain	No relief - pain may even ↑
6. Opposite testis	Normal (position and vertical)	May lie transversely
7. Epididymis	Could be felt	Impossible to differentiate
8. Fluid in secondary hydrocele	Serous	Serosanguinous
9. Doppler US or ^{99m}Tc scan	+ve blood flow	No blood flow

Acute Orchitis

- It usually occurs in eruptive fevers such as mumps and typhoid.
- The testis becomes uniformly enlarged, extremely painful and tender.
- Acute hydrocele may be present.
- Suppuration is unusual, but atrophy of the testis is rather more common.

Hernia Testis

- It results from a septic penetrating injury, or pyogenic infection of the testis.
- Infection leads to increased tension within the tunica albuginea with subsequent opening and herniation of the contents.
- There is a granulating mass herniating through an opening in the tunica albuginea and the skin of the scrotum.

Chronic Solid Swellings

Tuberculous Epididymo-orchitis

- It presents as one or more nodule in the epididymis (behind the testis).
- They are hard, nodular and slightly tender.
- A lax secondary hydrocele is present.
- The cord is thickened, and the vas deferens is beaded.
- If left untreated, the skin of the back of the scrotum may become adherent and an ulcer or sinus is formed posteriorly.
- Rectal examination reveals a thickened, irregular, indurated seminal vesicle on the same side.

Gumma of the Testis

- Syphilis is now a rare condition.
- It presents as a painless lump in the testis or an enlargement of the whole testis.
- It is hard in consistency, and usually associated with loss of testicular sensation and secondary hydrocele.
- It may ulcerate through the skin of the scrotum anteriorly.
- The epididymis and cord are normal.
- A previous history of exposure to venereal disease followed by the development of a hard chancre and rash may be obtained.

Tumors of the Testis

- Tumors of the testis are almost always malignant and affect young and adult men.
- The commonest types are seminoma (30–50 years) and teratoma (20–30 years).
- The usual presentation is:
    1. A painless swelling or sense of heaviness of the testicle.
    2. Rarely, it is painful simulating epididymo-orchitis.
    3. The patient may present by symptoms of metastases such as abdominal pains or swelling (para-aortic

lymph nodes), cough, dyspnea and hemoptysis (lung metastases), or bone aches (bone metastases).

- Clinical examination reveals:
  1. A purely scrotal swelling, usually not tender. It is firm-to-hard and smooth or irregular.
  2. Testicular sensation is lost.
  3. There may be secondary hydrocele.
  4. Para-aortic lymph nodes may be enlarged. Inguinal lymph nodes are involved only when the skin is affected.
  5. There may be gynecomastia in patients with teratoma. In addition, in many teratomata and some seminomata, the anterior hypophyseal sex hormone (Prolan A) is present in the urine in sufficient quantities to give a +ve Aschheim-Zondek test. A negative finding being of little value.

SWELLINGS OF THE SPERMATIC CORD (LOWER END)

Varicocele

- Primary varicocele is much more commoner on the left side.
- It causes a dragging sensation, and occasional hemato-spermia.
- The dilated, compressible bunch of veins feels like a "bag of worms" with the patient standing and a cough impulse may be felt.
- They empty on recumbency.

Hydrocele. Refer back.

Lipoma of the Cord. Refer back.

Inflammatory and Parasitic Conditions. Refer back

URETHRAL CONDITIONS

Periurethral Abscess

- It may form a swelling in the scrotum.

Point of Difference	Swellings in Body of the Testis		
	Mumps	Syphilis	Tumor
Age	Puberty or adolescence	Any age, usually 18-30 years	Any age, commoner after 30 years
History	Short history with pyrexia Previous contact with mumps Parotids enlarged	History of exposure to venereal disease. Usually has hard chancre and rash. Gummata elsewhere	Insidious onset. History of months. There may be pain or symptoms of metastases
Scrotum	Normal or red and hot	Normal or adherent in front. Later, ulcer with sharp edges and slough at base, or hernia testis	Normal or merely stretched till the growth has the size of a tennis ball ! when it may be invaded
Testis: Size and shape	Moderately enlarged, normal shape	Enlarged up to 2–3 times normal. May be nodular	↑ steadily and may reach 10-13 cm in diameter. First smooth, later nodular
Sensation	Tender and painful. Testicular sensation intact	Not tender or painful. Testicular sensation lost	Painful but not tender. Testicular sensation lost late
Tunica Vaginalis	Slight hydrocele in most	Hydrocele in 60%	Hydrocele early, later hematocele
Epididymis	Unaltered	Usually unaltered	Flattened
Spermatic Cord	May be tender	Normal	Usually normal, may have nodules of growth in lymphatics
Lymph Nodes	Not characteristically enlarged	Not characteristically enlarged	Para-aortic lymph nodes Inguinal lymph nodes if scrotum is invaded

- Tenderness, edema and fluctuation + history and evidence of urethral disease such as stricture, serve to make the diagnosis clear.

Primary Epithelioma of the Urethra

It is distinguished by the great pain and urethral obstruction.

Extravasation of Urine

- Usually develops in cases of rupture urethra. There is swelling of the perineum, scrotum, penis and lower anterior abdominal wall.
- In neglected cases, sloughing with urinary fistula may occur.

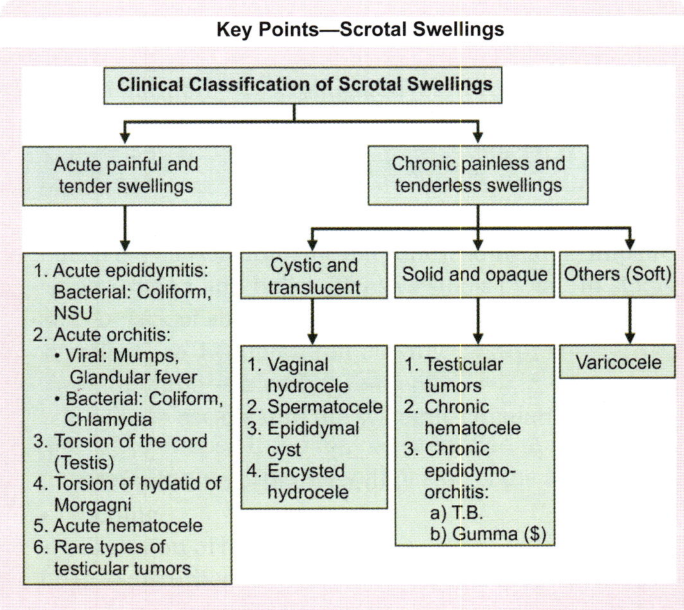

Diagnostic Algorithm

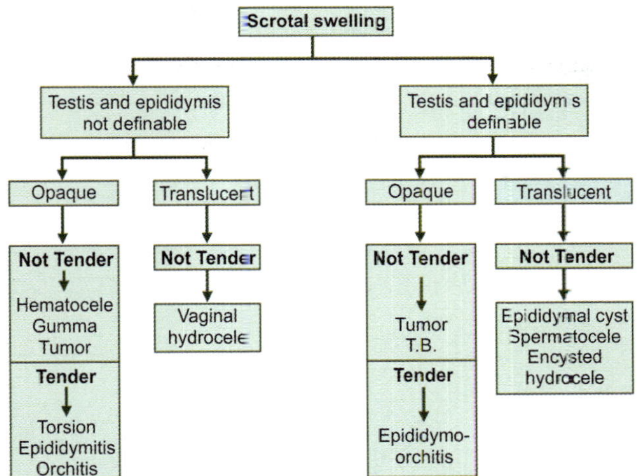

Special Investigations

1. **Aspiration** (Condemned Nowadays):
   - Hydrocele looks like urine.
   - Spermatocele or chylocele looks milky.
   - Early hematocele or malignant tumor reveals a blood-stained fluid.
2. **Ultrasound:** Painless, non-invasive imaging of the testicle.
3. **Doppler Ultrasound:** May confirm the presence of blood flow where torsion is thought unlikely.
4. **CT Scan:** Staging of testicular tumors.
5. **Surgery:** It may be the only way to confirm or exclude torsion in a high-risk group.
6. **Other investigations** according to the condition suspected:
   - Acute epididymo-orchitis .. Prostatic massage (may show gonococci in the smear).
   - TB epididymitis .... Urine analysis, IVU cystoscopy and special culture for TB.
   - Filariasis .... Blood examination (eosinophilia and microfilaria).
   - M.T. .... AZT (chorioepithelioma), lymphangiography or CT (LNs).

19. SWELLINGS OF THE POPLITEAL FOSSA

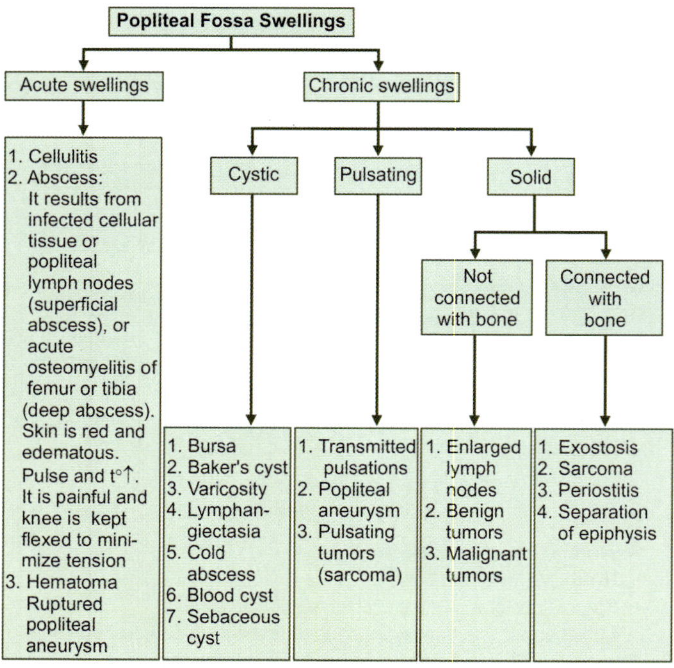

CHRONIC CYSTIC SWELLINGS

Bursa

1. Semimembranosus bursa: The bursa underneath the insertion of the semimembranosus muscle into the posterior aspect of the inner tuberosity of the tibia is often enlarged. It presents as a cystic translucent swelling on the inner side of the popliteal space. It becomes tense on extension and lax and hidden on flexion of the knee joint. It may communicate with the knee joint and become tender with acute infection of the joint. When a communication

does not exist, the bursa will not be reducible by pressure. In rheumatoid arthritis, it is common for fluid to pass from joint into bursa but not in the reverse direction, a ball-valve mechanism apparently operating.

2. The bursa under either of the 2 heads of the **gastrocnemius** muscle or those connected with the insertion of the **semitendinosus** may be enlarged similarly, but these are rare.

Morrant Baker's Cyst

- It is a herniation of the synovial membrane of the knee (**Figure 1.87**) and only occurs in connection with chronic inflammatory changes of the joint, most commonly in rheumatoid arthritis.
- In long-standing cases the hernial sac is much elongated, and may extend a considerable distance down the calf.
- Clinically, there is a soft cystic bulge near the midline behind the knee or in the upper calf. The underlying abnormality of the knee, with synovial effusion, will usually be obvious.

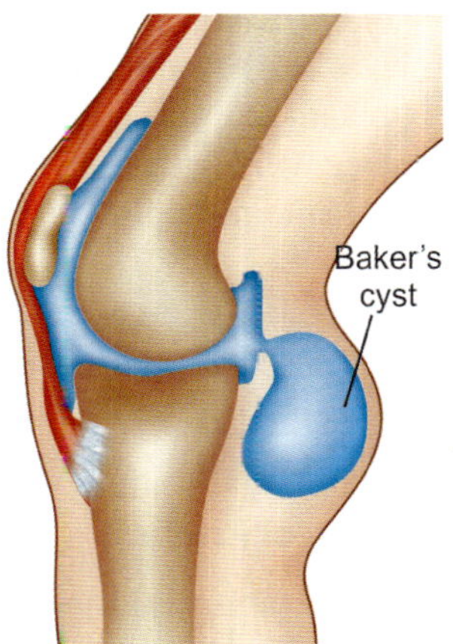

Fig. 1.87: Baker's cyst

Difference between Semimembranosus Bursa and Baker's Cyst

Criteria	Semimembranosus Bursa	Baker's Cyst
Etiology	Primary or secondary to a lesion in the knee joint (communicating type)	Secondary to osteoarthritis of the knee joint causing herniation of its synovial membrane
Site	Upper medial part of popliteal fossa between medial head of gastrocnemius and semimembranosus muscle	In the midline, with no relation to the semimembranosus muscle
Change of size	Becomes tense on extension of the knee and flaccid on flexion. May disappear on contraction of the semimembranosus muscle against resistance	Appears on extension but disappears with flexion of the knee
Treatment	Excision for the primary type and R/ of the cause in the knee for the secondary type	Treatment of the cause

Varicosity

- Varicose veins are often present in the popliteal fossa.
- The diagnosis presents no difficulties, as the veins in the lower part of the leg will also be varicose.
- These result from incompetent perforator of the short saphenous vein.
- Sometimes, they result from a tributary of the long saphenous vein.

CHRONIC CYSTIC SWELLINGS

Aneurysm of the Popliteal Artery

- It results from penetrating injuries (stabs, bullets, etc.) and is quite rare nowadays.

- There is a pulsating swelling in the depth of the fossa.
- Pressure on the femoral artery (above the aneurysm) stops pulsations and causes diminution in size of the swelling.
- There is a systolic thril, and may be an ischemic foot.
- Pulse at the ankle on the affected side may be smaller than that on the opposite, and delayed.
- There is edema of the leg and varicosities due to pressure on the popliteal vein.
- Movement of the limb is difficult due to pain and paresis.

Pulsating Tumors (Sarcoma)

- A soft vascular sarcoma growing from the end of the femur may be pulsatile, and over it a bruit may be heard, but the tumor is *not* as compressible as an aneurysm is and the effects on the distal pulse are not so marked.
- A radiograph will settle the diagnosis at once.

Transmitted Pulsations

- An abscess or a solid swelling lying over the popliteal artery may appear to pulsate, but the movement is heaving in character and *not* expansile.
- Pressure on the femoral artery stops pulsations but causes no ↓ in size of the swelling.
- Movement of the swelling, if possible, away from the line of the artery shows that the swelling itself in not pulsating.

CHRONIC SOLID SWELLINGS

Swellings Not Connected with Bone

Enlarged Popliteal Lymph Nodes

- *Popliteal lymphadenitis* results from septic lesions (e.g. a sore) in the back of the heel or calf. The swelling is lobulated, tender, firm, and lies in the middle of the popliteal fossa. It has an acute onset and may suppurate to form an abscess.

- Popliteal lymph nodes are a rare site for *TB* or *malignancy*.

Benign Tumors

- A *lipoma* may occur in the popliteal fossa. It has a long history and is well defined. It is soft in consistency and has a characteristic slippery edge.
- A *neurofibroma* of the lateral popliteal nerve presents as a fusiform swelling, lying obliquely behind the head of the fibula. Pressure on the swelling causes pain and tingling along nerve distribution. Usually there are other neurofibromata elsewhere.

Malignant Tumors

- Sarcomatous swellings, starting in the connective tissue of the popliteal fossa, or attached to one of the muscles, are rapidly growing and infiltrating.

Swellings Connected with Bone

Benign Tumors

a. Cancellous exostosis:
  - It may found, generally in children and young adults, growing from the region of the epiphyseal cartilage of the femur.
  - There may be others in other parts of the skeleton, or other members of the family.
  - The swelling is of slow growth, well defined, and rarely gives any trouble.
  - It is most found at the inner side of the popliteal fossa.

b. Medullary giant cell tumor:
  - It is prone to occur in the bones around the knee joint and may cause asymmetrical expansion of the

cortex, which may be so thinned out that an "egg shell crackling" sensation can be elicited.
- The X-ray shows the expansion and thinning of the cortex, absence of new bone formation, and the trabeculation.

Malignant Tumors

- These include *osteogenic sarcoma, fibrosarcoma and metastases.*
- Here, as in giant-cell tumor, enlargement of the bone is not usually confined to the popliteal fossa.
- Although there may be marked swelling, there is usually less effusion into the joint than in case of inflammatory lesions.
- Serological tests and biopsy should be done in all doubtful bony lesions.

Periostitis

- Popliteal necrosis with abscess formation may give rise to a big swelling.
- The signs of inflammation will usually be well marked and accompanied by constitutional manifestations and leukocytosis.
- Chronic periostitis, or chronic abscess of the bone, or central necrosis, may be extremely difficult to distinguish from a malignant growth.
- A radiograph should be taken, and if necessary, a biopsy.

Separation of the Epiphysis

- In the somewhat rare accident of separation of the lower epiphysis of the femur the lower fragment becomes displaced backwards, forms a prominence in the popliteal fossa, and presses on the vessels sometimes to a dangerous extent.
- It is unlikely that such a condition would present itself as a doubtful popliteal swelling for diagnosis.

20. CYSTIC SWELLINGS OF SKIN AND SC TISSUES

Cysts of the skin and SC tissues include: ***sebaceous cyst, dermoid cyst, ganglion and bursa.***

Sebaceous cyst is a cutaneous structure, while dermoid cyst is subcutaneous.

Ganglia and bursae have predilection to certain sites.

SEBACEOUS CYST

- *Age and sex:* It occurs mostly in adulthood and middle age (rare before adolescence), and affecting males > females.
- *Sites:* The most common sites affected are the scalp (**Figure 1.88**) and face, followed by the scrotum, shoulders, chest, back and abdomen. It *never* affects the palms and soles as they are devoid of sebaceous glands.
- The swelling grows slowly and is painless (unless infected), smooth, well-defined and cystic or doughy.
- There is a *punctum,* which is the opening of the occluded sebaceous duct.
- The swelling may be *indented* due to its doughy sebaceous material inside.

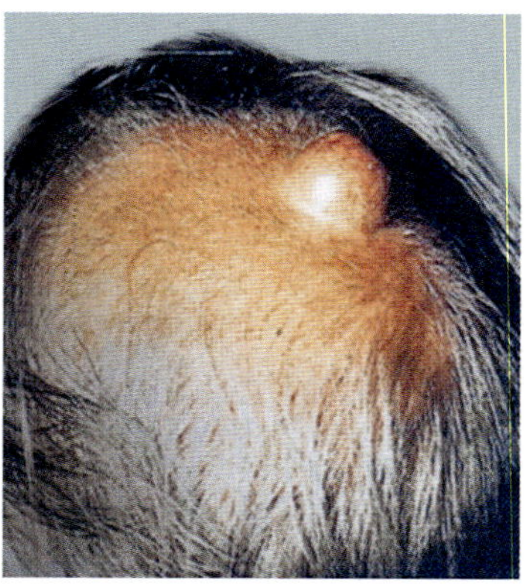

Fig. 1.88: Multiple sebaceous cysts of the scalp

- You *cannot* pinch the skin over it (it is intradermal), but it is mobile over the underlying structures.
- Squeezing causes the sebaceous material to come out through the punctum. Sometimes a cyst will discharge its contents through its punctum spontaneously and then regress or even disappear.
- It may present by any of its complications, which include:
  1. *Infection* (abscess formation).
  2. *Sebaceous horn.*
  3. *Cock's peculiar tumor* (ulcer on top of the sebaceous cyst simulating epithelioma).
  4. *Malignant transformation* (into sebaceous adeno-carcinoma).
  5. *Atrophy* of the hair follicles and baldness of the scalp.
- *It should be differentiated from:*
  1. Other diseases of sebaceous glands, e.g. sebaceous adenoma or adenocarcinoma.
  2. Dermoid cyst.

INCLUSION DERMOID CYST (SEQUESTRATION DERMOID)

- It may be noticed at birth, but usually first seen a few years later when it begins to fill up.
- The common sites affected are the post-auricular region (**Figure 1.89**), midline of scalp, pre-auricular (temporal) region, inner and outer canthus, midline of the chin, sublingual, supra-sternal, pre-sternal and pilonidal.
- The cyst is usually single, small (1–2 cm), ovoid or spherical, cystic or soft, with a smooth surface and well-defined borders. It may fluctuate but will *not* transilluminate (*opaque*). It is *not* pulsatile, compressible or reducible. The skin overlying is normal unless it is inflamed. It is *not* attached to the overlying skin.

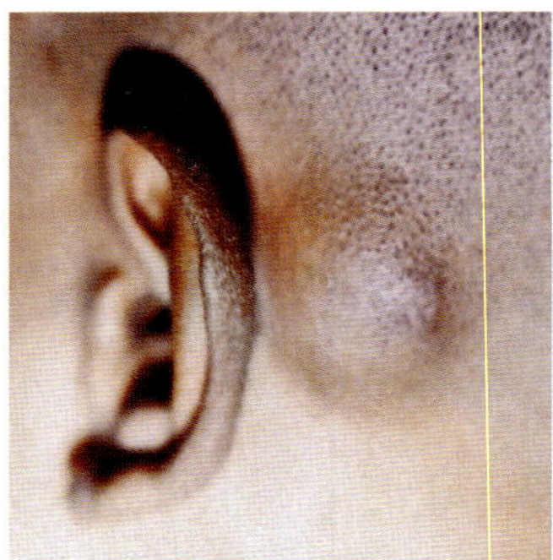

Fig. 1.89: Post-auricular dermoid cyst

Differences between a Dermoid Cyst and a Sebaceous Cyst

Criteria	Dermoid Cyst	Sebaceous Cyst
Age	Childhood and adolescence	Middle and old age
Site	At lines of embryonal fusion	Anywhere especially in scalp and face
Punctum	-ve	+ve
Pinching skin	+ve (SC location)	-ve (intradermal)
Consistency	Cystic or soft	Cystic or doughy (indented)
Multiplicity	Usually single	Commonly multiple
Extension	± intracranial (if in the scalp)	-ve

IMPLANTATION DERMOID CYST (ACQUIRED)

- It results from forcible implantation of epithelial cells in the SC tissues due to trauma, often a small deep cut or stab injury. However, the patient may not remember the initial injury.
- It is common in the palm of hands and fingers of gardeners.
- The cyst is usually small (0.5–1 cm), spherical, with a smooth surface and the skin overlying is often scarred from the previous injury.

- It is usually very tense (felt hard), and fluctuation may be difficult to elicit.
- It is *not* pulsatile, compressible or reducible, and *not* attached to the overlying skin.

GANGLION

- It is a cystic, myxomatous degeneration of fibrous tissue. That is why it is common around joints.
- Approximately, 90% of cases occur on the dorsal (**Figure 1.90**) and ventral (**Figure 1.91**) surfaces of the wrist joint and hand. It may occur on the dorsum of the foot.
- It is seen in all ages, but rare in children.
- It grows slowly and comes in all sizes, ranging from 0.5–5 cm.
- Spherical, with a smooth surface, not attached to skin and feels solid (tense cystic).
- Mobility is usually across the tendon and becomes restricted when the tendon is contracted.
- A ganglion may slip away between deeper structures when pressed, giving the false impression that its contents have reduced into the joint.
- Recurrence after treatment is common.

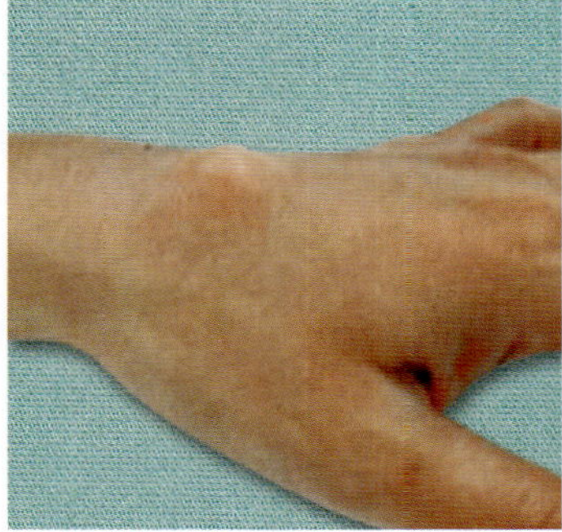

Fig. 1.90: Ganglion at the dorsum of the wrist

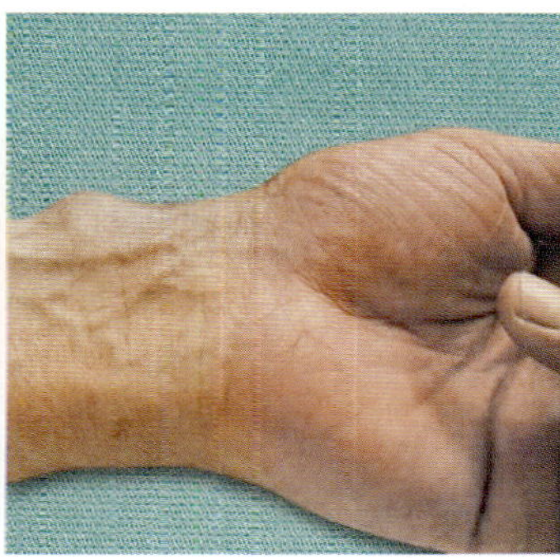

Fig. 1.91: Ganglion at the ventral surface of the wrist

SUBCUTANEOUS BURSA

- Bursae are uncommon in the young. They usually appear in the middle and late life due to prolonged friction between the skin and bone associated with the patient's occupation, or a deformity produced by injury or arthritis.
- There is usually pain and discomfort, and a crepitus may be noticed if the lining of the bursa is rough.
- Often multiple and symmetrical, e.g. both knees or elbows.
- The common sites are between the skin and olecranon (*student's elbow*) (**Figure 1.92**), between skin and head of first metatarsal (*bunion*), between skin and patella, i.e. pre-patellar (*housemaid's knee*), and between skin and patellar tendon, i.e. infra-patellar (*clergyman's knee*).
- It varies in size from few millimeters to 3-4 cm. Rapid growth is usually due to infection or trauma.
- Usually circular, with a smooth surface and indistinct edges.
- Skin overlying is thickened, white and cracked because of repeated friction.
- It is only tender if very tense or infected.
- It fluctuates and transilluminates (contains a clear viscid fluid).
- A *semimembranosus bursa* is the commonest swelling in the popliteal fossa (*Hamilton Bailey*). For details, refer back.

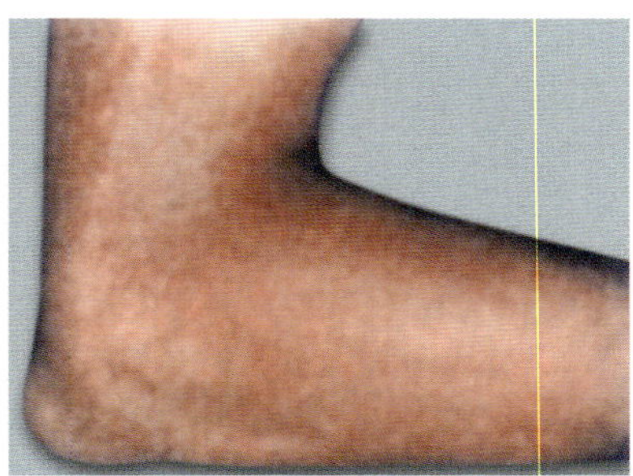

Fig. 1.92: Effusion in the olecranon bursa

21. SOLID SWELLINGS OF THE SKIN

CLASSIFICATION (*ACKERMANN*)

Origin	Benign Tumors	Malignant Tumors
Epidermis	• Papilloma (Achrochordon) • Seborrheic (Senile) keratosis • Actinic (Solar) keratosis • Cutaneous horn • Bowen's disease	• Basal cell carcinoma (BCC) • Squamous cell carcinoma (SCC)
Melanocytes	Moles (Pigmented nevi)	Malignant melanoma
Skin Adnexa		
A. Eccrine sweat glands	Eccrine poroma, cylindroma (turban tumor), syringoma, others	Eccrine sweat gland carcinoma, extra-mammary Paget's disease
B. Apocrine sweat glands	Cystadenoma	Cystadenocarcinoma
C. Sebaceous glands	Cystadenoma	Cystadenocarcinoma
D. Hair follicles	Keratoacanthoma, trichoepithelioma, tricholemmoma, pilomatrixoma	Tricho emmal carcinoma
Dermis		
A. Fibrous tissue (FT)	Fibroblastic tumors (Keloid)	Dermatofibrosarcoma protuberans
B. Histiocytes	Benign fibrous histiocytoma	Malignant fibrous histiocytoma
C. Nerve tissue	Schwannoma	Malignant schwannoma
D. Vascular tissue	Cutaneous (capillary) hemangioma, cutaneous lymphangioma	Kaposi sarcoma, angiosarcoma
E. Lymphoid tissue	–	Mycosis fungoides
Miscellaneous skin lesions	Warts, corns and callosities Pyogenic granuloma	Metastatic carcinoma

BENIGN TUMORS OF THE SKIN

Benign Tumors of the Skin Epidermis

Papilloma (Achrochordon = skin tag)

- *Synonyms*: Fibroepithelial polyp, fibroepithelial papilloma, squamous papilloma.
- *Age*: It can appear at any age, but is commoner in middle-aged and older persons.
- A pedunculated swelling of normal skin color, but may be pigmented, occurring anywhere on the skin, but mostly on the neck, trunk, face (**Figure 1.93**) and intertriginous zones. It is soft, solid and not fluctuant.
- Lymph nodes are *not* enlarged.

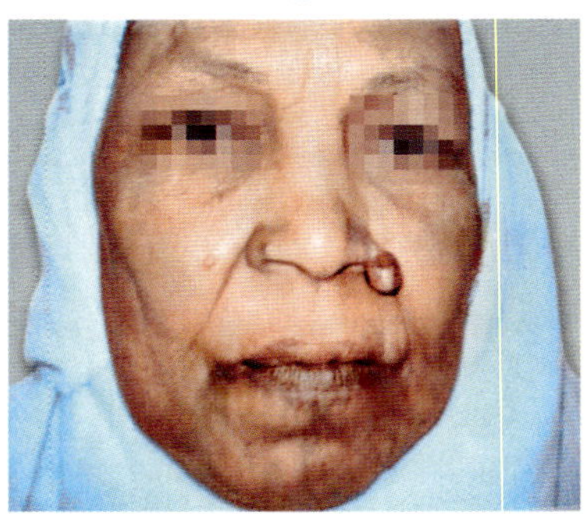

Fig. 1.93: Papilloma

Seborrheic (Senile) Keratosis

- *Synonyms*: Senile wart, seborrheic wart, verruca senilis, basal cell papilloma.
- It occurs more in advanced age (hence called "senile"), affecting both sexes equally.
- Raised slightly greasy skin lesions, gray to brown, occurring specially on the back (*not* on palms or soles). They vary in size, have a rough surface, and a harder consistency than normal skin. LNs are not enlarged.

Solar (Actinic) Keratosis

- Yellow gray, sometimes brown, patches, few mm to 1 cm in size, occurring most commonly on the back of fingers and hands, face and rim of ears. The keratinous layer is very hard and adherent to the underlying skin.
- If it turns malignant (SCC), it becomes adherent to underlying structures and local L.Ns become enlarged.

Cutaneous Horn (Cornu Cutaneum)

- A protruding skin lesion composed of keratin (*not a diagnosis)*. It resembles a *horn,* usually occurring on top of solar keratosis (Bowen's disease or epithelioma) and should therefore be excised and biopsied.

Bowen's Disease

- It is rare, but is mentioned because it is "precancerous". It presents as a cluster of flat, pink, papular patches, which are covered with crusts. The patches and the adjacent skin have a pale brown, thickened appearance.
- When crusts are removed, the papules can be seen to have a wet, oozy, bloody, papilloferous surface.

Moles (Pigmented Nevi)

- *Ethnic group:* More common in Caucasians living in hot countries (e.g. Australia).
- *Site*: Anywhere, but mostly on limbs, face and around mucocutaneous junctions (mouth and anus).
- *Color and size*: Varies from light brown to black. Amelanotic moles do exist. Mostly 1–3 mm in diameter.
- *Consistency*: Usually soft, being indistinguishable, by palpation, from surrounding tissues.

- *Shape and surface*: There are four clinical varieties of moles:
  1. Hairy Mole:
     - Flat or slightly raised above the level of skin, with hairs growing on its surface.
  2. Non-hairy (Smooth) Mole:
     - Smooth and not elevated, with no hair growing from its surface.
  3. Blue Nevus:
     - It lies deep in the dermis and is seen more in children.
     - Overlying skin is smooth and shiny.
     - It occurs more on face, dorsum of feet and hands and buttocks.
     - Rarely associated with malignant melanoma.
  4. Hutchinson Lentigo:
     - A large area of dark pigmentation is seen, commonly on the face and neck in *late adult life.*
     - Surface is smooth but there may be raised rough nodules, which become the site of *malignancy.*
- *Changes that Suggest that a Mole has Turned Malignant:*
  1. *Change in size*: The mole becomes wider and thicker, often changing from a flat plaque to a nodule.
  2. *Change in color:* It usually becomes darker (almost black).
  3. *Bleeding/ulceration:* Overlying epithelium becomes anoxic and ulcerates and bleeds on minor injury.
  4. *Itching.*
  5. *Local spread*: Halo, satellites, local lymph node metastases.
  6. *Distant metastases*: Pulmonary or hepatic metastases (uncommon).

Benign Tumors of Skin Adnexa

Cylindroma (Turban Tumor)

- It is a rare benign tumor that involves the scalp and forehead *without ulceration*.
- In 10% of cases, it occurs outside the head and neck. Some authors consider it *'locally malignant*" (*Hamilton Bailey*).
- It is reddish in color, lobulated with deep cervices, and devoid of hair of the head (**Figure 1.94**).
- Its appearance is very characteristic.
- It must be, nevertheless, distinguished from a *plexiform neurofibroma* (which is beneath the skin and as a rule is covered by hair unless ulcerated by repeated friction).

Keratoacanthoma

- It is a conical lump.
- About 1–2 cm in size.
- It is of normal skin color but with a necrotic brown or black center (looks like a *volcano*) (**Figure 1.95**).
- It usually affects the face and nose.
- The bulk of the lesion is firm and rubbery, but the central core is hard.
- If left untreated, it regresses over 2–3 months leaving behind a deep indrawn scar.

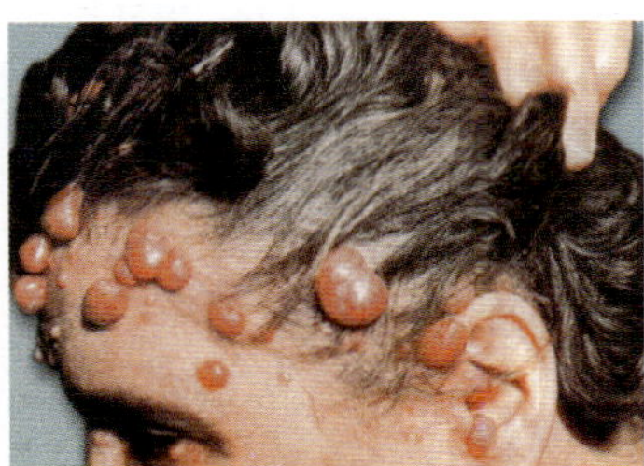

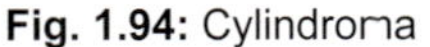

Fig. 1.94: Cylindroma

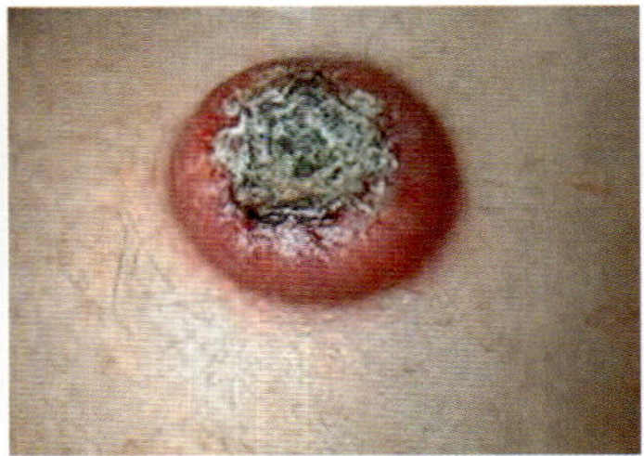

Fig. 1.95: Keratoacanthoma with a central dark core

Benign Tumors of the Skin Dermis

Fibroblastic Tumors (Keloid = Crab's Claw)

- *Factors Affecting its Occurrence*:
  1. Sites: Face, neck, ears, over sternum and in front of abdomen.
  2. Lines of skin tension (scars crossing skin creases).
  3. Race: It is more common in Nigroes.
  4. Age: It is less common in infants and in old people.
  5. Pregnancy: Incidence increases with pregnancy.
  6. Tuberculosis: It occurs more in patients with TB.
- *Characteristic Clinical Features* (**Figure 1.96**):
  The scar has the following features:
  1. It becomes raised above the surface.
  2. Pale pink in color, and firm in consistency.
  3. The surface may be lobulated or even claw-like.
  4. Margins are ill-defined and project irregularly.
  5. It continues to get worse even after years.
  6. It becomes very unsightly, tender and usually itchy.
  7. Recurrence is common whatever what you do.
  8. It never becomes malignant.

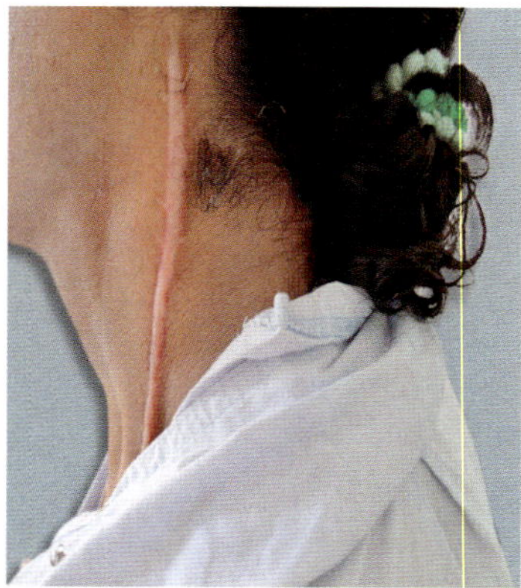

Fig. 1.96: Disfiguring keloid in the neck

Surface (Capillary) Hemangioma

Hemangiomata are *not* true tumors, but more or less localized congenital malformations or hamartomas. Types include:

- ***Strawberry nevus (Simple nevus, strawberry mark):*** It is a congenital intradermal hemangioma that is present at birth affecting both sexes equally. It is common in the head and neck (**Figure 1.97**), bright or dark red, protrudes from the skin surface, irregular, soft, compressible (but not pulsatile). The rate of refilling depends on the number of feeding arteries.
- ***Salmon pink patches (Stork bite):***
  - They are dull pink (salmon-colored), flat patches, present since birth and involve the facial region.
  - They usually disappear spontaneously (involuting). No treatment is required.
- ***Port-wine stain (Mother's mark):***
  - It is an extensive, non-involutional, intradermal hemangioma, present at birth, common on the face and junctions between the limbs and the trunk.

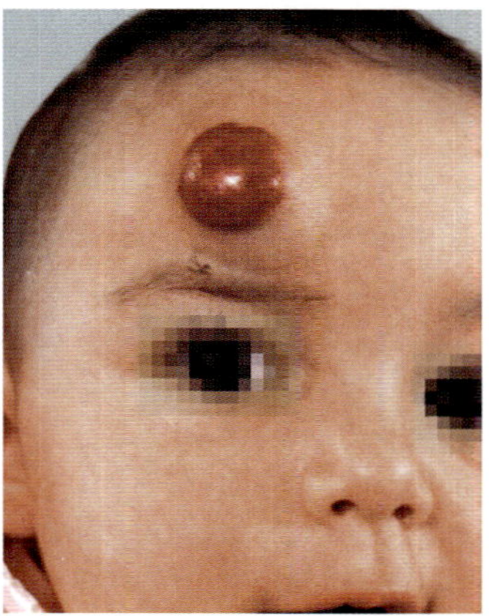

Fig. 1.97: Simple nevus

- It is purple-red (characteristic), starts flat and then becomes raised and nodular, and may be hairy.
- ***Spider nevus (Nevus araneus):***
  - Multiple small lesions that increase in number over years. Ask about alcohol consumption (may be associated with chronic liver disease).
  - Common on the upper half of the trunk, face and arms.
  - The central arteriole is bright red and the vessels radiating a little fainter.
- ***Sclerosing hemangioma:***
  - It does not look like a vascular growth. A nodule appears having the same color of the skin, firm, and not compressible.
  - A biopsy differentiates it from SCC, BCC and malignant melanoma.

Miscellaneous Benign Skin Lesions

Warts

- They are patches of hyperkeratosis that cause disfigurement or pain (when rubbed, become infected or lie in the sole, i.e. plantar warts).
- Multiple warts on the fingers may also interfere with fine movements.

Corns and Callosities

- A *corn* is a nodule of hyperkeratosis with a central corn of a dead cornified skin. They are tender.
- A *callosity* is a raised patch of grayish-brown hyperkeratotic skin over an area of excessive wear and tear. It is painless.

Pyogenic Granuloma

- It develops when chronic infection stimulates the capillary loops of granulation tissue to grow too vigorously to form a protruding, rapidly growing, painless lump.

- It *bleeds easily.*
- *It discharges* a serous or purulent fluid.

MALIGNANT TUMORS OF THE SKIN

Basal Cell Carcinoma (BCC)

- ***Age:*** It usually occurs in elderly people (mostly > 65 years), affecting men > women (2:1).
- ***Ethnic group:*** It is more common in fair-skinned people (e.g. Australia), and rare in dark-skinned races.
- ***Site:*** The majority (90%) is found in the middle 1/3 of the face bounded by a line joining the angle of the mouth to the ear lobule and a line from the outer canthus of the eye to the root of the helix (**Figure 1.98**). However, all skin is susceptible, particularly exposed areas (scalp, neck, arms and hands), *except soles and palms.*
  - It is (a) facial (95%), 90% in the middle 1/3 of the face, and 5% in the lower and upper thirds (including the scalp), and (b) *extra-facial* (5%) in the neck, arms and hands (exposed areas).

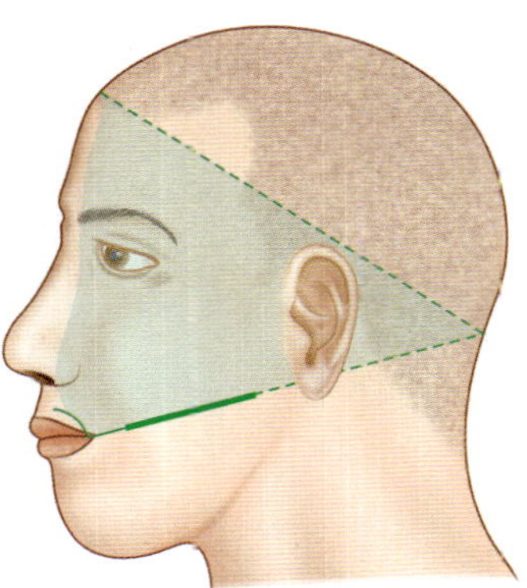

Fig. 1.98: Common sites of BCC

- Back of the ear, upper eyelid and lower lip are rarely affected.
- In the middle 1/3 of the face, the most common sites are: inner canthus, lower eyelid, tip of nose, ala nasi, outer canthus, dorsum of nose, glabella, and cheeks.

- ***Size:*** The ulcer or nodule is usually begins small but it can grow to a large size if neglected.
- ***Color:*** The raised part of the lesion is smooth, glistening and transparent, giving the impression that there are *pearly white* nodules just below the epidermis. These nodules also give the ulcer its typical "rolled edge". The surface of the nodular type is covered by distinct blood vessels, which may give it a *pink hue*. The whole lesion may be colored (*brown*) by excess melanin, simulating a mole or melanoma.
- ***Shape***: It starts as a nodule that later ulcerates. The ulcer has a raised rolled edge but not everted **(Figure 1.99)**. The center of the nodule can become large and look cystic. It is not cystic because it is solid and not fluctuant.
- ***Edge:*** The rolled edge is first circular but then becomes irregular.

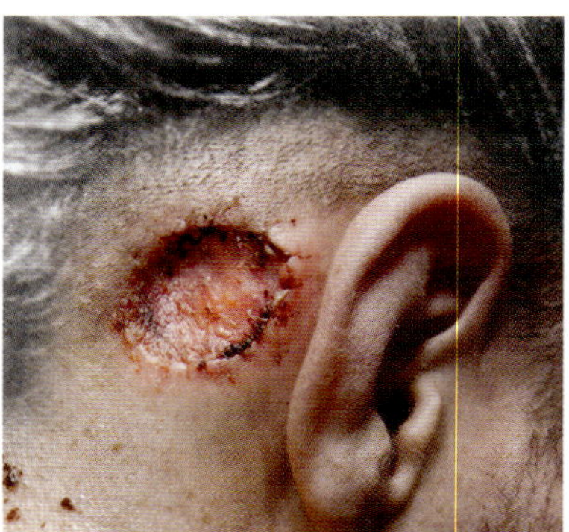

Fig. 1.99: BCC (retroauricular).
Note the raised and rolled-in edge (not everted)

- ***Base:*** It consists of the tissue into which the tumor is eroding (fat, muscle, bone, eye or brain), covered with granulation tissue. The base is usually not tender.
- ***Depth:*** Most BCCs are superficial and confined to the skin. However, neglected cases may erode deep into the face destroying the skin and bone and exposing the nasal cavity, air sinuses and even the eye and brain (rare).
- ***Lymph nodes:*** Local lymph nodes should *not* be enlarged (unless infected or transformed into a squamous cell carcinoma "SCC").
- ***Relations:*** Early lesions are freely mobile over deeper structures, later they invade deeply and become fixed.
- ***Epitheliomatous Transformation* (into a SCC) which is evidenced by:**
  1. Growth becomes rapid.
  2. Everted edges at least in a part of the ulcer.
  3. Induration extends beyond the base.
  4. Loss of the pearly white margin of the BCC.
  5. An enlarged lymph node, which becomes hard and fixed.
  6. Evidence of distant metastases.
  7. Biopsy (the surest diagnosis).
- ***Biopsy*** should be done to confirm diagnosis. It may be *excisional* in small lesions, or *incisional* in large lesions (it is taken from the edge and should include part of the lesion, and normal skin around it).

Squamous Cell Carcinoma (SCC)

- ***Age:*** The incidence of SCC with age.
- ***Occupation:*** Incidence with prolonged exposure to sunlight (sailors) and certain chemicals (engineers).
- ***Site:*** It is more common on exposed skin and skin subjected to repeated chemical or mechanical irritation.

The head and neck region is the most common site, specially the lower lip, ear and cheeks.

- ***Color:*** The everted ulcer edge is usually dark red-brown in color because it is very vascular.
- ***Shape and size:*** SCC begins as a small nodule. As it enlarges the center becomes necrotic, sloughs and the nodule turns into an ulcer, which is initially circular but can become of any shape as it enlarges.
- ***Discharge:*** If it becomes infected, the discharge becomes copious, bloody, purulent and foul.
- ***Floor:*** The ulcer floor may be covered with old coagulated blood, serum, or *necrotic material* (**Figure 1.100**).
- ***Edge***: It is everted because the excessive tissue growth raises it above and over the normal skin surface.
- ***Base:*** It is *hard and indurated.*
- ***Depth:*** Soft tissues are easily invaded and when they slough, they leave a deep ulcer.
- ***Relations:*** Depend on the extent of malignant infiltration, which causes the ulcer to become *fixed.*
- ***Local lymph nodes:*** These are often *enlarged*. Later, they become hard and fixed.
- ***Complications:*** Infection and bleeding are the most common. *All types of distant metastases are uncommon.*

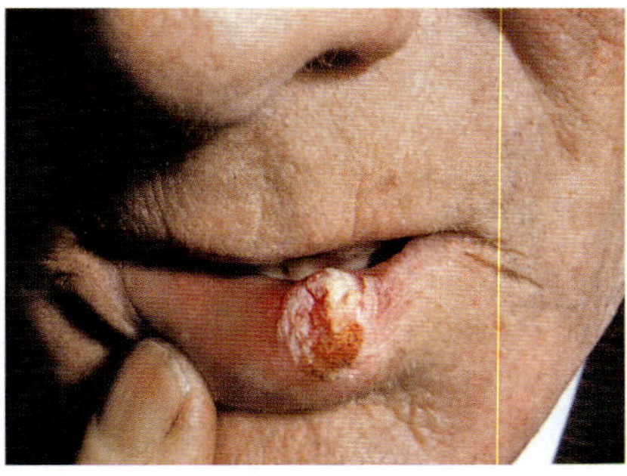

Fig. 1.100: SCC at the lower lip: Note the everted edge and necrotic floor

- ***Investigations:*** Biopsy, plain X-ray of related bone and investigations for distant metastases.
- **Marjolin ulcer:**
  - It is a SCC, which develops in a long-standing benign ulcer (usually venous), or scar (usually burn).
  - The edge is *not* always raised and everted, and other features may be masked by the pre-existing chronic ulceration or scarring. Unusual nodules or changes in a chronic ulcer or a scar should be suspicious.
  - It is slightly less malignant and slower growing than spontaneous SCC due to excessive fibrosis, but must be treated as vigorously.

Malignant Melanoma

- ***Age:*** Rare before puberty but can occur in children). It is most frequent between 30-50 years.
- ***Sex:*** It is 2–3 times more common in women than in men.
- ***Ethnic group:*** It is common in Caucasians and rare in Nigroes.
- ***Geographical distribution:*** It is more common in sunny areas (Australia and New Zealand).
- ***Occupation:*** Those who work out of doors, in regions with excessive sunlight, are particularly susceptible.
- ***Site*:** About 90% arise in junctional or compound mole, 10% arise de novo. The majority is found in limbs (sole, palm, subungual tissues) and head and neck. It may occur at mucocutaneous junctions (mouth and anus).
- ***Color*:** It varies from pale pinkish-brown to black (**Figure 1.101**). If rich in blood supply, they develop a purple hue.
- ***Shape and size*:** If neglected, it can become a florid tumor, protruding from and overlapping surrounding skin (**Figure 1.102**).
- ***Surface*:** When the covering epithelium dies from ischemic necrosis, the resulting ulcer is covered with a

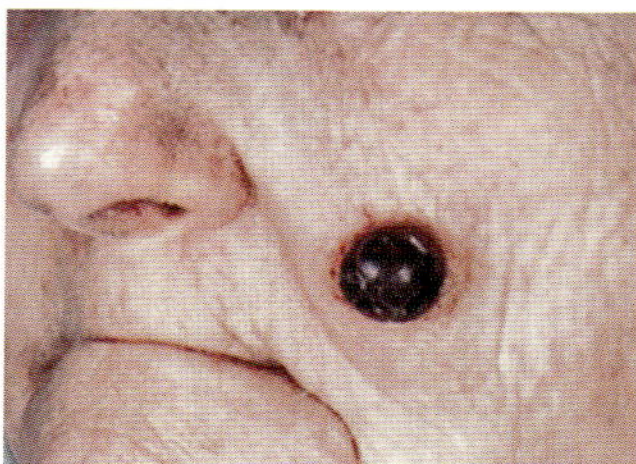

Fig. 1.101: Malignant melanoma at the left cheek.

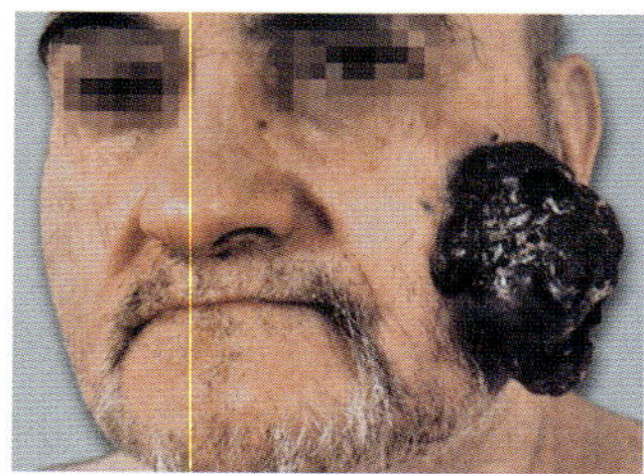

Fig. 1.102: A huge malignant melanoma of the "nodular type" in the left cheek of an old patient

crust of blood and serum. Bleeding and infection may make the surface of the tumor wet, soft and boggy.

- ***Consistency*:** Primary tumor is firm, but satellite nodules feel hard.
- ***Relations*:** The malignant tissue is intimately fixed to the skin.
- ***Regional lymph nodes*:** When involved, they are enlarged, hard, painless, mobile or fixed.
- ***Surrounding tissues***: There may be a halo, or satellite nodules around the primary lesion. If the tumor has been itchy, the surrounding skin may be excoriated.
- ***General examination:*** Malignant melanomas spread via lymphatics to the bloodstream and then to the lungs, liver and brain, resulting in *pleural effusions, hepatomegaly, jaundice and neurological abnormalities*.
- ***Investigations:***
  1. Biopsy (for diagnosis and microstaging of the degree of depth and thickness).
  2. Labeled-monoclonal antibodies for detection of deposits.
  3. CT-scan for distant metastases.

- ***Differential diagnosis:*** It has to be differentiated from ***other pigmented lesions***, mainly the following:
  1. *Moles (Pigmented nevi):* Junctional, compound, intradermal and blue nevi.
  2. *Pigmented BCC.*
     - Most common in middle age.
     - Blue-black.
     - Raised edges and capillary neovascularity.
  3. *Pigmented papilloma.*
  4. *Seborrheic keratosis:*
     - Occasionally black.
     - Usually 1 cm in size.
     - Typically appears raised, warty, greasy and as if being "stuck onto the skin".
  5. *Dermatofibroma:*
     - Occasionally dark brown.
     - Usually smooth.
     - Slightly raised and never contains hair.
     - It grows very slowly and never becomes malignant.
  6. *Pyogenic granuloma:*
     - A rapidly growing, pink nodule that results from minor trauma.
  7. *Subungual hemorrhage:*
     - Sudden onset, sharply defined under the nail bed.
     - In contrast, melanoma is of gradual onset and defined by poorly demarcated streaks extending along the axis of the nail and evacuating the blood.
     - With the passage of time, the entire subungual hemorrhage will migrate distally with clearing of the nail bed. Subungual melanoma, however, is a persistent lesion.
  8. Skin pigmentation with other diseases:
     a. *Cafe au lait patches:* Areas of pale brown pigmentation present since birth and often associated

with neurofibromatosis and sometimes pheochromocytoma. The pale brown, milk-coffee color is a relation of the small amount of melanin when compared to the normal mole. It does *not* turn malignant.

b. *Multiple circumoral moles associated with Peutz-Jegher syndrome:* It consists of multiple polyposis of endothelium of the stomach and small intestine and multiple small nodules on the skin of the face, particularly around the mouth, lips and buccal mucosa. These moles do *not* turn malignant.

Mycosis Fungoides

Definition

It is a distinct clinicopathologic type (T-cell malignant lymphoma).

Clinical Picture

- It presents with an *Inflammatory Premycotic Phase* (patch of thickening and reddening of the skin, which enlarges, rises up above the surrounding skin as a plaque (*Plaque phase*).
- It then progresses to a *Tumor phase,* which may ulcerate.
- The lesion may be multiple.

Metastatic Carcinoma

Common Sites

The commonest sites are the chest and abdomen, followed by the head and neck (in the scalp, it causes alopecia known as "alopecia neoplastica"). Metastatic carcinoma is rare in extremities.

Common Sources in Men:

- Lungs (25%)
- Large bowel
- Malignant melanoma
- Kidneys
- SCC of the oral cavity.

Common Sources in Women

- Breasts (70%)
- Lungs
- Melanoma
- Kidneys
- Ovaries.

Clinical Key Points—Swellings of the Skin

Diagnostic Features of the Four Common Surgical Skin Lesions

Skin Lesion	Duration of Growth	Physical Features
SCC	Few months	Nodule or ulcer with everted edge, occasional bleeding
BCC	Many months or years	Nodule or ulcer with rolled-in edge and permanent scab. No bleeding
Keratoacanthoma	Few weeks	Nodule with a central, hard, necrotic core. No bleeding. Spontaneous regression
Pyogenic Granuloma	Few days	Soft, red nodule that becomes covered with epithelium. Bleeds easily

Contd...

Contd...

Differential Diagnosis of Skin Lesions by Color (Browse)

Color	Skin Lesion
Black	Gangrenous skin, early pyoderma gangrenosum, early anthrax pustule
Brown-Black	Moles, malignant melanoma, pigmented BCC/SCC, pigmentation after bruise
Gray-Brown	Wart, seborrheic keratosis, keratoacanthosis, callosities
Yellow-White	Xanthoma, lymphangioma, pustules of furunculosis and hydradenitis
Red-Blue	Strawberry nevus, port-wine stain, spider nevus, telangiectasia, pyogenic granuloma
Skin color	Papilloma, early BCC and SCC, keloid scar, keratoacanthoma, pyogenic granuloma

Differential Diagnosis of Multiple Lesions (in the Body)

Skin and SC Tissues	Bone
1. Benign Lesions: Sebaceous cysts, moles (nevi), warts, acne vulgaris (face), pyogenic abscesses, lymph nodes, lipomatosis, neurofibromatosis. 2. Malignant Lesions: Secondary carcinomatous nodules, lymphoma (mycosis fungoides), malignant melanoma, basal cell carcinoma, Kaposi sarcoma, neurofibrosarcoma.	1. Multiple exostosis 2. Multiple myeloma 3. Multiple secondaries

22. SOLID SWELLINGS OF "SC" TISSUES

BENIGN TUMORS

Lipoma

- *Age:* Most common between 30–40 years, not common in children.
- *Sex:* More than 90% occur in women.
- *Course:* Slowly growing, painless lump, over many years.
- *Number:* It may be multiple (**Figure 1.103**).
- *Site:* Trunk, nape and limbs are common sites.
- *Skin overlying:* Normal, may show dimpling, or faint blue streaks (veins).
- *Size:* Lipomata come in all sizes.
- *Shape:* Spherical, may be flattened, or pedunculated (**Figure 1.104**).
- *Tenderness:* Lipomata are not tender.
- *Temperature:* Normal.
- *Edge:* Well-defined and lobulated, but slippery (slip-sign).
- *Consistency:* Soft (pseudofluctuant), no thrill, and dull on percussion.
- *Relations:* It can usually be moved in all directions, i.e. no attachments. It may be subfascial (**Figure 1.105**).

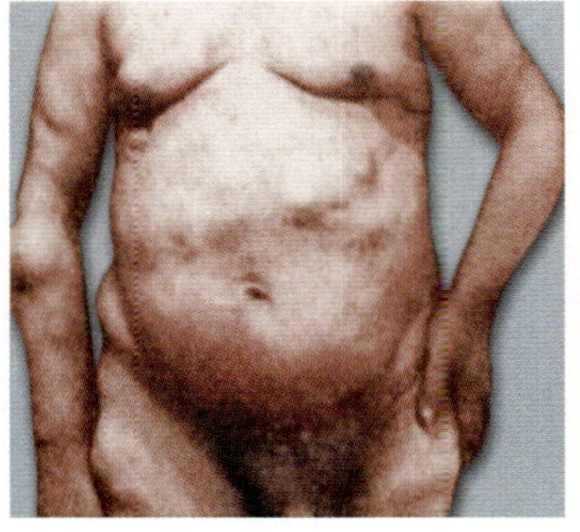

Fig. 1.103: Multiple SC lipomata

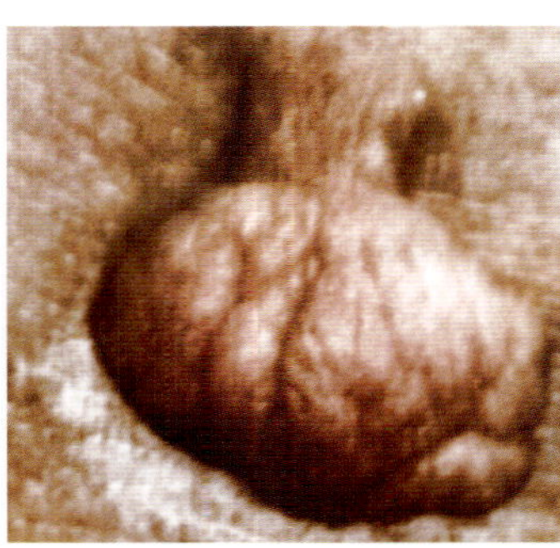

Fig. 1.104: Pedunculated lipoma

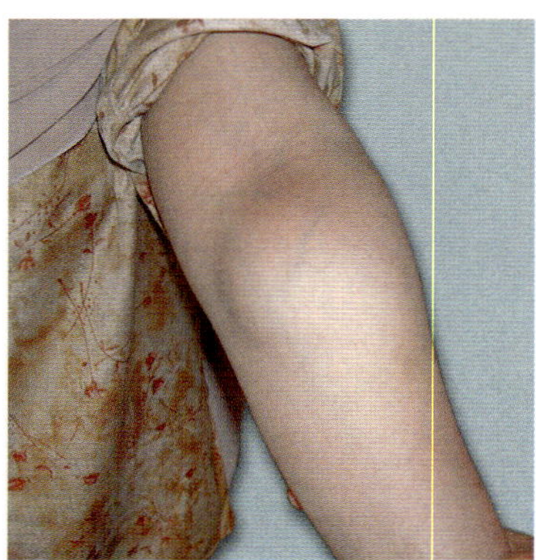

Fig. 1.105: Lipoma beneath the deep fascia in front of the elbow

- *Lymph nodes:* Not enlarged.
- *Local tissues:* Normal.
- *Complications:* It rarely turns into a liposarcoma. Dangerous sites are:
  1. The nape
  2. Back
  3. Retroperitoneum
- *Differential diagnosis:* It should be differentiated from:
  1. Other tumors of the SC tissues.
  2. Cystic or pseudocystic lesions such as:
     - Sebaceous cysts
     - Dermoid cysts
     - Cold abscesses.

Neurofibroma

- *Age*: It can appear at any age, but usually affects *adults*.
- *Multiplicity*: They are often *multiple*.
- *Site*: Can occur anywhere, but the *forearm* is the commonest site.
- *Size*: They are rarely > few cm in diameter.

- *Shape*: Fusiform, with their long axis lying along the length of the limb.
- *Surface*: Smooth.
- *Consistency*: Firm rubber, dull on percussion.
- *Relations*: Mobile and move freely at right angles to the course of the nerve to which they are connected.
- *Local tissues*: Normal. It rarely turns malignant.

Multiple Neurofibromatosis (Von Recklinghausen's Disease)

- *Definition*: Multiple neurofibromata (all over the body), familial and congenital, in which the following abnormalities can be elicited:
  1. Fibroepithelial skin tags.
  2. Cafe au lait patches (light brown pigmentation of the skin).
  3. Neurofibromata on major nerves particularly on the acoustic nerve (acoustic neuroma), and the sensory roots of spinal nerves.
  4. Persistent hypertension (pheochromocytoma).
  5. Malignant change in 5% of cases.
- *Clinical Examination:*
  1. The patient is covered with nodules of all sizes. Some are in the skin, some tethered to it, some in the SC tissues, and some become pedunculated.
  2. The nodules vary in consistency from soft to hard but each one is discrete with clear-cut edges.
  3. Neurological abnormalities are uncommon. It is important to test "hearing" and check the blood pressure (coexisting pheochromocytoma).

Cavernous Hemangioma

- It is a non-involuting hemangioma, which may occur anywhere, specially in the head and neck.

- It appears in the form of an elevated, bluish lesion that empties on pressure and refills after release of pressure.
- The skin over it is blue.

Lymphangioma

- It is an ill-defined, soft, spongy lesion that is partially compressible.
- The skin over it is whitish or faint blue.
- Sites: It is usually located in the neck, shoulders, axillae, buttocks and groin.
- It has to be differentiated from hemangioma.

SOFT TISSUE SARCOMA (STS)

Liposarcoma

- It may be malignant from the start or on top of lipoma particularly in the back, nape (and retroperitoneum).
- It occurs most frequently in old patients, and in men > women.
- It is hot, vascular (dilated veins on the skin overlying), tender and grows rapidly.
- Signs of dissemination may be detected.
- It is liable to recur after excision.

Fibrosarcoma

- It is more common in men, mostly in old patients, but may be seen in children and adults (35–55 years).
- It may occur anywhere, but is more common in limbs (thigh and arms), and tends to grow slowly but can reach a large size, with apparent dilated veins and warmer skin overlying.
- The surface is usually smooth, and the edge is ill-defined, except in slow-growing tumors (well-defined).

- It is firm or hard, possibly with cystic areas. If very vascular, it pulsates and a thrill or bruit may be elicited.
- When invasion reaches the muscle, it may be moved transversely only when the muscle is relaxed.
- On rare occasions, regional lymph nodes may be enlarged. Distant metastases occur in 20%, mainly to the lungs.

Malignant Fibrohistiocytic Tumors

Dermatofibrosarcoma Protuberans

- It is a rare tumor that occurs equally in males and females.
- It tends to occur in young adults.
- It presents as one or more red or bluish dermal nodules **(Figure 1.106)**.
- Initially, they grow slowly, but if untreated, they may suddenly enlarge and ulcerate.
- It is so aggressive locally that a safety margin (2 cm) should be taken during its resection in order to avoid recurrence.
- Amputation may be required.
- Death has been reported.

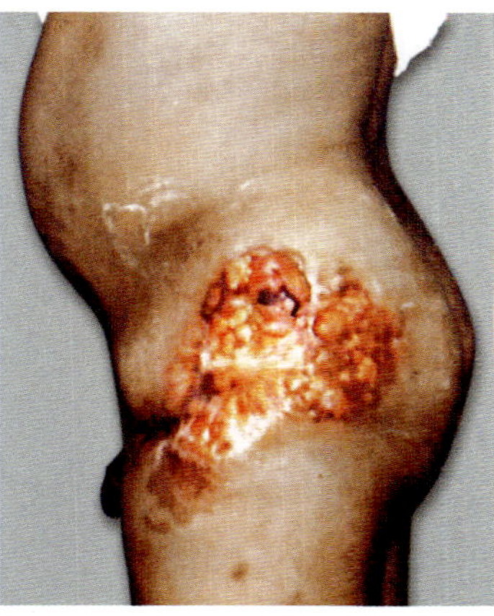

Fig. 1.106: Dermatofibrosarcoma protuberans of the groin

Malignant Fibrous Histiocytoma

- It is the most common STS that occurs in adults, affecting men > women.
- More than 5% occur in skeletal muscles of the lower limbs, particularly the thighs.
- It may be pigmented. The pigment is derived from blood and merges into the surrounding tissue.
- They are very malignant and local recurrence after resection occurs in 50% of cases and metastases in > 40%.
- Spread may be hematogenous or to regional lymph nodes.

Key Points — Soft Tissue Sarcoma

- Prognosis is poor because of aggressive local invasion and early hematogenous spread. It depends on the stage and grade of the disease.
- Distant metastases are usually to the lungs, but infrequently, STS spreads to local lymph nodes.
- When feasible, pulmonary resection is recommended for pulmonary metastases.
- Distal lesions have a better cure rate than proximal lesions.
- About 80% of all local recurrences following surgery occur within 2 years.
- About 80% of patients who develop distant metastases do so within 5 years after resection of primary tumor.
- Death results from uncontrollable local recurrence or metastases to lungs, liver or other sites.

23. BONE SWELLINGS

SWELLINGS AT THE END OF LONG BONES

- Traumatic
- Inflammatory
- Benign Tumors
- Locally Malignant Tumors
- Malignant Tumors
- Bone Cysts
- Generalized Bone Disease

Traumatic

Malunion

History of fracture, which united in a bad position, i.e. angulation, rotation, or over-riding.

Excessive Callus Formation

A hard mass develops around the fracture site 3–4 weeks after fracture.

Inflammatory

Osteomyelitis

a. *Acute osteomyelitis*:
    - Onset is acute with severe pain and tenderness, high fever and swelling of bone and surrounding tissues (DD: cellulitis is superficial in the skin and SC tissue).
    - Fluctuation indicates a deep abscess formation (DD: rheumatic arthritis: swollen joint, limited movement, bone is free).

b. *Subacute and chronic stages:*
    - Clear history, exacerbations and remissions. Bone is thickened with one or more sinuses.

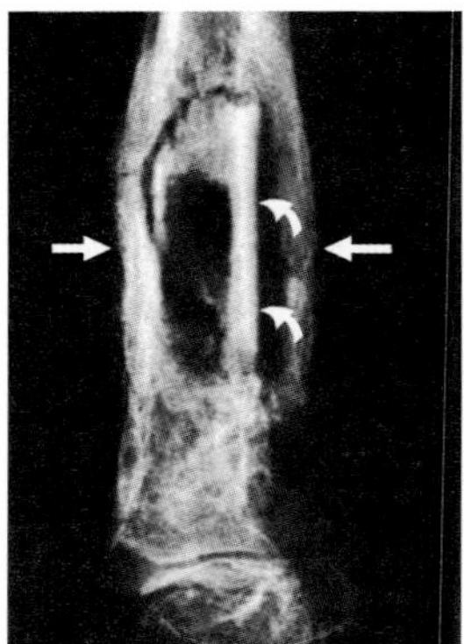

Fig. 1.107: Chronic osteomyelitis. The involucurum (straight arrows) surrounds the sequestrum (curved arrows).

- The chronic sclerosing type and cases with periostitis may simulate malignant disease.
- Plain X-ray **(Figure 1.107)** shows the sequestrum (appears as a denser shadow than the rest of the bone) and involucrum (subperiosteal new bone thicker and denser, and with several holes in it known as "cloaca"). When the sequestrum is separated, it can be removed; separation being tested by passing a probe through a cloacum and feeling a click, or by X-ray.

Brodie's Abscess

- *Definition*: It is a localized form of chronic osteomyelitis of the metaphysis of a long bone, caused by a Staphylococcus of low, or of attenuated virulence.
- *Sites*: The most frequent sites are the lower end of the tibia, the upper end of the tibia, the lower end of the femur and the upper end of the humerus, in that order.
- *Clinical picture*: There are recurrent attacks of pain, fever, and thickening with tenderness over the bone, without marked external swelling.

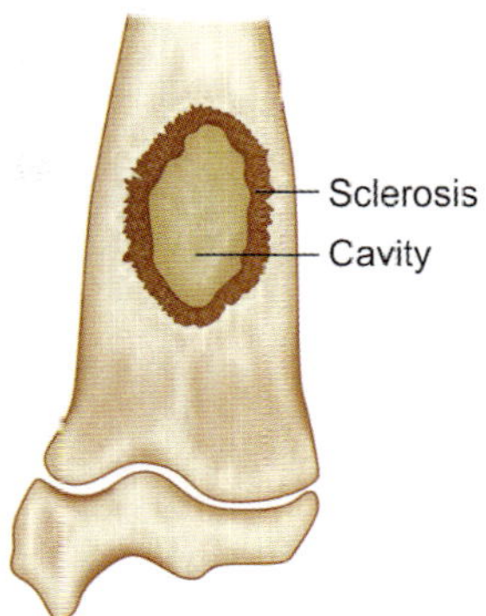

Fig. 1.108: Brodie's abscess

- *Plain X-ray:* It shows a cavity with bone sclerosis around, but without a sequestrum inside as shown in **Figure 1.108**.

Benign Tumors

Osteochondroma (Solitary Exostosis)

- *Age*: It is common, especially in adolescents.
- *Sites*: Approximately 50% are located at the lower metaphysis of the femur, or the upper metaphysis of the tibia.
- A hard, well-defined swelling, stationary or very slowly growing and stops growth after union of epiphysis (18–20 years).
- It may be solitary, or part of generalized exostosis.
- It is capped by cartilage, which in turn sometimes surmounted by an adventitious bursa.
- Usually large in size, lobulated with many soft areas resulting from degeneration.
- It may turn malignant (*chondrosarcoma*).
- *Plain X-ray:* It is diagnostic showing a bony stalk arising from the metaphysis and usually pointing away from the

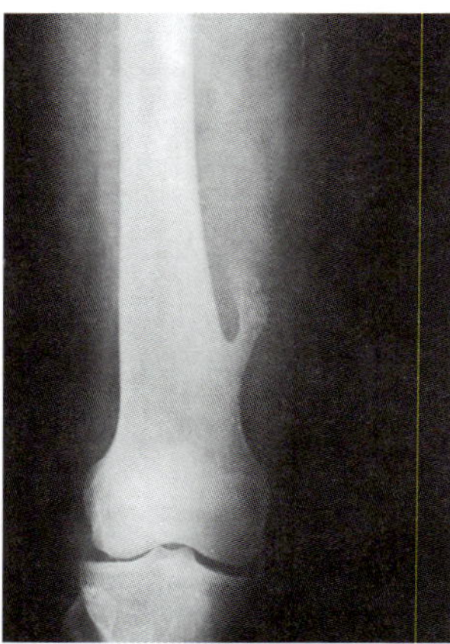

Fig. 1.109: Osteochondroma at the lower end of the femur

adjacent epiphysis (**Figure 1.109**). The end of the stalk is irregular and covered with a cartilaginous cap of varying thickness.

Locally Malignant Tumors

Osteoclastoma (Giant Cell Tumor)

- It is a disease of adults (20–40 years), males and females being affected equally.
- It may attain a huge size causing dull aching pain.
- It occurs at the lower end of the femur, upper end of humerus, lower end of radius, upper end of the tibia (**Figure 1.110**), and clavicle. It starts at the site of the epiphysis and may extend and destroy the joint.
- The edge is well-defined, consistency is hard, and the tumor gives the characteristic egg-shell crackling sensation due to the thin shell of bone.
- *Plain X-ray:* It shows soap-bubble appearance and the presence of new bone formation shutting off the

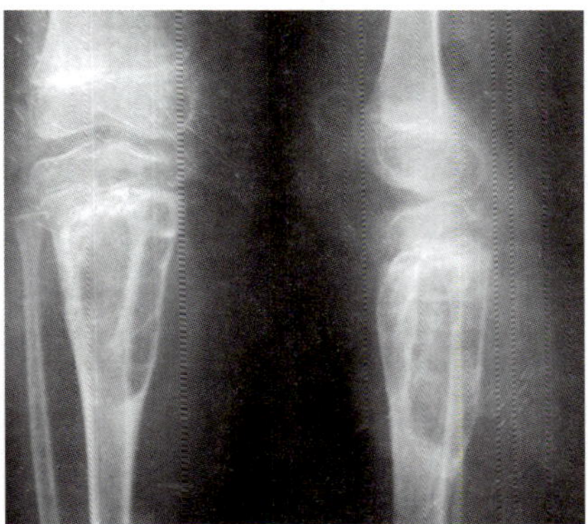

Fig. 1.110: Giant cell tumor of upper end of tibia causing bone expansion

medulla of the bone from the tumor (medullary plug or operculum). Absence of this plug indicates malignant change or the presence of secondaries.

Malignant Tumors

Primary Tumors

a. Osteogenic Sarcoma:

- It is the most serious disease, which occurs in children and teenagers (10–20 years), more in males.
- *Sites*: About 90% occur at the lower end of the femur and upper end of the tibia. The upper end of the humerus is the third common site.
- It occurs in the *metaphysis* and spares the extreme end of the bone (condyles of the femur and tibia).
- History of mild trauma and severe unremitting pain months before appearance of the swelling.
- The edge is ill-defined. Dilated veins indicate high vascularity, which may cause pulsations.
- Pulmonary metastases occur regularly and comparatively early; they are sometimes present when the patient first attends.

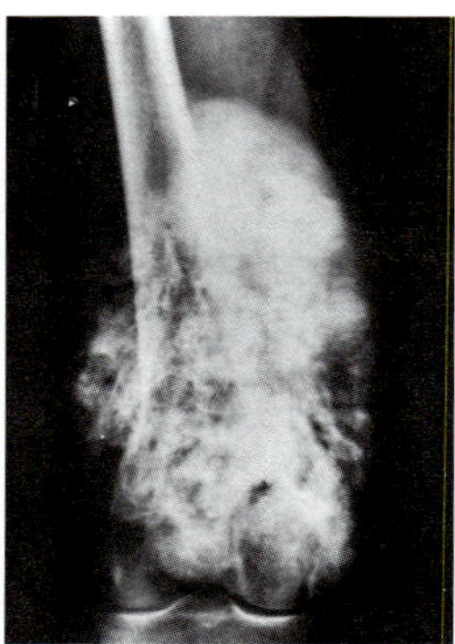

Fig. 1.111: Osteogenic sarcoma

- *Plain X-ray* shows irregular bone destruction (but still the ghost of the original shaft is seen in the tumor), and new bone formation, outside and inside the bone, subperiosteal at the edge of the tumor, known as *Codmann's triangle,* and around the raised periosteal vessels at right angles to the bone, known as *sunray appearance* (**Figure 1.111**).

Differences between Osteogenic Sarcoma and Osteoclastoma

Point of Difference	Osteogenic Sarcoma	Osteoclastoma
• Age	• Teenagers	• Adults
• Pain	• Severe and persistent for months before appearance of the swelling	• Just dull ache with a huge mass
• Site of origin	• Metaphysis	• Epiphysis
• Rate of growth	• Very rapid	• Less rapid
• Edge	• Ill-defined	• Well-defined
• Joint involvement	• Never involved	• Commonly involved
• Plain X-ray	• Bone destruction, new bone formation, Codmann's triangle, and sunray appearance	• Destruction of the medullary plug and invasion of the shaft

Differences between Osteogenic Sarcoma and Sclerosing Osteomyelitis

Point of Difference	Osteogenic Sarcoma	Sclerosing Osteomyelitis
Pain	Severe and precedes the swelling	Usually at night when legs are covered and there is congestion
Vascularity	Markedly vascular	Lacks vascularity due to end arteritis
Course	Very rapid deterioration	Better prognosis

b. ***Malignant Osteoclastoma:***
   - The tumor is ill-defined, rapidly growing and secondaries may be evident.
   - *Plain X-ray* shows destruction of the medullary plug (operculum) and shaft invasion.

c. ***Chondrosarcoma:***
   - Age: 10–40 years.
   - It may be primary, but most commonly, occurs on top of a chondroma.
   - The pelvis is the commonest site, and about 75% are situated in the trunk, or the upper end of the femur or humerus.
   - It grows slower than osteogenic sarcoma, but may attain a huge size, pain is less and metastases occur later.
   - *Plain X-ray* shows irregular bone destruction, clear areas of tumor tissue that may show calcifications (**Figure 1.112**), and reactive bone formation under the periosteum.

Secondaries

- These are the commonest bone tumors after adolescence.
- Usually present with pain or pathological fracture that draws attention to the swelling.

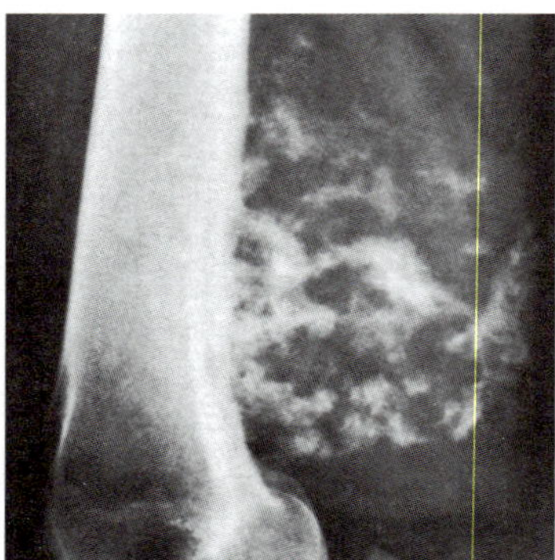

Fig. 1.112: Prominent dense calcification in a large exostotic chondrosarcoma

- The common sites are the upper end of the femur and humerus.
- The common sites of the primary are carcinoma of the breast, thyroid, and prostate, hypernephroma and bronchogenic carcinoma.
- *PXR* shows bone destruction (osteolytic lesions), no new bone formation (except in metastases from the prostate which shows dense new bone, i.e. osteosclerotic).
- Evidence of primary tumor and metastases elsewhere (e.g. chest) should be searched for.

Bone Cysts

Aneurysmal Bone Cyst

- *Definition:* It is an expansile osteolytic lesion with a thin wall, containing blood-filled cystic cavities. The term aneurysmal is derived from its radiologic appearance.
- *Pathophysiology*: Trauma is considered an initiating factor in the pathogenesis of some cysts in cases involving acute fracture. The lesion is a component of, or arises within, a pre-existing bone tumor in about 1/3 of cases. Aneurysmal

bone cysts may be purely intraosseous, arising from the bone marrow cavity. They may be extra-osseous, arising from the surface of bones, eroding adjacent cortex, and extending into the marrow space.

- *Sex:* It occurs more in females.
- *Age:* Between 10–30 years (peak at 16 years). About 75% of patients < 20 years.
- *Sites:* Long bones (most common is the metaphyseal region of knees); also, flat bones.

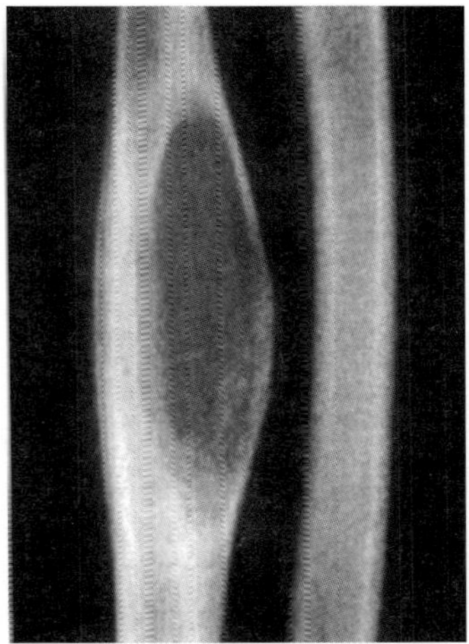

Fig. 1.113 Aneurysmal bone cyst of radius

- *Plain X-ray:* Metaphyseal if unfused, metaepiphyseal after fusion, lytic, expansile, thin continuous rim, thin internal bony strands (**Figure 1.113**). Sometimes, the exclusion of fractures or complications is difficult by plain X-ray. *MRI* is diagnostic in such cases.

Solitary Bone Cyst

- It is the commonest benign neoplasm (H. Bailey) that results from disordered growth at the epiphysis, the swelling appearing in the metaphysis.
- It may be large enough to be noticed as a swelling, but usually presents in childhood as a spontaneous fracture, the fact that a cyst is the cause being noticed on X-ray.
- The most frequent sites are the upper end of the humerus, femur and tibia.

Hydatid Cyst

- It is rare, and usually affects the femur or humerus.
- It presents with little pain or pathological fracture.
- Serological tests are positive and may be evidence of hydatid disease elsewhere.

Generalized Bone Disease

Rickets

- *Age*: 6 months – 2 years.
- Generalized bone deformities due to softening, e.g. genu valgum, genu varum, pigeon chest, etc.
- Greenstick fractures may occur.
- Metaphysis becomes broad and cup-shaped, showing a swelling at the end of long bones.

Multiple Exostosis

- These are osteochondromata (**Figure 1.114**).
- They are common around the knee, ankle, shoulder and wrist.
- Even flat bones may be affected.

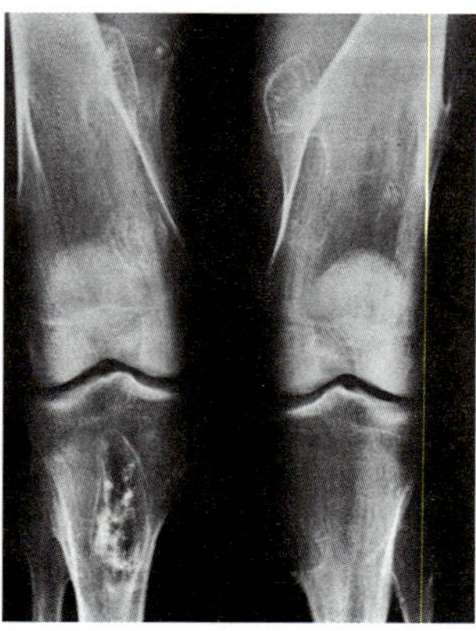

Fig. 1.114: Multiple exostosis. Bilateral involvement of distal femurs and proximal tibias

SWELLINGS AT THE MID-SHAFT OF LONG BONES

Diffuse Osteomyelitis or Diaphysitis

- The whole shaft of the bone is diffusely inflamed with sequestration.

Syphilis

- It is rare nowadays and is usually painless, except occasionally, particularly at night (a marked feature).
- Plain X-ray shows bone sclerosis and dense new bone formation (characteristic feature) (**Figure 1.115**).
- It may occur in 2 forms:
  a. A localized gumma, which may break down to involve the skin.
  b. Diffuse thickened bone with rounded borders (cucumber bone). Sometimes, several layers of bone are deposited under the periosteum leading to anterior thickening of the tibia (sabre tibia).

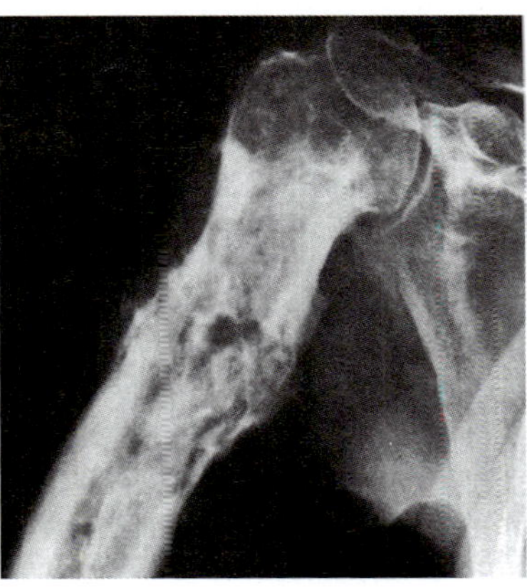

Fig. 1.115: Diffuse lytic destruction of the proximal humerus with reactive sclerosis and periosteal new bone formation

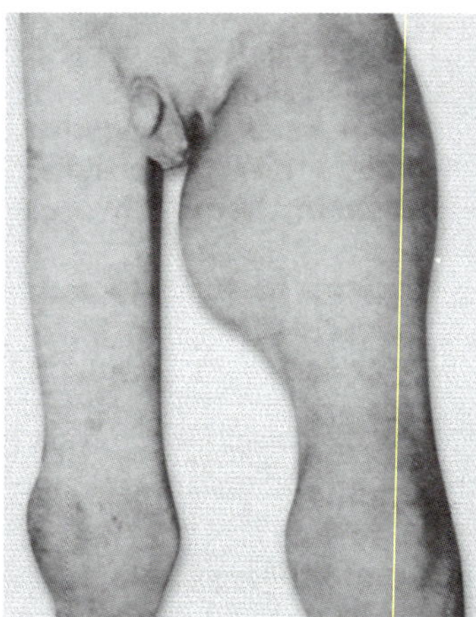

Fig. 1.116: Ewing's sarcoma

Ewing's Tumor

- It is one type of reticulum cell sarcoma, which is more common in young girls.
- It affects the middle of the shaft (**Figure 1.116**).
- It starts with pain and fever, malaise, with a red, hot and tender swelling, with leukocytosis.
- Fluctuation may appear and on incision, necrotic material, resembling pus, comes out (often mistaken with inflammation).
- *Plain X-ray* shows central destruction resembling onion peel (diagnostic).

Secondaries

- These may occur in the middle of the shaft and present with pain and pathological fractures. A swelling appears later.
- *Plain X-ray* shows complete destruction of the bone substance without new bone formation.
- The primary malignant disease should be looked for.

MULTIPLE BONE SWELLINGS

- Secondaries
- Multiple Myeloma
- Multiple Exostosis
- Multiple Enchondromata
- Generalized Bone Disease
- Syphilis
- Osteitis Fibrosa Cystica

Secondaries

- Bone metastases occur from carcinoma of thyroid, breast, kidney, prostate, bronchus, uterus, testis and GIT.
- Bones commonly affected are vertebrae, ribs, sternum, and upper end of the humerus and femur.
- The patient is usually an adult, presenting with pain, or spontaneous (pathological) fracture, which may be the first indication of the disease. Diagnosis is confirmed by discovering the primary tumor.

Multiple Myeloma (Plasma Cell Myeloma)

- This rare disease affects adults, most frequently between 50–70 years, with a male preponderance.
- Pain that becomes worse by movement, coughing or sneezing and multiple swellings are the main symptoms. The swelling feels firm, rubbery and is rather tender.
- The most frequent sites by order are the rib or skull, followed by the clavicle or sternum.
- Spontaneous (pathological) fractures occur frequently, more often in a vertebra than elsewhere.
- As the disease advances, general lymphadenopathy, together with enlargement of the liver and spleen, is usual. An invariable finding, even in early case, is anemia. A few patients suffer from a bleeding tendency, and attend first with epistaxis, bleeding gums, hemoptysis or hematemesis.

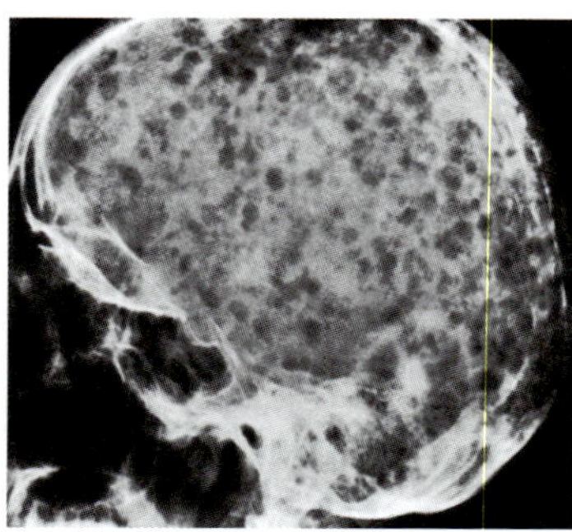

Fig. 1.117: Multiple myeloma of skull showing rounded punched out holes

- There may be Bence-Jones proteins in urine (when urine is heated to 50–60°C, coagulation appears, but disappears as temperature increases, to reappear again on cooling).
- Plain X-ray is diagnostic: It shows the typical lesion as rounded, punched out holes occurring in the marrow, varying in size greatly, but usually between 0.5–2.5 cm (**Figure 1.117**).

Multiple Exostosis

- An osteoma (exostosis) presents as a pedunculated bony outgrowth from the metaphysis.
- With growth in the length of the bone, the metaphysis shifts its position but the exostosis remains stationary and appears to have grown from the diaphysis.
- Multiple exostosis in diaphyseal aclasis (hereditary multiple exostosis):
  - Aclasis in Greek means breaking.
  - It appears in childhood.
  - During adolescence, the patient may show bowing of forearms with ulnar deviation of the hand, often associated with a short stature.

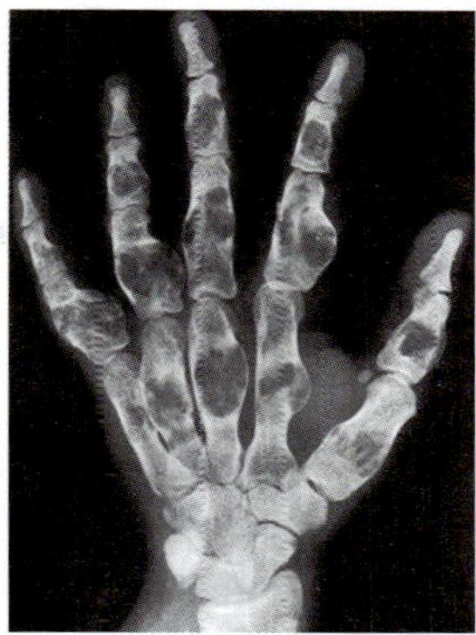

Fig. 1.118: PXR shows multiple, globular, lucent filling defects

Multiple Enchondromata (Ollier Disease)

- Hamartomata of cartilage within bone.
- A non-hereditary disorder
- It usually presents during childhood or adolescence.
- The femur and tibia are most commonly affected. It may affect the wrist and hands. The affected extremity becomes shortened (asymmetric dwarfism).
- The lesion is diaphyseal, lytic, expansile, and with a thin sclerotic rim. Plain X-ray is diagnostic **(Figure 1.118)**.
- It may degenerate → chondrosarcoma.

Mafucci Syndrome

It is a rare syndrome which consists of *multiple enchondromata* (40–50% → chondrosarcoma) + *multiple cavernous hemangiomata* (may degenerate → angiosarcoma).

Generalized Bone Disease

Paget's Disease (Osteitis Deformans)

- It is a slowly progressive disorder of one bone (monoostotic) usually tibia (**Figure 1.119**), femur, or sometimes

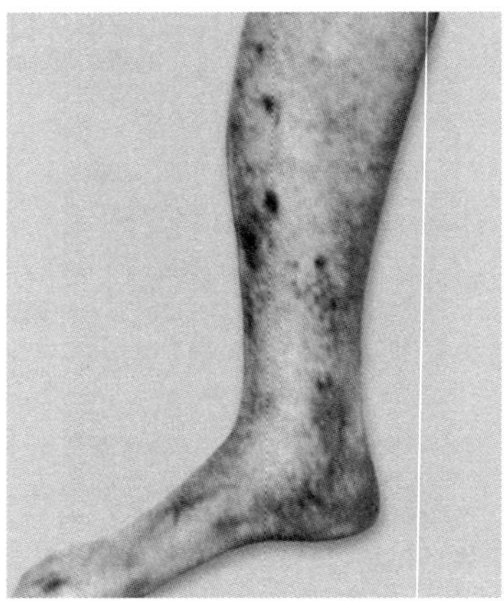

Fig. 1.119: Paget's disease involving the tibia only. Note the bone is actually bent

clavicle. It may affected many bones (generalized) which become thickened and spongy with a tendency for bending.

- The patient is about 40 years, presenting with pain in the affected bone, deformity resulting from bending of bones (e.g. bowing of legs, kyphosis), or thickening of bones, especially the tibia and skull.
- Serum alkaline phosphatase is raised. Plain X-ray shows thickening of bones with ↓ density of the cortex assuming a spongy texture.
- Complications include *pathological fracture* especially of the upper femur or upper tibia and *supervention of sarcoma*.

Rickets

- The disease usually presents in infants or children due to vitamin D deficiency.

- Clinically, characteristic abnormalities develop in the skeleton:
  - The costochondral junctions enlarge to cause the "*richitic rosary*".
  - The long bones bow under the body weight.
  - The skull develops frontal bosses.
  - The pelvis becomes *triradiate*.

Syphilis

- The SC bones are commonly affected such as the skull, clavicle, sternum, ulna and tibia.
- Characteristically, the disease affects the central segment of the bone. The patient gets a deep boring pain particularly when the part is warm. On examination, the bone is thickened. In some cases, the gumma might soften and break down to form a typical syphilitic ulcer.
- Other syphilitic lesions, +ve WR reaction, and sclerosis of bone on X-ray confirm diagnosis.

Osteitis Fibrosa Cystica (von Recklinghausen's Disease of Bone)

- It is a relatively rare manifestation of hyperparathyroidism, recurrent renal calculi being the more usual.
- Cystic degeneration affects several bones in adults, particularly the mandible. Pain, fractures, and possible localized expansion draw the attention to the affected bone.
- Serum calcium is very high. On radiology, the bone shows small clear cystic spaces and the skull may have a characteristic homogenous ground glass pattern.

Key Point — Bone Swellings

In answering the most important question, "benign or malignant"?, this table may prove helpful:

Benign	Malignant
Swelling often large Painless Local temperature normal Slow growth	Bone not greatly enlarged Often painful Warmth to touch Rapid growth or recent enlargement of long-standing swelling

Swelling at the Lower End of Radius

1. Osteoclastoma
2. Osteomyelitis
3. Brodie's abscess
4. Malunited Colles fracture

Swelling at the Upper End of Fibula

1. Osteoclastoma
2. Secondaries
3. Osteochondroma
4. Osteomyelitis

Bone Swellings According to their Prevalence at Certain Age Groups

Age Group	Common Swellings
From birth until 3 years	Intra-uterine fracture with callus (including those due to osteogenesis imperfecta), rickets, scurvy, congenital syphilitic epiphysitis.
From 3 until 15 years	Fracture, calcified subperiosteal hematoma, acute osteomyelitis, TB, congenital syphilitic periostitis, localized fibrocystic disease, multiple exostosis, Ewing's tumor, Aneurysmal bone cyst, non-osteogenic fibroma, benign chondroblastoma.
From 15 until 25 years	Fracture, calcified subperiosteal hematoma, chronic osteomyelitis, TB rib, osteoma, osteo-chondroma, chondroma, angioma, osteogenic sarcoma, Ewing's tumor
From 25 to 40 years	Fracture, onset of acromegaly, TB rib, acquired syphilis, osteoclastoma, periosteal fibrosarcoma, generalized fibrocystic disease (von Recklinghausen's disease).

CHAPTER

2

Differential Diagnosis of Organomegaly

1. HEPATOMEGALY

ETIOLOGIC CLASSIFICATION OF HEPATOMEGALY

Causes	Examples
1. Congenital	• Riedel's lobe • Polycystic disease
2. Traumatic	• Subcapsular hematoma
3. Inflammatory	• Infective hepatitis • Portal pyemia • Leptospirosis (Well's disease) • Actinomycosis
4. Parasitic	• Amebic hepatitis and abscess • Hydatid disease
5. Neoplastic	• Primary tumors • Secondary deposits
6. Cirrhosis	• Portal, biliary, cardiac, metabolic (e.g. hemochromatosis)
7. Hemopoietic disease and Reticulosis	• Hodgkin's disease • Non-Hodgkin lymphoma • Leukemia

CLINICAL CLASSIFICATION OF HEPATOMEGALY

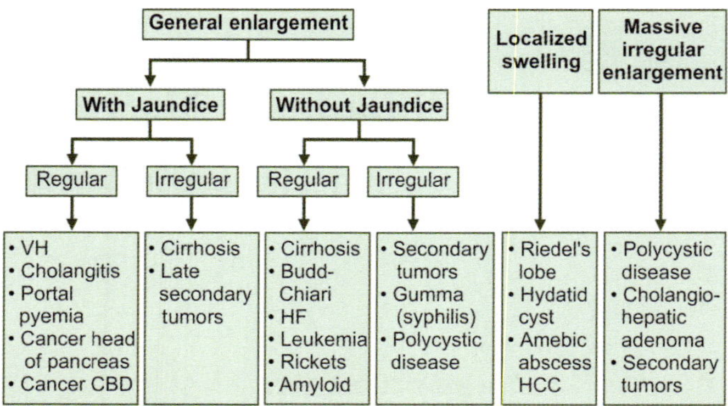

VH: viral hepatitis, CBD: common bile duct, HF: heart failure, HCC: hepatocellular carcinoma (hepatoma)

Characteristic of a Hepatic Swelling

1. It is an intra-abdominal swelling that lies just beneath the AAW.
2. It lies in the right hypochondrium, but may extend to the epigastrium or downwards to the right iliac fossa.
3. You cannot get above it.
4. It moves with respiration.
5. It is dull to percussion, which is continuous with the normal dullness of the liver.
6. Swelling characteristics (tenderness, surface, edge, consistency, etc.) depend on the cause.

Clinical Approach

A useful approach is to determine whether the swelling is localized or generalized.

If it is a Localized Swelling

- *Is it solid* (Riedel's lobe and hepatoma) *or cystic* (e.g. hydatid disease and liver abscess)?
- *Is it tender*? e.g. Amebic abscess is tender.

If it is a Generalized Swelling:

- Is it smooth (regular)? e.g. obstructive jaundice.
- It is irregular? e.g. liver cirrhosis and secondaries.

CHARACTERISTIC CLINICAL FEATURES ACCORDING TO CAUSE

Liver Cirrhosis

- The liver is slightly enlarged, firm in consistency, and its surface may be finely nodular. It is not tender.
- It is associated with manifestations of portal hypertension such as esophageal varices and splenomegaly, or manifestations of liver failure (End-Stage Liver Disease, ESLD) such as palmar erythema **(Figure 2.1)** and spider nevi.

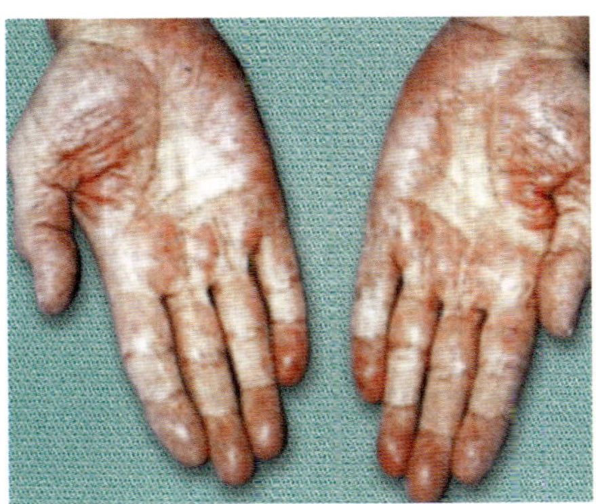

Fig. 2.1: Palmar erythema

Liver Malignancy

- The *liver* can be markedly enlarged. It is hard in consistency, very painful and tender, and its surface shows multiple nodules.

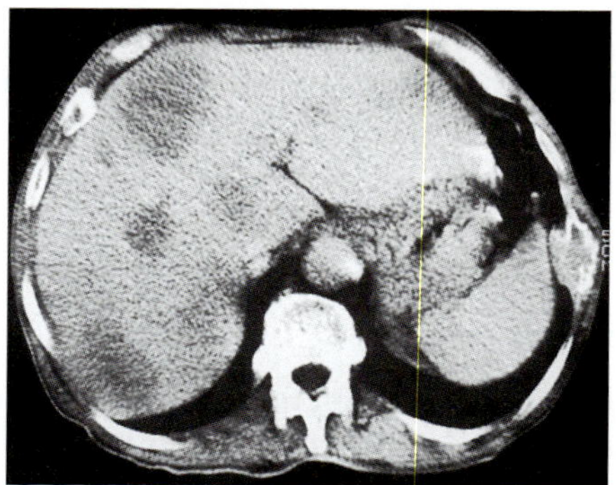

Fig. 2.2: CT multiple hepatic lesions

- Symptoms include pain due to tumor necrosis, anorexia and rapid loss of weight. Cachexia may be present.
- In case of secondaries, the primary tumor (GIT, breast, melanoma) may be evident.
- CT may show a solitary or multiple lesions, most commonly secondaries **(Figure 2.2)**, rather than multiple hepatomas.

Amebic Liver Abscess

- The liver is tender and shows asymmetrical enlargement. It is smooth, firm and displaced downwards.
- There is history of amebic dysentery. Symptoms include fever, rigors, sweating, anorexia, loss of weight and pain in the right hypochondrium, often referred to the right shoulder.
- Examination reveals tenderness and rigidity in the right hypochondrium + basal lung crepitations and pleural effusion (dullness on percussion).
- The abscess may point in the epigastrium, giving rise to a swelling, mobile with respiration.

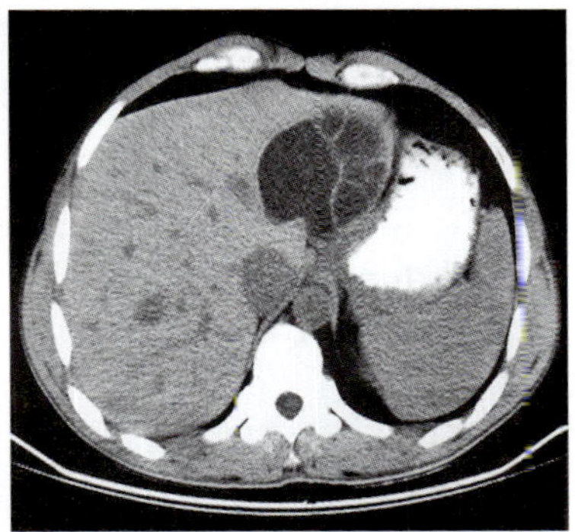

Fig. 2.3: CT liver showing hydatid cyst (multiloculated)

Hydatid Cyst

- There is a *mass*, smooth and painless, in the right hypochondrium, mobile with respiration. If present in the upper part of the right lobe, it causes downward displacement of the liver.
- There is history of contact with dogs and coming from an endemic area (sheep-rearing).
- Symptoms include epigastric discomfort and sensation of pressure. Pain is rare and usually denotes complications.
- A hydatid thrill is rarely elicited on examination.
- Serological tests should be done for confirmation of diagnosis, in addition to US and CT scan **(Figure 2.3)**.

Infective Hepatitis

- The *liver* is tender, and examination reveals symmetrical enlargement and a smooth surface.
- Symptoms include malaise, anorexia and fatigue. Arthritis and urticaria are common in HBV (due to circulating immune complexes).
- There may be jaundice (50% of cases) and splenomegaly (20% of cases).

- Diagnosis is based on clinical examination and laboratory findings.

Congestive Heart Failure

- The *liver* shows symmetrical enlargement, moderate or severe, and a smooth surface.
- It is very tender; however, tenderness is less marked in chronic heart failure.
- Evidence of congestive heart failure present.

2. SPLENOMEGALY

CAUSES OF SPLENIC ENLARGEMENT

Etiology	Example
1. Traumatic	Subcapsular hematoma.
2. Infective	
– Bacterial	Typhoid, paratyphoid, typhus, anthrax, TB, septicemia, abscess.
– Spirochetal	Weil's disease, syphilis ($).
– Viral	Infectious mononucleosis (IMN), psittacosis, chicken pox.
– Protozoal	Schistosomiasis, Malaria, kala-azar.
– Parasitic	Hydatid cyst (echinococcosis).
3. Non-parasitic cysts	Congenital (Polycystic disease), Acquired (True solitary cyst).
4. Neoplastic	• BT: Hemangioma, lymphangioma, hamartoma, lipoma, fibroma. • MT: Primary fibrosarcoma, HD, lymphosarcoma, primary and metastatic solid tumors
5. Hematologic	• Hemolytic anemia (congenital, acquired). • Thrombocytopenic purpura (idiopathic, thrombotic). • Hypersplenism (Primary, Secondary). • Polycythemia rubra vera. • Lymphomas and leukemias (myeloid leukemia, lymphatic leukemia).
6. Congestive	• Portal hypertension, infective endocarditis, mitral stenosis, vinyl chloride-induced congestion. • PV occlusion (thrombophlebitis, neoplastic), splenic vein thrombosis.
7. Infarction	• Emboli from: bacterial endocarditis, L.A. during atrial fibrillation associated with mitral stenosis, or L.V after myocardial infarction. • Splenic artery/vein thrombosis in polycythemia and retroperitoneal malignancy.
8. Metabolic	Rickets, porphyria, amyloidosis, Gaucher's disease, Niemann-Pick disease, Hand-Schuller-Christian disease, hemosiderosis, hyperlipemia.
9. Collagenic	Still's disease, Felty's syndrome.

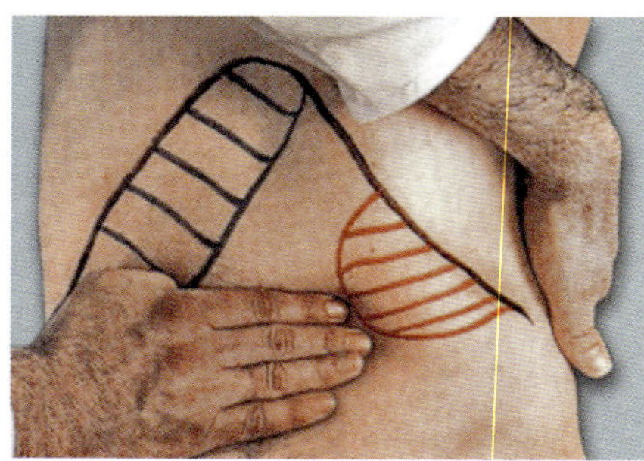

Fig. 2.4: Clinical examination of the spleen. The lower pole is felt (in the left hypochondrium)

Examination of Splenomegaly (or Splenic Swelling)—Characteristics

Site: In the left hypoch-ondrium. It may extend to the umbilical region and even downwards to the right iliac fossa (RIF) (i.e. it grows downwards, forwards and medially) **(Figure 2.4)**.

Size: Measured in fingerbreadths below the left costal margin + extent of dullness of upper pole.

Shape: Oblong.

Surface: Smooth, irregular, or nodular.

Edge: Sharp or rounded. The anterior border is sharp with one or more notches. The hand cannot be insinuated between it and the costal margin.

Consistency: Soft, firm, or hard.

Tenderness: Tender or not? e.g. it is tender in typhoid.

Mobility: It moves up and down with respiration. Mobility should also be tested from side-to-side.

Percussion over the spleen: Dull. A splenic swelling is continuous with splenic dullness.

CHARACTERISTIC FEATURES OF COMMON CAUSES OF SPLENOMEGALY

Bilharzial Splenomegaly

- It is the commonest abdominal swelling in Egypt.
- The patient usually gives a history of bilharziasis.
- The spleen is usually moderately enlarged; however, it may reach the RIF.
- It is firm, smooth, not tender, and the notch is preserved.
- The liver may be enlarged (early) or shrunken (late), firm with sharp borders.
- The blood picture shows signs of hypersplenism.

Malarial Splenomegaly

- The spleen is moderately enlarged and tender in acute cases, with rounded borders. It is soft and difficult to feel the notch.
- Positive history of malaria, and blood film show anemia, leukopenia with relative monocytosis. The parasite is detected in the RBCs.
- In chronic malaria, the spleen is markedly enlarged and firm in consistency, but less tender.

Typhoid Splenomegaly

- It is slightly enlarged, soft (liable to rupture spontaneously), and tender.
- Other manifestations of typhoid are present.

Leukemic Splenomegaly

- The spleen is markedly enlarged, firm or hard in consistency, in an old patient. The anterior border may show depressions due to infarctions. It may also show pitting under the examining finger.

- Marked leukocytosis. Differential count shows predominant myelocytes in chronic myeloid leukemia, and predominant lymphocytes in chronic lymphatic leukemia.
- Short duration.
- Other manifestations of chronic leukemia.

Lymphoma

- The spleen is enlarged, and hard in consistency.
- It is irregular (fine irregularity in Hodgkin's disease, and coarse or bosselated in Non-Hodgkin lymphoma).
- Other manifestations of lymphoma.

Amyloidosis

- The spleen is very markedly enlarged, firm and associated with macroglossia, together with hepatomegaly.
- The patient always exhibits chronic suppuration (usually chronic suppurative lung disease).

Causes of a Tender Spleen

- Splenic abscess, perisplenitis.
- Splenic vein thrombosis, splenic artery embolism, splenic infarction.
- Malaria, typhoid, SABE (subacute bacterial endocarditis).
- Viral hepatitis.

CHAPTER

3

Differential Diagnosis of Lymphadenopathy

CLINICAL APPROACH

For proper diagnosis and differential diagnosis of lymphadenopathy, one has to answer 3 main questions:

1. **Is the swelling a lymph node?**
   Multiplicity, anatomical site ± primary focus (of infection or tumor) is suggestive of lymph nodes till otherwise proved.
2. **Is it a primary or secondary disease?**
   Primary disease such as lymphoma or secondary to a primary malignant tumor or to a septic focus such as tonsillitis may be the cause of lymphadenopathy.
3. **Is the swelling localized or generalized?**
   Each may be due to infection (acute or chronic), malignancy, or others.

Etiology	Localized Lymphadenopathy	Generalized Lymphadenopathy
A. Infections	1. Non-specific: • Acute • Chronic 2. Specific: • Caseating tuberculous (TB) lymphadenitis.	1. Infectious mononucleosis (IMN). 2. Lymphadenoid tuberculous (TB) lymphadenitis. 3. Syphilis (Secondary stage).

Contd...

Contd...

	• Syphilis (primary stage) • Filarial lymphadenitis • Lymphogranuloma inguinale • Cat scratch disease (chlamydial)	
B. Malignancy:	1. Early Hodgkin lymphoma. 2. Metastases	1. Late Hodgkin lymphoma 2. Non-Hodgkin lymphoma 3. Leukemia
C. Others	Iatrogenic (post-vaccinal).	1. Systemic lupus erythematosis 2. Sarcoidosis

1. LOCALIZED LYMPH NODE ENLARGEMENT

A. INFECTIONS

Non-specific Inflammation

Acute Non-specific Lymphadenitis

- Affected lymph nodes become enlarged, tender and firm within a few days, accompanied by fever and malaise.
- If suppuration occurs (usually due to Staphylococcus), an acute abscess results.
- Skin overlying may show redness, edema, adhesions, scar, sinus, or ulcer.
- The primary focus is evident such as acute tonsillitis.

Chronic Non-specific Lymphadenitis

- It occurs in association with chronic infection as in chronic tonsillitis, pediculosis of the scalp (cervical lymphadenopathy), or individuals who walk barefoot (inguinal lymphadenopathy).
- Lymph nodes are enlarged, firm, slightly tender ± abscess formation. Lymph nodes do not become matted, nor adherent.

Specific Inflammation

Tuberculous (TB) Lymphadenitis

- The most common lesion of clinically apparent lymphadenopathy is the *cervical region* (Scrofula) where a draining sinus may form that communicates with the skin (scrofuloderma).
- Tuberculous cervical lymphadenitis is a common problem in Egypt. It is predominantly a disease of children and young adults; however, no age is immune. It affects mainly the upper deep cervical lymph nodes (primary TB).

- Natural history: Affected LNs are enlarged, but remain discrete, then they coalesce and breakdown to form TB pus, which may then perforate the deep fascia and present as a cold abscess. The skin overlying may breakdown and a sinus is formed.
- Apart from the enlarged lymph nodes, the child is healthy without other evidences of TB.
- Lymph nodes (usually upper deep cervical) are enlarged and usually matted due to periadenitis, painless, but slightly tender and firm, but may be cystic due to caseation and cold abscess formation, or hard due to calcification.
- Presence of a TB ulcer or sinus confirms the diagnosis of TB.
- Cord-like structures can be felt between the enlarged nodes due to TB lymphangitis.

Primary Syphilitic Lymphadenitis ($)

- It is an infective granuloma caused by "*Treponema pallidum*".
- In genital chancres, regional LNs (inguinal) become enlarged, painless, firm and shotty.
- In extra-genital chancres, regional lymph nodes become greatly enlarged, may be tender, fleshy and discrete.
- *In the third stage of syphilis,* "septic" lymphadenitis may arise from infection of the tertiary syphilitic lesion.

Filariasis (Varicose LNs)

- These are peculiar to the inguinal lymph nodes and result from lymphatic obstruction by filariasis.
- They feel soft and tortuous like a varicocele.
- Other manifestations of filariasis are evident.

Lymphogranuloma Inguinale (LGI) or Venereum (LGV)

- Inguinal lymph nodes become enlarged and form "*buboes*" which gradually soften and produce abscesses and sinuses. The primary lesion on the glans penis, or in the vagina, or on the cervix simulates herpes.
- In LGI, a lymph node enlarges in one or both groins. The infection spreads to other nodes, and often the external iliac group becomes involved. Soon peri-adenitis occurs, the mass in size, and the overlying skin becomes purple. Untreated, the lymphadenopathy proceeds to liquify, and the mass breaks down and discharges thick white pus. The resulting sinus persists for months or years. In the late stages, elephantiasis and rectal stricture are liable to occur.
- *Diagnosis* is confirmed by *Frei's Intradermal Test and biopsy.*

Cat Scratch Disease (CSD)

- *Causative Organism.*
  Recently, the causative organism is believed to be a bacterium known as "*Bartonella henselae*" which consists of pleomorphic gram -ve rods. It is a member of the oral flora of many cats.
- *Clinical Picture:*
  Fever, malaise, pustular lesions that subside, and after 2-4 weeks regional lymph nodes (axillary, cervical, inguinal) become enlarged (painless). Suppuration often occurs but the pus is sterile.
- *Diagnosis*:
  It is usually reached by unilateral involvement of lymph nodes, history of cat scratches, a positive intradermal skin test to cat scratch antigen, and excision biopsy.

B. MALIGNANCY

Early Hodgkin Disease

- More often localized to a single axial group of nodes (cervical, mediastinal, para-aortic), and orderly spread by contiguity (loco-regional).
- It is more common in males and young adults, but may occur at any age group.
- The patient commonly presents with painless progressive lymph node enlargement in the cervical, and may be associated with generalized symptoms such as malaise, fever, weight loss or pruritis.
- Lymph nodes vary greatly in size. They are smooth, *firm or elastic, painless, discrete and mobile.*

Metastatic Lymphadenopathy

- Lymph nodes are the most common site of metastatic malignancy due to lymphatic extension from a primary lesion in their draining areas. They sometimes constitute the first clinical manifestation of the disease (occult primary).
- Metastatic lymph nodes are common with carcinoma and malignant melanomas, and rare with sarcomas.
- Sites of *occult* primary tumors:
  - *Head and Neck:*
    - Nasal sinuses (e.g. maxillary sinus)
    - Nasopharynx (fossa of Rosenmolar)
    - Hypopharynx
    - Pyriform fossa (larynx)
    - Papillary carcinoma of the thyroid gland.
  - *Chest, abdomen, pelvis (infraclavicular):*
    - Breast
    - Bronchus
    - Stomach

- Testis
- Prostate.

- *Characteristics of metastatic lymph nodes (secondary):*
  - Enlarged
  - Irregular
  - Stony hard
  - *Fixed* (at first mobile, but become fixed in a short time)
  - Painless at the beginning, but later become painful, may ulcerate and fungate through the skin in neglected cases.
- *Diagnosis:*
  - Short history
  - Characteristic clinical features of the enlarged lymph nodes
  - Evidence of the primary tumor.
  - Biopsy of a whole lymph node, which is the *surest* method of diagnosis.

2. GENERALIZED LYMPH NODE ENLARGEMENT

A. INFECTIONS

Infectious Mononucleosis (IMN)

- It is a benign, acute infective disease of an incubation period of 7–10 days, caused by *Epstein Barr (EB) virus.*
- IMN occurs chiefly in adolescents and young adults of either sex.
- It occurs either sporadically or in epidemics.
- The common presenting features are:
  1. Tiredness, malaise, headache, anorexia, fever and enlargement of superficial lymph nodes, particularly the posterior cervical group. Enlarged lymph nodes tend to be *painful, tender, bilateral and symmetrical.*
  2. Petecheal hemorrhages at junction of the soft and hard palate may occur early followed by sore throat.
  3. A maculopapular rash often appears during the first 10 days in adults.
  4. Epigastric and subcostal tenderness is common and reflects hepatitis.
  5. The spleen is often palpable.
  6. Pain in the right iliac fossa may result from mesenteric lymphadenitis.
  7. Rarely, there may be signs of meningitis or encephalitis.
- *Diagnosis:*
  1. Lymphocytosis.
  2. Heterophil antibodies.
  3. "Monospot test".
  4. Biopsy (it should be differentiated from lymphoma). Leukemia should also be excluded (bone marrow biopsy).

Secondary TB (Due to Blood-Borne Infection)

- Usually due to active TB (widespread + other active foci in the body).
- TB toxemia.
- Affected lymph nodes:
  - *Discrete or matted.*
  - *Fleshy in consistency.*
  - *Rarely become caseous.*
  - They are usually found in *chains*, as several groups are affected especially lower deep cervical lymph nodes.

Secondary Stage of Syphilis

- Nodes all over the body (generalized) become *enlarged, painless, firm/hard, discrete and shotty*.
- Enlargement is most marked in the "epitrochlear, mastoid and occipital" lymph nodes.
- There is always a diffuse rash, mucus patches, condylomata and a positive Wasermann reaction (WR) .

B. MALIGNANCY

Advanced Stages of Hodgkin Disease

- Several groups of lymph nodes are involved, but usually of different size as they appear at different times.
- The spleen and liver are often palpable and firm.
- *Pressure effects* may occur due to compression by the enlarged lymph nodes and Hodgkin's deposits causing d*yspnea, dysphagia, jaundice or paraplegia*.
- *Generally*, there may be progressive weakness with anemia and loss of weight, pruritis and skin eruptions, Pel-Ebstein fever, alcohol intolerance, malabsorption (gastrointestinal lymphoma), and bony deposits.

Non-Hodgkin Lymphoma (NHL)

- *Lymph nodes enlargement* (mass) rapidly increasing in size.
- *Pressure symptoms,* e.g. "mediastinal syndrome" due to diffuse spread in the mediastinum involving the lungs, trachea and great blood vessels.
- *Systemic symptoms*: GIT symptoms (due to affection of the stomach, intestine and colon), renal manifestations (50%), and nervous system and skeletal affection.
- *Local examination:* Lymph nodes *are:*
  - *Enlarged, of variable sizes and consistencies*
  - *Matted together*
  - *Invade the skin early*
  - *They are usually painless,* but may be painful, and associated with high persistent fever, particularly in children (to the extent that the term "acute lymphoma" has been recently introduced).
- *General examination*: May reveal:
  - Pleural effusion, splenomegaly, hepatomegaly and/or ascites.
  - SVC syndrome.
  - Spinal compression syndrome or meningeal involvement.

Leukemia

- Lymph node enlargement is:
  - Generalized from the start
  - Bilateral and symmetrical (nearly of the same size)
  - Elastic
  - Discrete
  - Mobile.

- Not attached to surrounding structures causing no pressure symptoms unless confined to a limited space such as the thoracic inlet.

- The spleen and liver are enlarged.
- There is tenderness over the bones, more evident over the sternum.
- The patient is pale due to marked anemia.
- There may be bleeding from the gums or nose.
- The leukocytic count is characteristically high (over $100{,}000/mm^3$).
- Bone marrow biopsy settles the diagnosis.

OTHER CAUSES

Sarcoidosis (Boeck's Sarcoid, Benign Lympho-granulomatosis)

- *Definition*:
  It is a *non-caseating* granulomatous disease of *unknown etiology* and affecting any tissue, mainly liver, spleen, lymph nodes, lungs, skin, bones and joints.
- *Clinical Presentation*:
  Sarcoidosis may be entirely *asymptomatic* and discovered only incidentally at autopsy or as bilateral hilar adenopathy on chest X-ray obtained for other reasons. Alternatively, it may present with *isolated* cutaneous or ocular lesions, peripheral lymphadenopathy or hepatosplenomegaly with *insidious onset* of respiratory difficulties or constitutional symptoms (fever, night sweats, weight loss), or with an *acute onset* accompanied by fever, erythema nodosum and polyarthritis.
- *Diagnosis*:
  Biopsy is essential for diagnosis.

Connective Tissue Diseases Involving Lymph Nodes

Systemic Lupus Erythematosis (SLE)

- *Etiology*
  It is a collagen disease that has an immune type of tissue injury.
- *Clinical Picture*
  It is characterized by erythematous skin eruptions with multisystemic affection of joints, lungs, glomeruli, and occasionally lymph nodes, mostly the cervical nodes.

Rheumatoid Arthritis

- *Clinical Picture*
  Generalized lymphadenopathy occurs in many patients with rheumatoid arthritis and may be accompanied by weight loss, anemia and fever.

CHAPTER

4

Differential Diagnosis of Ulcers

1. CLASSIFICATION OF ULCERS

DEFINITION

An ulcer is a *"break in the continuity of covering epithelium whether skin or mucous membrane".*

PATHOLOGICAL CLASSIFICATION

1. Non-Specific:	1. Traumatic • Mechanical • Physical • Chemical	 • Pressure of splint or dental tongue ulcer • Electric or X-ray burn • Caustics
	2. Arterial	• Atherosclerosis • Buerger's disease • Raynaud's disease
	3. Venous	• Varicose ulcer • Post-phlebitic ulcer
	4. Neurogenic	• Bed sores • Perforating ulcer
	5. Metabolic ulcer	• Gout (ulceration of a tophi) • Diabetes mellitus (DM).

Contd...

Contd...

2. Specific	1. Tuberculosis (TB) 2. Syphilis ($) 3. Soft sore 4. Meleney's ulcer 5. Actinomycosis 6. Mycotic (fungal)	
3. Malignant	1. Squamous cell carcinoma (SCC) 2. Basal cell carcinoma (BBC) (Rodent ulcer) 3. Malignant melanoma 4. Sarcomatous ulcer 5. Metastatic ulcer	

NON-SPECIFIC ULCERS

Traumatic Ulcers

- *Site:* Chin of the tibia, malleoli and back of heel (skin close to bones).
- The *edge* is sloping (or serrated). The *floor* is covered with granulation tissue and the *base* is firm, mobile or fixed.
- *Draining lymph nodes* are free, but may be enlarged if infected.
- Generally, they heal quickly and do not become chronic unless infected or ischemic.

Ischemic Ulcers

- *Site:* Toes, dorsum of the foot or the heel (pressure areas).
- *Edge* is punched out (patch of dry gangrene which sloughs).
- *Other ischemic changes* in the LL (dry pale skin, cold, loss of hair, fissuring of nails, and absent pulses).
- *Very painful ulcer* + *History* of intermittent claudication or rest pain.

Venous Ulcers

- The *edge* is sloping.
- The *base* is rough and fibrous.

Varicose Ulcer	Post-Phlebitic Ulcer
• Painless callous ulcer. • On the medial aspect of lower leg. • Never penetrate the deep fascia. • Pigmentation or eczema around it. • Varicose veins in the limb.	• Painful. • Situated on the lower leg. • Always penetrates the deep fascia. • A complication of the post-phlebitic leg after operation or parturition,..etc.).

Neurogenic (Trophic) Ulcer

- *Site*: Sole or heel, or base of 1st and 5th toes, sacrum or greater trochanter (pressure sites).
- *Painless*: The surrounding areas have a normal blood supply.
- May have punched-out *edges* and a sloughing *floor*.
- The *Base* is firm and mobile, but rarely fixed.
- *Discharge*: Slight serous (healing ulcer) or purulent with a bad odor.
- ***Perforating ulcers*** occur behind the head of the 1st metatarsal starting as a callosity under which suppuration occurs and discharges pus from a hole, which gradually burrows through the flexor tendon to the bone or joint resulting in a cavity filled with offensive matter. Finally, the track becomes lined with skin rendering healing impossible.

Tropical Ulcer

- *The edge* is raised. *Discharge* is copious and serosanguinous.
- It refuses to heal and retains its same size for months and years.

- In some cases, it spreads widely destroying the soft parts so much as to require *amputation*, in others it heals after a long period with a parchment-like pigmented scar.

Gouty Ulcers

- *Sites*: They occur over gouty deposits. The *MP joint* of the big toe is a favorite site.
- The *floor* is covered with white chalky deposits, which are the uric acid crystals.
- There is evidence of acute gouty arthritis.

SPECIFIC ULCERS

Tuberculous Ulcer (TB)

- *Site:* Neck, axilla, groin (due to bursting of caseous lymph nodes resulting in the formation of a *painful* ulcer). Also on the dorsum of the tongue (Secondary to pulmonary TB).
- *The edge* is undermined (similar to bed sores only) (**Figure 4.1**).
- *Floor* is pale and covered with granulation tissue.
- The *base* is slightly indurated.
- *Surrounding tissues* are bluish and slightly edematous.

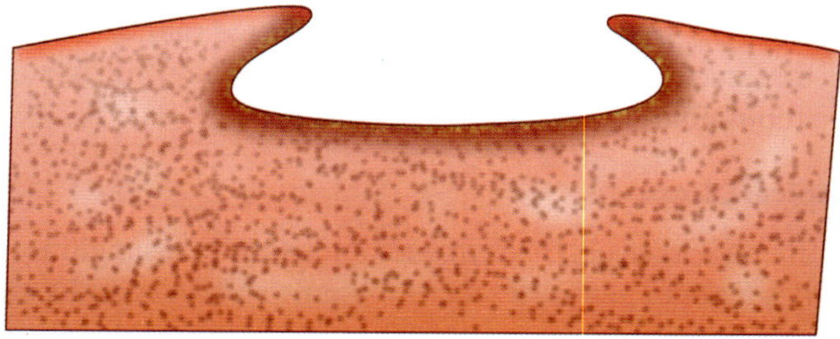

Fig. 4.1: TB ulcer with undermined edge

- ***Lupus vulgaris (cutaneous TB)*** *(Lupus = wolf because it spreads):*
  - It occurs in children and young adults in the face and arm.
  - Starts as superficial ulcer, which tends to heal at the center but remains active at the periphery.
  - Press the ulcer firmly with a glass slide or tongue depressor → pressure will remove the surrounding hyperemia and apple-jelly-like nodules (TB papules) become apparent.

Syphilitic Ulcer ($)

1ry $ • ***Hard Chancre (Hunterian Chancre = 1ry Syphilitic Sore):***
  - Painless ulcer with sloping edge and indurated base (feeling like a button), usually oval and exudes a discharge that is often blood-stained.
  - It occurs after 3–5 weeks from infection.
  - Inguinal lymph nodes become shotty (small and hard), firm, discrete, mobile and with no tendency to soften or suppurate.
  - Extra-genital chancres (upper lip): May not be indurated and regional lymph nodes in size.
  - Spirochetes must be seen under the microscope by dark ground illumination.

2ry $ • ***Mucus Patches:*** White patches of thick epithelium.
  - *Condylomas:* Flat-topped, raised, white and hypertrophic epithelium. Occur at mucocutaneous junctions, e.g. corner of mouth, anus and vulva.
  - There is often generalized lymphadenopathy, specially epitrochlear and suboccipital.

3ry $ • ***Gummatous Ulcers:***
  - Usually seen over SC bones (sternum, tibia, ulna and skull).

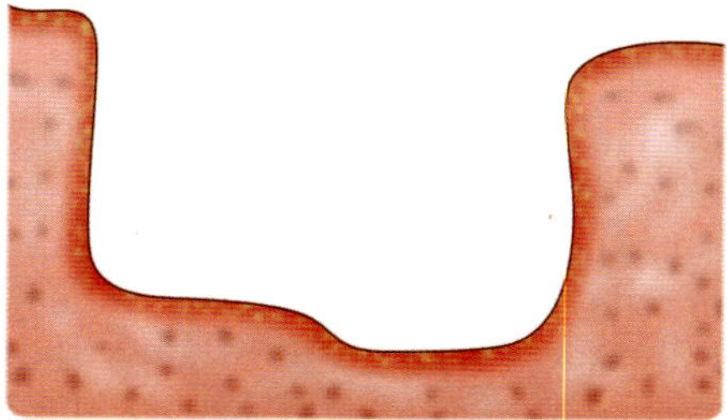

Fig. 4.2: Gummatous ulcer with punched out edge

- Also in the testis, upper part of leg and at the sterno-mastoid.
- Lymph noes are seldom involved unless secondary infection occurs.
- WR is positive.
- Punched out edge (**Figure 4.2**) (may be seen in varicose ulcer and trophic ulcers specially perforating ulcer associated with DM).
- The base is covered with wet wash-leather (Chamois leather) slough, which contains one or more islands of normal tissue which escaped necrosis.
- A healed gumma ends in a circular "tissue-paper" scar (similar to Yaws).

Soft Chancres or Soft Sores (Ducrey's)

- Appear within 3–6 days after inoculation (infection with *Haemophilus ducreyi*) as *painful*, non-indurated ulcers (multiple due to autoinoculation) that occur on genitalia or adjacent parts (buttocks and perianal).
- The ulcers have edematous edges and yellowish slough discharging copious purulent discharge. The complete absence of induration led to the term "soft sore".
- Lymph nodes are similar to acute lymphadenitis (i.e. firm and tender) with tendency to suppuration.

Meleney's Ulcer

- Mostly found in the postoperative wound either for perforated viscus or drainage of empyema thoracis, and rarely on the dorsum of the hand.
- Results from *symbiotic action* of *micro-aerophilic non-hemolytic streptococci + hemolytic Staphylococcus aureus.*
- Undermined ulcer with a lot of granulation tissue in the floor, surrounded by deep purple zone, which in turn is surrounded by a zone of erythema. It is painful, toxemic and the general condition deteriorates without treatment.

Actinomycosis

- It leads to marked induration of the skin and subcutaneous tissue over the lower jaw and neck with the development of multiple sinuses.
- The discharge contains the typical characteristic sulfur-like granules (colonies of the microorganism).

Fungus Infections

- Blastomycosis sporotrichosis is a common example.
- The fungus is always found in the scrapings.

MALIGNANT ULCERS

Squamous Cell Carcinoma (Carcinomatous Ulcer)

- It can hardly be mistaken, especially after eversion and induration of the edge have been observed **(Figure 4.3)**.
- The base is hard and the floor is necrotic.
- Painless ulcer (unless infected) and bleeds on touch.
- Occurs anywhere (lips, cheeks, tongue, anus).
- In the face, it is more common in lower lip and upper eyelid, in contrast to rodent ulcer.
- Draining lymph nodes are enlarged, hard and mobile in early cases, but later become fixed.

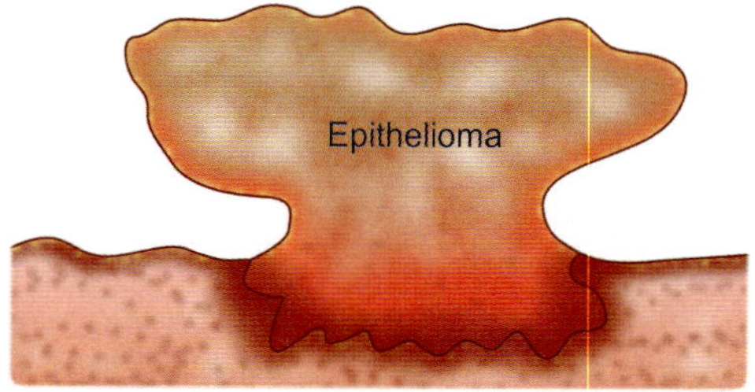

Fig. 4.3: SCC with everted edges

- **Marjolin's ulcer**:
  It is a squamous cell carcinoma start occurs on top of:
  1. A previous chronic scar.
  2. Previous burn.
  3. Any chronic non-specific ulcer such as a venous ulcer.

Basal Cell Carcinoma (Rodent Ulcer)

- Particularly if early, the features of malignancy are not nearly so obvious.
- *History*: It starts as a papule or nodule (sometimes multiple). When the patient scratches it, it bleeds and forms a scab. When the scab fall off, it leaves an ulcer behind.
- *Site*:
  Being situated above a line joining the angle of the mouth with the lobule of the ear should alert the clinician to the diagnosis.
- Its outline is circular, it edge is raised and heaped-up (**Figure 4.4**), and often shows nodules possessing a peculiar pearl-like luster. Minute venules in the edge are characteristic.
- *Lymph nodes* are usually *not* involved. Their enlargement may denote carcinomatous change or secondary infection.

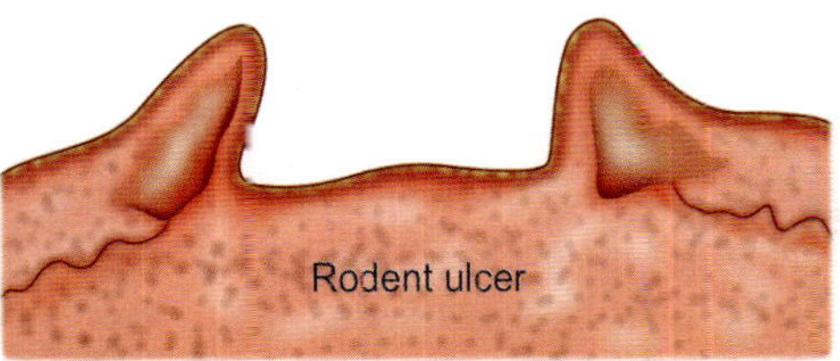

Fig. 4.4: BCC with rolled-in edges

Malignant Melanoma

- The most frequent site in the foot is in the soft skin of the instep. Unfortunately, the lesion in its early stage is asymptomatic and unnoticed until ulceration occurs.
- When suspected, the regional lymph nodes (groin) and the liver must be palpated for secondaries (enlarged and hard).
- Pigmented floor and skin nodules around the ulcer **(Figure 4.5)**.

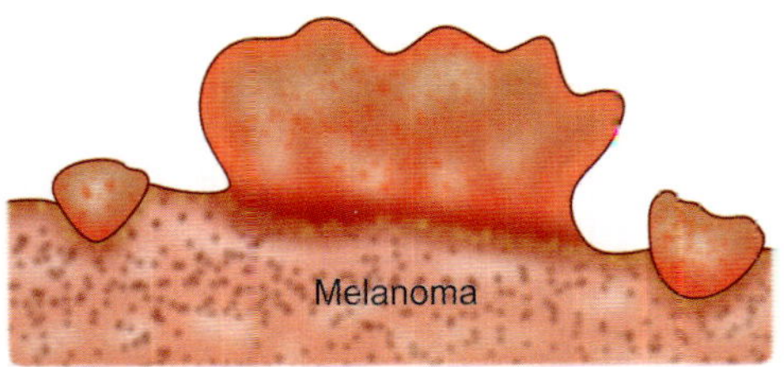

Fig. 4.5: Melanoma with skin nodules around the ulcer

Ulcerating Sarcoma or Carcinoma

- The swelling underneath the ulcer is evident.
- The tumor itself may fungate through the ulcer.
- Such ulcers lack the everted *edge* of the squamous ulcer.
- The *floor* is made of nodules of tumor tissue.
- The draining *lymph nodes* are hard and fixed.

Table 4.1: Differential diagnosis of the different types of ulcers

Criteria	Traumatic	Varicose	Trophic	Tuberculous	Syphilitic (3ry)	Epithelio-matous	Rodent (BCC)
Site	Anywhere, but common on legs	Common on medial aspect of lower leg	Usually over bony prominences in the sole or over the heal	Usually over TB nodes in the neck, axilla or groin. May occur over TB bone	Upper 1/3 of leg and near knee, mouth, tongue and nose. May occur due to softening of gumma (tibia, sternum, ulna, skull)	Common on face, tongue, lips. May occur in LL on top of chronic venous ulcer, scar, burn or sinus of chronic osteomyelitis (Marjolin)	Common on the middle third of the face (lower eyelid and upper lip). May be extra-facial in 5%
Size	Variable	Variable	Usually small	Usually small	Variable	May be large	May be large
Shape	Round or oval	Round or oval	Round or oval	Round or oval	Round or oval. May be circinate or serpiginous.	Usually irregular	Round or oval at the beginning then becomes irregular
Skin Around	Healthy	May be eczematous and pigmented	Heaped-up, white and desquamated	Bluish in color	May be coppery		

Contd...

Contd...

Edge	Punched (active), sloping (healing)	Punched-out or sloping	Punched-out	Undermined	Punched-out	Everted	Inverted or rolled-in. Beaded
Floor	Covered with pus and slough, or red healthy GT (healing ulcer)	Covered by granulation tissue (GT)	Covered with very little granulation	Covered with dirty granulation tissue	Covered by a wash leather slough	May be heaped-up and raised above the surface of skin or deeply excavated	May be deep reaching cartilage or bone (rodent).
Base	Soft	± indurated and callus and fixed to underlying bone	Formed of a sinus which may lead to a joint or bone	Usually formed of a sinus track leading to the underlying TB lesion	May be indurated and fixed to underlying bone	Hard and indurated	Firm
Draining LNs	May be acutely inflamed	May show non-specific inflammation	-	Usually already tuberculous		Enlarged and malignant (stony hard and fixed)	May be enlarged due to secondary infection or epitheliomatous transformation

2. ULCERS OF THE FACE

CLASSIFICATION

Ulcerative Infective Lesions		Ulcerating Tumors
A. Non-specific	B. Specific	
1. Chronic non-specific ulcer 2. Infected sebaceous cyst 3. Molluscum sebaceum	1. Tuberculosis (TB) 2. Syphilis ($) 3. Leishmaniasis 4. Leprosy 5. Actinomycosis 6. Anthrax	1. Rodent ulcer (BCC) 2. Epithelioma (SCC) 3. Malignant Melanoma 4. Metastatic Mass Ulceration 5. Infiltrating deeply seated tumor, which invades the skin and ulcerates

I. ULCERATING INFECTIVE LESIONS

Non-Specific Ulcers

1. Chronic Non-specific Ulcer

a. Exuberant Type (Hypertrophic granulation tissue):
   - Warty-like lesion
   - Soft
   - Granulating tumor
   - Bleeds easily.

b. Flat Type:
   - Painful
   - Irregular margin
   - Floor covered with granulation tissue
   - Firm base
   - Purulent or serous discharge
   - Persistence of the cause maintains its chronicity.

2. Infected Sebaceous Cyst

Long history, irregular edge, floor covered with purulent exudate, painful and firm base, hair follicle or punctum could be seen, infected sebaceous-like material can come out on squeezing.

3. Molluscum Sebaceum

Warty lesion that forms a superficial ulcer with umbilicated center, hard in consistency, long history, does not spread, lymph nodes are not enlarged, may heal spontaneously (usually disappears within 2 months leaving behind a fibrous scar), and should be differentiated from SCC.

Specific Ulcers

1. *Tuberculous Ulcers:*
   - These ulcers are painful.
   - *Site*: TB ulcer is common in the neck due to break down of LNs, in the maxillary region due to TB of underlying bone, and in the skin of the face due to lupus vulgaris.
   - *Outline*: Irregular.
   - *Edge*: Undermined and bluish, with characteristic apple-jelly nodules (in lupus vulgaris) around it.
   - *Floor*: Pale, soft, covered with unhealthy granulation tissue.
   - *Discharge*: Serous or watery.
   - Scarring may be present.
2. *Syphilitic Ulcer*:

(a) Chancre (1ry syphilis)	(b) Gumma (painless) (3ry syphilis)
• Site: It occurs on the lips, nose, or eyelids • Surrounded by marked edema • Associated with enlarged lymph nodes • Swab examination shows spirochetes	• Site: Common in frontal region • Margin: Circular or serpiginous • Edge: Punched out (steep sides) • Floor: Wash-leather • Skin Around: shows pigmentation and scar • Fixed to bone and plain X-ray shows bone sclerosis • Other stigmata of syphilis are present • WR reaction is positive

3. *Leishmaniasis (Oriental Sore)*:
   - A slowly progressive, painless, ulcer that may occur anywhere in the face (exposed to mosquito bites).
   - May be raised above the surface and have a cauliflower-like appearance.
   - The flat form is less common.
   - Microscopic examination shows "Leishmania Donovani Bodies".
4. *Actinomycosis:*
   - Multiple sinuses with sulfur-like granules (colonies of the organism).
   - Diffuse dense fibrosis around the openings.
   - Spreading in nature.
5. *Anthrax*:
   - It affects mainly wool workers and horse workers.
   - Localized painful area of induration.
   - Multiple sinuses, covered with yellow necrotic slough.

II. ULCERATING TUMORS

A. Basal Cell Carcinoma

- It occurs in old and middle age
- The middle third of the face is the commonest site (90%), other sites in the face and scalp (5%), and extra-facial (5%)
- It may be multiple
  1. *Non-ulcerating Phase*:
     - Painless, flat nodule in the skin.
     - Not attached to deep structures.
     - Long duration.
  2. *Ulcerating Phase*:
     - Superficial Type: Beaded raised, or rolled-in edge, firm base, floor shows granulation tissue ± attempts of epithelization, lymph nodes are not enlarged.

- Penetrating Type: In addition to the previously mentioned signs there is infiltration of deeper structures (bone and cartilage).

B. Squamous Cell Carcinoma (Epithelioma)

- Seen in old or middle age
- Painless
- Everted edge
- Hard base
- Necrotic floor that bleeds
- Fixation to surrounding structures
- Lymph nodes may be enlarged and hard
- It may occur on top of a chronic benign ulcer, chronic scar or burn (Marjolin ulcer).

C. Malignant Melanoma

- Ill-defined mass in the skin that ulcerates
- Pigmented floor
- Skin nodules around the ulcer
- Lymph nodes are enlarged and hard
- Metastases in the liver or elsewhere (with melanin pigments).

D. Fungating Malignancy

- Painless
- Hard in consistency
- Its base is elevated above the surrounding tissue level
- Floor is covered with necrotic masses and is made of nodules of tumor tissue
- Discharge is purulent or serosanguinous
- Draining *lymph nodes* are hard and fixed.

3. ULCERS OF THE LIPS

CRACKED OR FISSURED LIPS

- Occurs as a fissure in the mid line, in cold weather as the skin becomes hardened.
- It is very painful, tender and bleeds easily.
- The lesion heals quickly with medical R/, but if becomes chronic, it may require excision.
- *Cracked corner of the mouth* occurs most commonly due to vitamin deficiency.

MALIGNANT ULCER

- Most patients are over 60 years of age, men being affected > women (8:1).
- It may start as a small crack or fissure, as a small nodule, or as a warty papillomatous growth. It then becomes a typical malignant epitheliomatous ulcer or a papillary wart-like mass.
- *Site*: Lower lip > upper lip, more to one side of the midline ± upper lip by implantation (kissing ulcer).
- *Skin* over the lump may show evidence of premalignant change (blistering, thickening, leukoplakia).
- *Size*: The initial lesion is usually small, but the ulcer may become large if neglected.
- *Shape*: It starts as a small lump, which ulcerates in its center.
- *Tenderness*: It is *not* tender, but *bleeds* easily on touch.
- *Edge*: Everted (typical of SCC).
- *Floor*: Necrotic, covered with a thin, soft, friable, gray-yellow slough.
- *Discharge*: Thin, watery and slightly blood-stained. It is usually infected.
- *Base*: Hard and indurated.

- *Depth*: The ulcer is initially shallow but can infiltrate deep into the lip.
- *Relations*: It is invariably fixed to the underlying SC structures, and only very late to the gum and jaw.
- *Lymph nodes*: They may be enlarged by inflammation (tender) or malignancy (hard) which occurs later than in case of cancer tongue.

SYPHILITIC ULCER

It is very rare nowadays, but may present as:

- *Primary chancre:* Common on upper lip (opposite to cancer). It has a smooth ulcerated surface with inflammation of the lip substance. It may resemble carcinoma but differentiated by (1) being more common on upper lip, (2) more rapid course, (3) early LN involvement, (4) more smooth and less warty, (5) younger age, (6) good response to medical R/, and (7) biopsy.
- *Secondary syphilis:* Mucus patches on the lips similar to those of the tongue and buccal mucosa.
- *Third stage of syphilis:* Gummatous ulcer with serpiginous margins, punched out edges and wash leather floor.
- *Congenital $ (Rhagades):* Cracks and mucus patches may leave scars radiating from angles of the mouth.

DYSPEPTIC (APHTHOUS) ULCERS

- *Painful* erosions on the inner surface of the lips and cheek and may be also on the tongue.
- Short history.
- Ulcers are small may be *multiple,* with whitish *floor,* hyperemic *margins,* sloping *edge* and soft *base.*
- *Lymph nodes* are not enlarged.

TRAUMATIC (DENTAL) ULCERS

- They mostly occur at the side of the tongue and the lip due to trauma by a broken tooth or ill-fitting dentures.
- The ulcer is *painful,* with sloping serrated *edges,* elongated shallow *floor* with granulation tissue and soft or mildly indurated *floor.*
- It heals within a few days when the cause is removed; otherwise it should be *biopsied* to exclude cancer.

N.B.

Leukoplakia is not an ulcer, but whitish patches of thickened mucosa that may precede (precancerous) or accompany cancer (SCC).

4. ULCERS OF THE TONGUE

CAUSES OF TONGUE ULCERS

Traumatic	Inflammatory	Dyspeptic	Malignant
1. Dental ulcers 2. Frenulum ulcers	1. Herpetic ulcers 2. Tuberculous ulcers 3. Syphilitic ulcers 4. Chronic superficial (non-specific) glossitis 5. Ulcerative stomatitis	Aphthous ulcers (Metabolic or Dyspeptic)	1. Epithelioma 2. Lymphoepithelioma 3. Adenocarcinoma 4. Basal cell carcinoma 5. Malignant melanoma

A. TRAUMATIC ULCERS

Dental Ulcers

- *Site*: Mostly at the side of the anterior 2/3 of the tongue opposite a broken tooth or ill-fitting dentures.
- It is *painful*, with sloping serrated *edges*, elongated shallow *floor* covered with granulation tissue, and soft or mildly indurated *base*. Lymph nodes may be enlarged (firm and tender).
- It heals in few days when the cause is removed; otherwise, it should be *biopsied*, particularly if there are features suggestive of malignancy (SCC).

Frenulum (Pertussis) Ulcer

- *Cause*: It is due to trauma of the frenum of the tongue by the teeth during coughing.
- *Site*: In the frenum or on the under surface of the tongue on either side of the frenum of children (6–8 months old due to eruption of lower teeth) with whooping cough.

B. INFLAMMATORY ULCERS

Herpetic Ulcers

- *True herpes linguis:* It is due to Herpes Simplex in patients with low resistance as after pneumonia. It either occurs alone in the tongue and angles of the mouth, or as a part of herpes of branches of the trigeminal nerve. It presents with severe unilateral pain followed within a few hours by vesicles which burst to become small, multiple and painful ulcers.
- *Herpetic ulcers in children* are *not* herpes but superficial blisters on upper and under-surfaces of the tongue.

Tuberculous Ulcers

- *Cause*: Active TB of the chest, or infected milk (causing ulcers, or diffuse fibrosis - woody tongue).
- *Site*: Mostly at the tip (**Figure 4.6**) and sides of the tongue.
- May be multiple.
- Painful.
- Shallow ulcers with undermined edges.
- Yellowish floor.

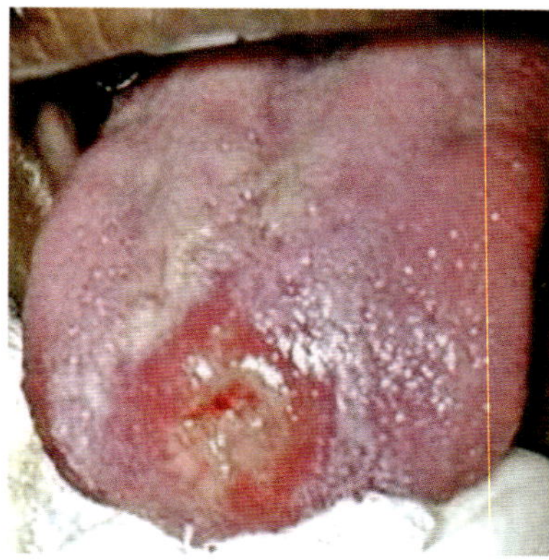

Fig. 4.6: TB ulcer at the tip of the tongue

- Soft base.
- Presence of pulmonary TB should point to the true diagnosis.

Syphilitic Ulcers

- *Primary chancre*: More common in men. Occurs at the tip of the tongue, submental and submandibular lymph nodes are enlarged, serologic tests are +ve and spirochetes are detected in discharge from the sore.
- *Secondary syphilis:* Mucus patches + snail track ulcers at the sides of the tongue (multiple, small, round, *painful*, with sharply cut edges and grayish white floor) + Hutchinson's warts or condylomata.
- *Tertiary (third stage) syphilis*: *Gummatous ulcer*—at the midline of the dorsum of the tongue. It is painless, single, with clear-cut *edges* and wash-leather *floor*. Leukoplakia or diffuse fibrosis may also be present.

Chronic Superficial Glossitis

- It may be associated with chronic repeated non-specific ulcers, usually on the dorsum. Ulcers are superficial, small and painful. They are associated with fissures or vesicles and have a unilateral distribution.
- Chronic superficial glossitis has the following clinical stages: Hyperkeratosis with hypertrophy of papillae, white patches (*leukoplakia*), red patches due to loss of papillae (painful), cracks or fissures in the red patches, small projections (carcinoma in situ), and finally, epithelioma (squamous cell carcinoma).

Ulcers in Connection with Stomatitis (Ulcerative Stomatitis)

- Septic infection of the mouth due to alkalis, acids or mercury may be associated by the formation of small vesicles, which on bursting give rise to superficial ulcers on the tongue, inner surface of cheek and gums.

- Tongue ulcers may occur in *small pox, chicken pox, pemphigus*. Diagnosis depends on skin eruptions not the ulcers.

C. DYSPEPTIC (APHTHOUS) ULCERS

Characteristic Features

- It is the commonest type.
- Short history.
- Painful erosions at the tip and sides of the tongue due to dyspepsia.
- Ulcers are small, multiple, with whitish floor, hyperemic margins, sloping edge and soft base **(Figure 4.7)**.
- The lymph nodes are not enlarged.
- It is usually self-limited.

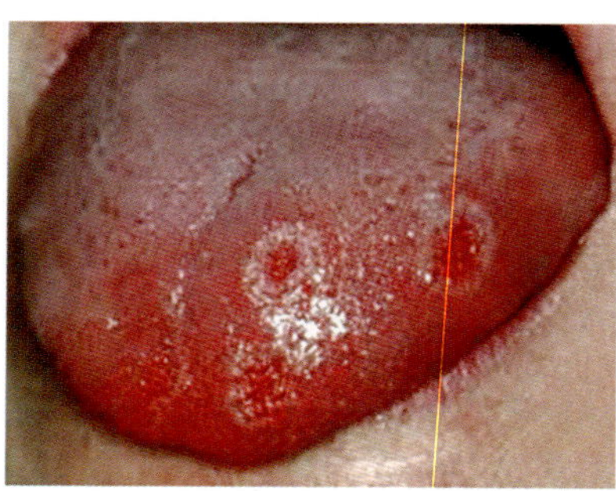

Fig. 4.7: Multiple dyspeptic ulcers

D. MALIGNANT ULCERS

Types

1. *Epithelioma*: The most common.
2. *Lymphoepithelioma* (in the posterior 1/3 of the tongue).
3. *Salivary adenocarcinoma* (from minor salivary glands).
4. *Basal cell carcinoma.*
5. *Melanoma.*

Epitheliomatous Ulcer

- The epitheliomatous ulcer occurs more in men and is rare below the age of 45 years. It has a raised nodular everted edge (**Figure 4.8**), necrotic floor that bleeds easily, and a hard indurated base. The commonest site is the anterior 2/3 of the tongue. The patient has a foul smell of breath and may be limited or deviated protrusion of the tongue
- Regional lymph nodes are usually enlarged (hard, mobile or fixed), with or without infiltration of deeper tissues.

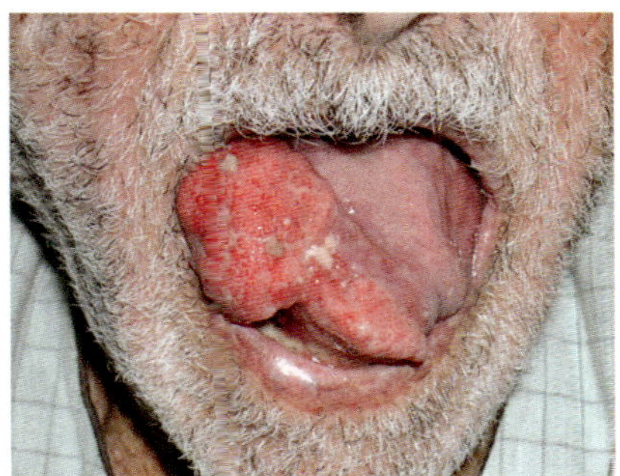

Fig. 4.8: Epitheliomatous ulcer at the side of the tongue

Key Points — Cancer Tongue

Any tongue ulcer occurring in a middle-aged man, and lasting for > 2–3 weeks, should always awaken suspicion of malignancy.

Causes of early spread of carcinoma of the tongue?

1. Rich blood supply.
2. Rich communicating lymphatics.
3. Continuous movement of the tongue.

Causes of death?

1. Severe cachexia.
2. Chest infection:
   - Pneumonia.
   - Bronchiectasis.
   - Lung abscess.

3. Severe hemorrhage from erosion of a blood vessel.
4. Suffocation (lesions in the posterior 1/3 of the tongue).

Causes of secondaries on the other side of the neck?

1. Lesions at the tip of the tongue (draining on both sides).
2. Lesions near the midline.
3. Diffuse type of tongue cancer.
4. If lymph nodes on the same side were removed before, or blocked by cancer, leading to retrograde spread.

5. SCROTAL AND PENILE ULCERS

SCROTAL ULCERS

Tumors of the Scrotum

1. *Epithelioma of the scrotum:* Most commonly seen among chimney sweeps, paraffin, tar and chemical workers. It starts as a small SC nodule that enlarges and forms an irregular ulcer that bleeds easily on touch. It extends both radially and vertically into the tissues of the scrotum to involve the testis later. Inguinal lymph nodes are enlarged, first due to inflammation and later due to malignant infiltration.
2. *Papilloma of the scrotum:* It may be the starting point of malignant change. A small amount of foul discharge is present often forming a scab, which on removal leaves an ulcer with indurated, everted edges with the gradual progress of a cutaneous epithelioma.

Fistulae

- Fistulae may occur in the scrotum and cause ulceration.
- They occur in association with TB or syphilis of the testes, or may follow urine extravasation, peri-urethral abscess, or burrowing from rectal suppuration.

Syphilis of the Scrotum

1. *Primary chancre:* There is often only slight induration of the ulcer compared with that of a penile chancre, but the edge is raised and rolled. Inguinal lymph nodes are enlarged and discrete. After 5-6 weeks, secondary symptoms of syphilis appear.
2. *Mucus tubercles.* May be present on the scrotum, usually on the femoral aspect. They may extend directly from the anal area. Other signs of syphilis are obvious making diagnosis easy.

Testicular Diseases

In some cases, extension of disease in the testicle may involve the coverings of the scrotum, and may even perforate them to form a scrotal ulcer. This occasionally occurs with:

1. *Testicular abscess:* Uncommon but may occur from direct extension from the urethra (via seminal vesicles and vas deferens) or from hematogenous spread in cases of scarlet fever, mumps and typhoid fever.
2. *TB of the testis:* May be primary or more commonly secondary to genitourinary TB elsewhere. The ulcer is most likely on the *posterior* aspect of the scrotum. Evidence of TB in the testis, prostate or seminal vesicles.
3. *Gumma of the testis:* Usually present on the *front* of the scrotum. The whole testis is enlarged and painless. The cord is not thickened. There is history of $ and other tertiary lesions, e.g. gummatous periostitis.
4. *Malignant disease of the testis*: Seminoma or teratoma rarely causes ulceration because they are usually removed beforehand. They may cause ulceration through a scar of a biopsy.

Suppurating Cysts of the Scrotum

- Exceptionally, a *sebaceous cyst* in the scrotal skin may suppurate and leave an ulcer with raised edges simulating epithelioma.
- History and biopsy settle the diagnosis.
- They are less common than epithelioma.

Infected Hematocele

- It may form an abscess, which bursts through the scrotal coverings.
- It may resemble a gumma.

Irritants and Corrosives (Mustard Gas)

- It caused the most troublesome ulcerations in the scrotum (and elsewhere) during the First World War.

Behcet's Syndrome, Herpes Simplex, Candidiasis

- *Behcet's syndrome* causes painful ulcerations of the scrotum and penis, unlike those of the vagina and vulva, which are often painless and missed. It may be accompanied by abscesses or herpes-like lesions of the scrotum.
- *Herpes simplex*, both types I and II, may cause vesicular lesions less commonly, and very rarely *candidiasis*.

PENILE ULCERS (SORES)

Balanitis

- If inflammatory processes are allowed to continue under the prepuce, ulceration of the mucous membrane covering the glans or lining the prepuce will occur, accompanied by a stinking, purulent discharge.
- Multiple shallow ulcers are formed and rapidly coalesce causing discomfort and edema of the prepuce.

Herpes Genitalis

- It may occur as part of Herpes Zoster (less common than Herpes simplex), which is unilateral.
- It starts as a patch of erythema on the inner surface of the prepuce or glans, followed by vesicles and pustules that ulcerate when rubbed by clothes.
- It should be differentiated from a soft sore or syphilitic chancre.

Soft Sores (Chancroids) of the Penis

- It occurs from infection during sexual intercourse. Incubation period is short. Vesicles appear in 2 days.

- Soft chancres are usually deeper (than herpes), with marked edges; their bases are sloughing, and they are usually accompanied by a bubo, which is exceptional with herpes.

Syphilitic Chancre

- It is the initial lesion of syphilis that generally appears about 25 days after infection as a reddened patch, which becomes raised above the surface of the mucous membrane, with distinctly indurated margins. The central part breaks into an ulcer.
- The ulcer is usually single, indurated, raised, and is accompanied by the typical multiple, discrete inguinal lymph nodes. Dark ground illumination shows the *Treponema pallidum* in the discharge expressed from the sore.

Granuloma Inguinale (Granuloma Venereum)

- It is a chronic granulomatous ulceration that affects the perineum, inguinal region and penis in the Tropics.
- The penile lesions starts as a papule that breaks forming a superficial ulcer. Examination of the discharge shows capsulated bacteria (*Donovan bodies*), which are believed to be the cause. *Lymph nodes are not involved.*

Lymphogranuloma Venereum (Lymphogranuloma Inguinale)

- The penile lesion appears after an incubation period of about one week as a papule, vesicle or ulcer and tends to disappear by time, but *inguinal lymph nodes are markedly enlarged* and tend to breakdown and form sinuses.
- It is due to a filterable organism (*Chlamydia group*) and can be diagnosed by CFT, demonstration of specific skin

reactivity and biopsy. Rectal stricture and effusions into joints are other lesions caused by this disease.

Gummatous Ulceration of the Penis

- It occurs occasionally from disintegration of a small gumma of the glans or prepuce, frequently on top of an old scar. It may be mistaken for a chancre but absence of induration and history of onset settle the diagnosis.

Tuberculous or Lupoid Ulceration of the Penis

- Very rare and is generally associated with advanced TB elsewhere.
- TB ulcers are usually multiple and painful.

Epithelioma

- It is the commonest malignant tumor of the penis. An epitheliomatous ulcer in size gradually in spite of treatment.
- It has a hard indurated base, everted edges and necrotic floor + enlarged inguinal lymph nodes. Biopsy proves diagnosis.

Papillomata (Venereal Warts or Condylomata Acuminata)

- They occur on the glans mainly the corona and contiguous surface of the prepuce.
- They are simple papillomata, usually multiple, and the base is not indurated unlike epithelioma.

Injury (Bite !)

- It is an uncommon cause of penile sore. History helps reaching the proper diagnosis.
- A case of epithelioma of the penis following a bite from a pig has been reported (*Sir Eric Riches*).

6. ULCERS OF THE LEG

The lower leg is the seat of an ulcer many times more often than the whole of the rest *of the surface of the body.* ***Venous ulcers*** *are the commonest ulcers of the lower limb.* ***Ischemic ulcer*** *is a remote second. However, there are other causes of leg ulcers, which should be born in mind.*

CAUSES OF CHRONIC LEG ULCER

I	**Vascular:** A. Arterial B. Venous C. Capillary	 • Atherosclerosis, Thromboangiitis obliterans, A-V fistula, Collagen vascular disease (PAN), Raynaud's disease. • Post-phlebitic (CVI), VVs (primary), post-injection reaction • Chronic lymphedema
II	Traumatic	• Thermal burns • Irradiation • Insect bites • Decubitus (bed sores) • Sports
III	Infective	• Bone: Acute osteomyelitis, adherent fracture site • Pyogenic ulcer (staphylococcal abscess → skin necrosis) • Synergistic gangrene (Meleney's ulcer) • TB and syphilitic ulcer (Gumma on outer side of the leg) • Tropical disease (Leishmaniasis)
IV	Neoplastic	• Primary skin tumor: SSC, BCC, malignant melanoma, Kaposi sarcoma • Leukemia • Secondary: metastatic • Marjolin ulcer: malignant transformation of venous ulcer

Contd...

Contd...

V	Neuropathic (Neurotrophic)	• Spinal Cord lesions (Syringomyelia) • Peripheral Neuropathy: Tabes dorsalis, diabetes mellitus (DM), peripheral neuritis, alcoholism
VI	Cryopathic	Chilblains - Cold injuries
VII	Self-Inflicte:	In psychologically disturbed patients
VIII	Systemic/ Metabolic	• Ulcerative colitis • Felty's syndrome (congenital hemolytic anemia) • Collagen disease • Diabetes mellitus • Avitaminosis.

DIAGNOSTIC APPROACH

A useful approach is to find out if the ulcer is *painless or painful, acute or chronic* and whether the patient is *diabetic or not,* as follows:

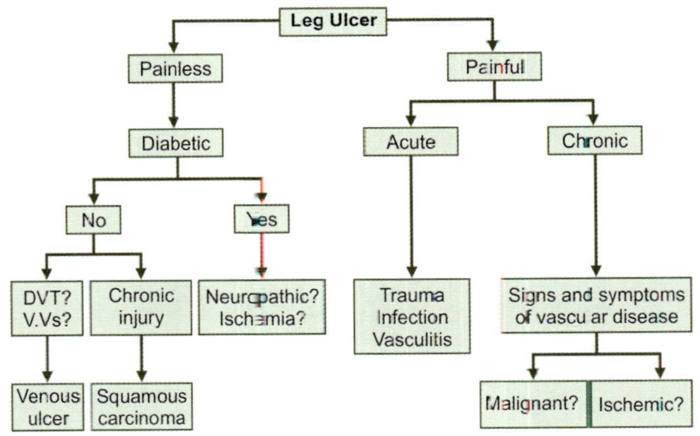

VENOUS ULCER

As a rule, venous stasis ulcer = 90% of lower limb ulceration. Venous ulcers either coexist with incompetent superficial (varicose) veins, and are accurately termed "*varicose ulcers*", or more commonly, develop secondary to DVT (*post-thrombotic or post-phlebitic ulcers*).

A. Varicose Ulcers

- Associated with primary varicose veins.
- *Site*: In front of the medial malleolus (they tend to ride long saphenous vein "LSV"; however, a considerable portion lie behind and above the medial malleolus). Less commonly, it occurs on the lateral aspect of the leg (small saphenous vein "SSV").
- *Floor and edge*: The ulcer is shallow, never penetrates the deep fascia and has irregularly shaped shelving edges, which are often characterized by a thin, blue line of growing epithelium (**Figure 4.9**).
- *Base:* The ulcer base can be formed of pink granulations, pale granulations, and slough.

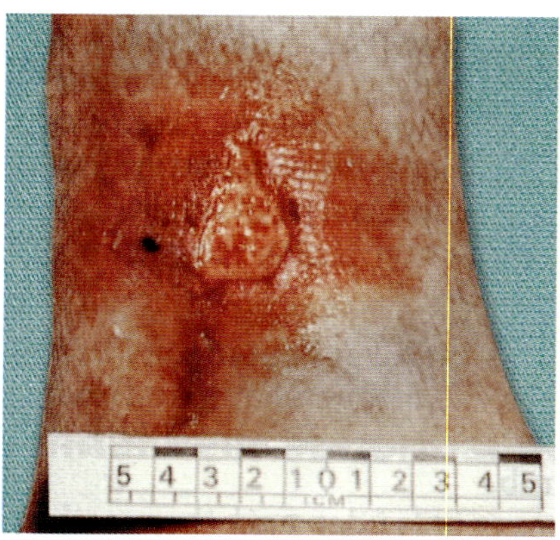

Fig. 4.9: Acute venous ulcer. Note the surrounding lipodermatosclerosis. The ulcer is shallow and never deep

- *Size:* The size is variable and in long-standing cases the ulcer may encircle the limb.
- *Painless* but considerable infection and involvement of the saphenous nerve in scar tissue cause pain.
- Varicose ulcers commonly follow trauma and are associated with edema and dermatitis, and in long-standing, with eczema and hyperpigmentation. Often one or more large feeding veins can be seen proceeding towards the edge of the ulcer.
- *These are now known to be rare as most venous ulcers are post-phlebitic.*

B. Post-phlebitic Ulcers (Post-thrombotic Ulcers = Blow Out Syndrome)

- *History*: Often there is history of DVT after child birth, abdominal operation, or a leg accident.
- *Site*: Similar to varicose ulcers (ulcer-bearing area = gaiter area = area of highest pressure).
- *Ulcer description*: They do not differ in description from varicose ulcers (they are shallow ulcers **(Figure 4.10)**, with

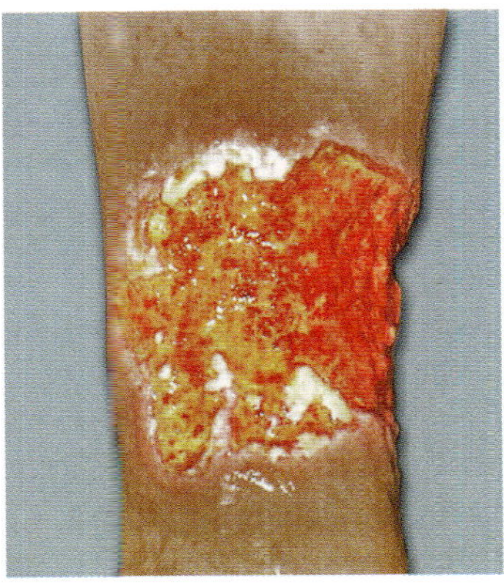

Fig. 4.10: Post-phlebitic ulcer with hyperpigmentation and dermatitis

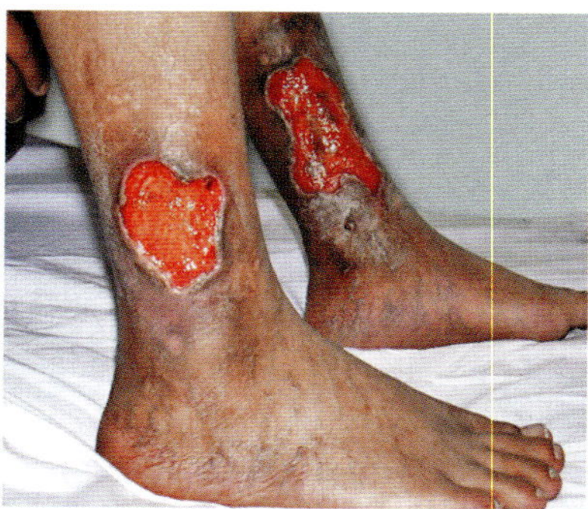

Fig. 4.11: Bilateral post-phlebitic ulcers

circular or serpiginous outline, shelving edges and bluish erythematous margins) **(Figure 4.11)**.

- In contrast to varicose ulcer
  1. Pain is fairly a constant feature.
  2. Varicose veins are lacking in spite of a very careful search for them.
  3. Skin is firm and seems to be tethered to underlying structures.
- Extensive induration, which often extends half way up the calf, producing a characteristic shape of the leg (Inverted Beer-Bottle) may be present.

C. Carcinoma Secondary to Venous Ulcer (Marjolin Ulcer)

- In a few neglected cases of venous ulcer, carcinoma develops, in which even too often the diagnosis is written on the face of the ulcer.
- It is a classical squamous cell carcinoma with everted edges, hard base and necrotic floor (**Figure 4.12**).
- It should be routine to examine the groin for neglected *lymph nodes.*
- It is essential to biopsy any ulcer with a suspicious *everted edge* in any part of its circumference.

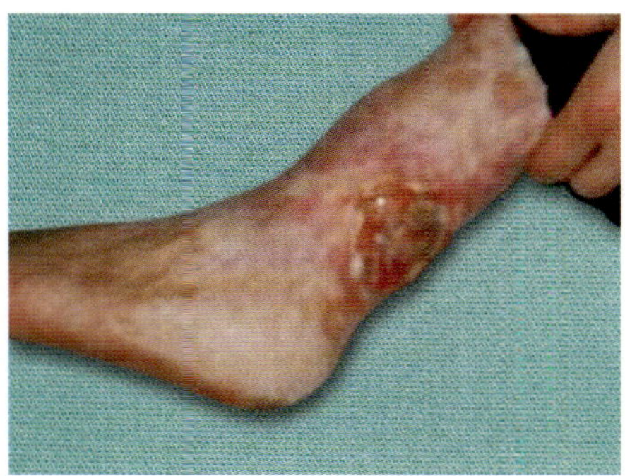

Fig. 4.12: Marjolin ulcer

ARTERIAL ULCER

Characteristic Features

- *Incidence:* It is *rare* when compared with venous ulcer.
- *Age and sex:* Men and women, usually over 60 years of age, are affected equally.
- *Pain:* It is extremely painful (unless there is associated diabetic neuropathy).
- *Tenderness:* The ulcer and surrounding tissues are very tender.
- *Temperature:* The surrounding tissues are usually cold because they, too, are ischemic.
- *Site:* Most commonly in areas exposed to *trauma* (e.g. lateral malleolus) and at *bony prominences* (e.g. heel and heads of metatarsals) (**Figure 4.13**).
- *Size:* Any size from small deep lesions 1-2 mm to large flat ulcers on the lower leg 10 cm in diameter.
- *Edge:* Punched out (square-cut) because there is no attempt at healing by surrounding tissues.
- *Base*: It may contain gray-yellow sloughing tissue and is often infected. The tissue forming the base has a good blood supply but it is not sufficient to support the growth of red healthy granulation.

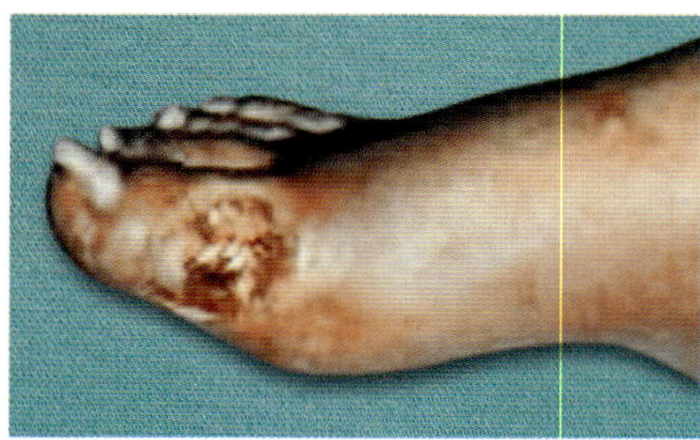

Fig. 4.13: Ischemic ulcer at the head of the first metatarsal. The ulcer is deep to the deep fascia and may penetrate to the bone

- *Depth*: The ulcer is deep. Not only does it penetrate the deep fascia but also, not uncommonly tendons are exposed in its base. In advanced cases the bone itself is exposed (penetrating or perforating ulcer).
- *Discharge*: It is either clear fluid (serum) or pus. It is rarely blood stained.
- *Local Tissues*:
  1. Absent pulsations of pedal arteries.
  2. Foot is cold.
  3. Often there is a history of intermittent claudication and sometimes discoloration of one or more toes, in which event the onset of gangrene is imminent
  4. Varicose veins are likely to be absent, but their presence does not exclude the diagnosis.
  5. It is essential to examine the nerves of the limb.

Differences Between Venous and Arterial Ulcers

Point of Difference	Venous Ulcer	Arterial Ulcer
• Etiology	Venous (varicose veins, post-phlebitic)	Arterial (ischemia)
• Site	Gaiter area	Pressure points
• Depth	Superficial	Deep
• Edge	Sloping	Punched out (square-cut)

Contd...

Contd...

• Healing	Heals readily (conservative R/)	Difficult to heal
• Pain	On sitting, standing	On walking, rest pain (advanced)
• Bleeding	Bleeds much	Does not bleed much
• Associated features	Varicose veins, eczema, pigmentation.	Ischemic manifestations.

TRAUMATIC ULCER (FOOTBALLER'S ULCER)

- It occurs over the *shin* in otherwise healthy males due to knocks from any cause (football).
- May be multiple and may attain any size. If it gets infected it becomes adherent to the bone.
- In the ***active ulcer***, *edges* are punched out and the *floor* is covered with pus and necrotic tissue, but in the ***healing ulcer***, edges are sloping and the floor is covered by red granulation tissue— The *base* of the ulcer is usually soft.

TUBERCULOUS ULCER

Primary TB of the skin occurs at the upper part of the *calf* leading to ulceration while secondary *TB* of the skin occurs over deeply seated TB of the bone, joints or lymph nodes causing ulceration that has the following features:

- Multiple in number and small in size.
- *The skin* around the ulcer is *bluish* in color.
- *Edges* are undermined.
- Floor is covered by unhealthy granulation tissue ± painless enlarged inguinal lymph nodes, but the ulcer itself is painful.
- *Diagnosis* can be verified by biopsy (including the ulcer edge).

GUMMATOUS ULCER (SYPHILIS—THIRD STAGE)

- It starts as dusky red, painless nodules, that coalesce and breakdown leading to ulcer formation (*painless*).
- *Site:* It may occur anywhere but usually in the middle two-fourths or upper 2/3 of the leg .
- *Edge*: It is unquestionably *punched out* (very characteristic).
- *Margin:* Serpiginous.
- *Floor* is covered with the characteristic wet *wash-leather* (chamois leather) slough, which may contain one or more "islands" of normal tissue that have escaped the necrosis.
- *Base:* Indurated (but less than that of malignancy).
- A healed gummatous ulcer gives a circular "*tissue-paper*" scar, which is strong evidence of a previous syphilitic infection.
- The scar of Yaws is similar and has to be differentiated.
- The characteristic punched-out appearance of gummatous ulcer is seen sometimes in:
  1. Gravitational or a varicose ulcer.
  2. Trophic ulcers, particularly perforating ulcer of the foot associated with tabes dorsalis and other diseases of the CNS or diabetic neuropathy.

MELENEY'S ULCER (MELENEY'S GANGRENE; PYODERMA GANGRENOSUM)

- This was originally described in relation to infected abdominal and thoracic operated wounds, which are still its commonest situations. However, the infection may occur on the leg (or in the hand) arising either *de novo* (particularly in ulcerative colitis) or, more usually, as a complication of a previously existing ulcer, which is usually varicose.
- It starts by erythema and induration, leading to multiple areas of gangrene and ulceration.

- The onset is very rapid and the most important clinical characteristic is *burrowing*, which may extend 2 cm beneath the apparently healthy skin; the *margins* therefore are extensively *undermined*.
- The ulcer is *painful and tender.*
- It shows a tendency to spread wider in an alarming fashion.

PARASITIC ULCER (ORIENTAL SORE—LEISHMANIASIS)

- It is due infection with a protozoal parasite (*Leishmania tropica*).
- It starts by a papule which soon ulcerates leading to the formation of a shallow ulcer, that has a long and slowly progressive course, and if left untreated leaves an ugly pigmented scar.
- Once suspected, *biopsy* (from the ulcer margin) shows the characteristic *Leishmania donovani* bodies.

LEG ULCERS IN THE TROPICS

Yaws

- The primary sore sometimes is found on the leg or foot (but more often on the buttocks of young children before they walk) as an infected abrasion on which the causative organism *Treponema pertenue* can be found.
- It heals in a few weeks. In the tertiary stage, multiple deep ulcers, which also contain the *spirochete*, are present. They are painless and in the course of healing form "tissue-paper-like" scars.

Diphtheric Desert Sore

- Diphtheric infection (*Corynebacterium diphtheriae*) starts as a papulopustule and within a few days, the top of the papule becomes necrotic and an ulcer forms.

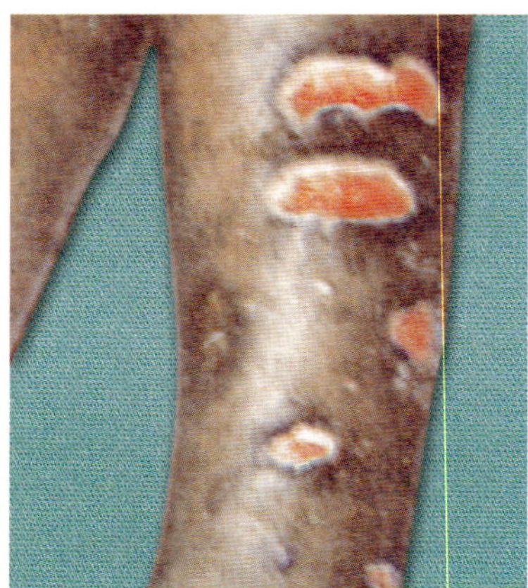

Fig. 4.14: Multiple diphtheric ulcers

- It slowly enlarges, until it attains a diameter of 1–2 cm.
- Ulcers may be multiple (**Figure 4.14**).
- Uncommonly the ulcer floor is covered by typical diphtheric membrane, which is removed with difficulty.
- The ulcer runs a chronic course.
- The patient may show signs of peripheral neuritis due to toxin produced.

Tropical Ulcer (Chronic Phagedenic Ulcer)

- It is due to infection by Vincent's organisms.
- It starts as a papulopustule, which in a few hours becomes surrounded by a zone of inflammation with induration and enlarged, painful, tender lymph nodes. In 2–3 days, the pustule burst and an ulcer forms and extends. The interior of the ulcer is brown, its edges are undermined, and zone of skin in the immediate vicinity is infiltrated and raised. There is a copious serosanguinous discharge with a vile odor and considerable pain, but with comparatively slight constitutional symptoms.

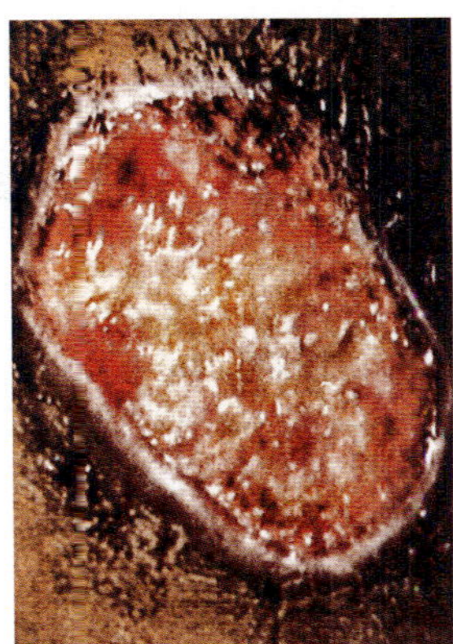

Fig. 4.15: Tropical ulcer on the lower aspect of the left leg

- The ulcer may remain stationary in size for months or even for 1 or 2 years; but in others, it may assume "phagedenic characteristics" (Phagedena in Greek means "to eat"); it then can become so large with great destruction of the soft parts of the leg **(Figure 4.15)** and foot as to call for amputation.

NEUROPATHIC ULCERS (TROPHIC - PERFORATING ULCERS)

- *Etiology*: These ulcers occur due to loss of sensation resulting from peripheral neuropathy (as in diabetes mellitus), spina bifida, tabes dorsalis, and leprosy.
- *Site*: They usually occur over bony prominences as they are exposed to more pressure, e.g. over the heads of the first or fifth metatarsal, or over the heel.
- The *edges* are sloping but the center of the ulcer is deeply perforating, and may reach the bone (**Figure 4.16**).
- The surrounding skin is usually heaped, and cornified with impairment (or even total loss) of sensation.
- It penetrates deep, usually causing suppuration, which may extend to bones and joints.

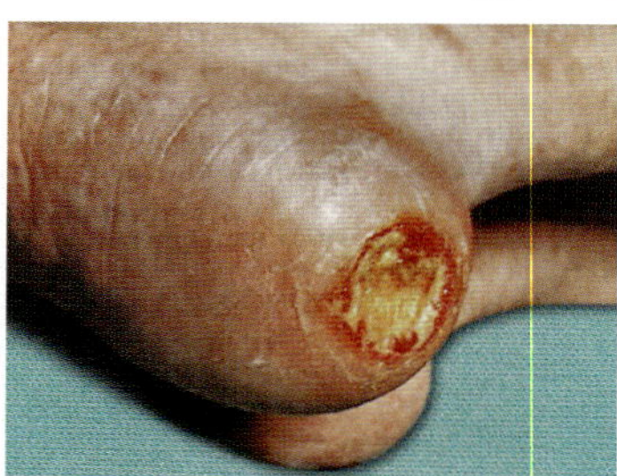

Fig. 4.16: A trophic ulcer at the heel of a bedridden patient. Ulcers at the heel are difficult to heal

- **N.B.** ***In diabetes mellitus:***
  The ulcer, which usually proceeds to *gangrene* could result from:
  1. Ischemia (microangiopathy).
  2. Neuropathy (peripheral neuritis).
  3. Sepsis.

MALIGNANT ULCERS

Squamous Cell Carcinoma (SSC)

- It arises most commonly in the face, tongue, lips, but may occur in the lower limbs.
- It arises *de novo* or *on top* of a scar, burn, varicose ulcer, or sinus of chronic osteomyelititis.
- Its shape is irregular and may attain large sizes. The base is indurated and may be fixed to underlying structures. The edge is characteristically everted and the floor may be heaped up and passed above the surface of the skin, or it may be deeply excavated, or necrotic (**Figure 4.17**).
- Lymph nodes are enlarged and show malignant features (hard and painless).

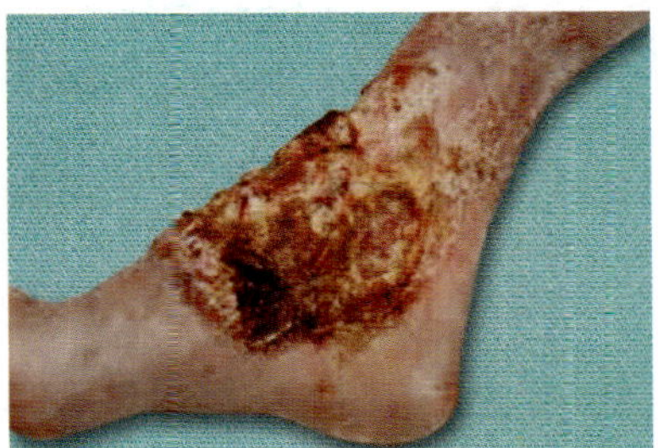

Fig. 4.17: A malignant ulcer (SCC) of the leg. Note the everted edges and necrotic floor

Basal Cell Carcinoma (BCC)

- Uncommon on the legs.
- Rolled-in edges.
- Pearly white.
- Locally malignant.
- Lymph nodes are *not* enlarged.

Malignant Melanoma

- It is an ulcerated malignant melanoma, occurring on an already present nevus.
- The commonest site is the sole of the foot and the big toe.
- There is pigmentation of the ulcer.
- There may be satellite nodules around the ulcer with secondary lymphatic spread.

Fungating Tumors

- These ulcers occur in case of fungation of malignant tumors such as soft tissue sarcoma and melanoma.
- The base is elevated above the surrounding tissue level.
- The floor is covered with necrotic tissue and is made of nodules of tumor tissue.

- *Discharge* is purulent or serosanguinous.
- It is an ulcerated malignant melanoma, occurring on an already present nevus.
- Draining lymph nodes are usually enlarged, particularly in the presence of infection, which renders them tender.
- Biopsy of the original tumor settles the diagnosis.

LEG ULCER COMPLICATING BLOOD DISEASES

- Ulcer of the leg is common is *sickle cell anemia*.
- It also occurs, too frequently to be coincidental, in *acholuric jaundice, Mediterranean anemia* and *Felty's syndrome.*
- Therefore, examine the spleen for enlargement when the cause of the ulcer is not perfectly clear.

LEG ULCER IN RHEUMATOID ARTHRITIS

- This is peculiar to patients with severe crippling arthritis and occurs among those 20% in whom SC nodules are plentiful (***Allison***). This seems to suggest that it is due to breakdown of a nodule.
- The ulcer(s) varies in size, is punched-out, shallow (its floor being formed of subcutaneous tissue) and clean.
- As a rule: "It is without surrounding edema or palpable induration, but is encircled by a dark-red flush, is situated on the lower third of the leg and is painful and slow to heal".

LEG ULCER ASSOCIATED WITH OSTEITIS DEFORMANS

- As both Paget's disease of bone and venous ulcer are common conditions, often the ulcer is a coincidental venous ulcer. On the other hand, a small, deep ulcer situated right over the *convexity of the anteriorly bowed tibia* strongly suggests that the ulcer is an example of this clinical entity.

- The *base* of the ulcer is bone, to which the edges are adherent densely. Consequently it is extremely resistant to treatment.

ARTEFACT ULCER (FACTITIOUS ULCER; AUTOMUTILATION ULCER)

- A self-induced ulcer of the leg, which is not exceedingly rare, is encountered in a highly neurotic individual or in a litigant desirous of obtaining compensation. The mode of production varies.
- The ulcer is always in an accessible site, often on the anterior or the lateral surface of the leg.
- Possible diagnosis is suggested by the unusual shape or an unusual, or even an artificial, appearance; commonly the ulcerated surface looks so pink, clean and healthy that the clinician is amazed that under treatment it remains stationary, or even in size. Signs that suggest neurosis can be very valuable for diagnosis.

Key Points — Leg Ulcers

Clinical Key Points Differentiating "Pain" in: Arterial, Venous and Non-vascular leg ulcers

Criteria	Arterial Ulcer	Venous Ulcer	Non-vascular (joints, spinal, neuromuscular)
Pain during activity	Walking (rest pain in advanced stages)	Sitting, standing	Lying, walking (e.g. hip joint arthrosis)
Typical features	Pain depends on workload, reproducible	Heaviness, tiredness, swelling	Paresthesias, joint pain
Localization of pain	Calf, thigh and/or buttocks	Lower leg, calf	Radicular pain, dorsal aspect of leg, lateral thigh
Improves by	Stopping walking	Walking in most instances, leg elevation	

CHAPTER 5

Differential Diagnosis of Pain

1. PAIN IN THE TONGUE

Pain in the tongue may result from an obvious lesion such as an ulcer; however, it may be an insistent complaint when there is no superficial evidence of abnormality. The conditions that have to be considered include the following:

I. PAIN UNDERNEATH THE TONGUE OR DEEPER

Injury to the Fraenum Linguae

- Injury to the fraenum by a fish-bone or other sharp object, or lower incisor teeth in whooping cough, may cause a visible abrasion or a definite ulcer.
- The injured part is painful and tender.

Inflamed Ranula

- Ranula is not painful unless it becomes inflamed.
- It is an asymmetrical red smooth swelling in the floor of the mouth under the tongue to one side of the fraenum.
- It may result from obstruction of one of the ducts of the sublingual salivary glands, but more often it is a retention cyst arising in one of the many mucus glands in the floor of the mouth.

Calculus in the Duct of the Submandibular Salivary Gland

- It may cause discomfort or pain, recurrent or constant according to the degree of inflammation.
- X-ray and enlargement of the gland with food intake settle the diagnosis.
- The calculus can frequently be palpated bimanually in the floor of the mouth and is occasionally seen to protrude through the duct orifice.

Foreign Body in the Tongue

- It is uncommon (e.g. fish-bone).
- Diagnosis rests on history or detection of the foreign body by palpation or radiology.

Myositis of the Tongue

It is seldom if ever a localized condition; it may, however, be a prominent feature in polymyositis.

II. PAIN UPON THE SURFACE OF THE TONGUE

Bitten Tongue

Pain may persist after a tongue-bite even when no obvious bruising or breach of the surface can be detected.

After General Anesthetic

Patients often complain of soreness of the tongue resulting from the use of tongue forceps or of a mouth-gag.

Injury by a Tooth or Dental Plate

It may cause a local painful site upon one side of the tongue; pain being increased by tongue movement in speaking, eating or swallowing. It needs to be watched to be certain that it disappears after the offending irritant is smoothed down or removed, otherwise an epithelioma is considered.

Glossitis

Antibiotic glossitis may arise from infection with Monilia albicans after broad spectrum antibiotics or from vitamin deficiencies resulting from suppression of normal gut flora. Glossitis may also occur and cause pain in Lichen planus, Behcet's disease, erythema multiforme, or pemphigus vulgaris.

Congenital Fissured Tongue (Scrotal Tongue)

The tongue is thick, deeply fissured, and usually symptomless. If food particles lodge in the fissures infection may arise and thus cause pain.

Geographical Tongue

It shows red denuded patches of irregular outline, which often change their position. It causes anxiety rather than pain.

Smoking

Smoking and the effect of hot liquid or food may cause acute pain in the tongue lasting for days after the cause has ceased to act.

Epithelioma of the Tongue

It starts as a fissure, nodule or ulcer, usually on the lateral border of the tongue. At first painless, it becomes painful as it invades and becomes grossly septic. The pain often radiates to the ear via the lingual branch of the trigeminal nerve supplying the tongue along its auriculotemporal branch. Ulceration is accompanied by bleeding; hence, the typical picture of late disease is an old man spitting blood with a plug of cottonwool in his ear.

2. PAIN IN THE BREAST

When pain in one breast is the chief symptom the first step is to palpate both breasts to detect an early carcinoma. Unfortunately, pain does not occur as an early symptom in carcinoma of the breast, and by the time it is pronounced there may be an obvious stony-hard tumor. Other causes of pain in the breast are (Harold Ellis):

PREGNANCY

Pain in the breast due to intrauterine or ectopic pregnancy is bilateral and associated with other signs of pregnancy. Suggestive indications are dark brown color of nipples, broad areola and swollen Montgomery's glands.

MENSTRUATION

Pain in the breast, which precede menstruation, is also bilateral and recur periodically before each menstrual cycle.

THE ONSET OF PUBERTY

Pain may occur in one breast before the other. The breast is enlarged, tender, painful and indurated but never suppurates. It results from *pubertal (hormonal) mastitis* that requires no treatment.

LACTATION

Milk engorgement during lactation results in an enlarged, tender, painful breast with fever and predisposes to abscess formation.

CRACKED/INFLAMED NIPPLE

It results from trauma to the nipple during suckling and predisposes to breast abscess formation due to the entrance of infection via the ducts (Staphylococcus) or lymphatics (Streptococcus).

BREAST ABSCESS (Acute Suppurative Mastitis)

Pain is throbbing and associated with hard and pitting edema that softens *very late* so that fluctuation may be detected **(Figure 5.1).** Fever is hectic due to attacks of septicemia. Aspiration reveals pus. Axillary lymph nodes are enlarged, painful and tender, but not hard.

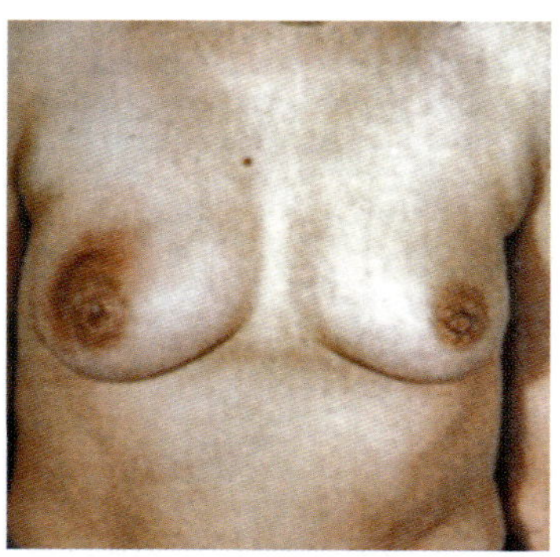

Fig. 5.1: Non-lactational right breast abscess

OTHER CAUSES OF MASTITIS

These include *acute mastitis* such as plasma cell mastitis (mammary duct ectasia), or *chronic mastitis* (non-specific, or specific).

TUBERCULOSIS (TB) OF THE BREAST

It may be bilateral and pain usually results from an infected cold abscess. Sinuses may be seen. Axillary lymph nodes are enlarged and may be caseous. Signs of TB toxemia may be present.

OTHER INFLAMMATORY LESIONS OF THE BREAST

Examples include *sarcoidosis* or *foreign body reaction* (e.g. breast prosthesis).

GALACTOCELE (MILK CYST)

It occurs in a lactating breast behind an obstructed duct as a single, painless swelling deep to the areola, with a milky discharge on squeezing the breast. It becomes painful with more engorgement and when infection commences.

FIBROCYSTIC DISEASE

Pain may shoot to the shoulder. It is aggravated by menstruation (one week before the menstrual cycle) and movement of the arm and is relieved one week after the cycle and also by pregnancy and lactation. It is associated with a swelling (lobular, lobar or nodular) and nipple discharge which is usually whitish but may be altered by blood. Axillary lymph nodes may be enlarged and tender but *never hard.*

ACUTE CANCER OF PREGNANCY AND LACTATION (MASTITIS CARCINOMATOSA)

The breast becomes diffusely swollen, painful, tender and hot on palpation, with dilated veins on the overlying skin so that it may be mistaken for acute mastitis. However, there is *no* pyrexia, *no* leukocytosis, *no* response to antibiotics, *no* tender lymph nodes (though enlarged), besides it is a rapidly growing and spreading tumor.

AFTER EFFECTS OF A BLOW OR INJURY

History of trauma is usually positive but sometimes the injury is forgotten. Hematoma or bruising is evident. Traumatic mastitis may follow local irritation by tight bras.

LESIONS OUTSIDE THE BREAST

These include *myocardial infarction, intercostal neuralgia, H.Z* and *Teitze's disease.*

ANXIETY STATE

It may cause pain in the breast, which is magnified because of fear from cancer particularly if the patient has a positive family history of breast cancer.

Key Points — Pain in the Breast

Thorough clinical examination is mandatory and sometimes a **mammography** is required particularly in a sophisticated, anxious patient to reinforce the negative clinical findings. Should the slightest nodule become palpable, its removal for microscopic examination is justified. If no abnormality could be found and the patient's mind is set at ease by the absence of further developments, the pain will often completely disappear.

3. PAIN IN THE ABDOMEN

Acute abdominal conditions may result from medical or surgical causes, abdominal or extra-abdominal, or may be divided according to the underlying **pathology** or **mechanism** causing acute abdominal pain, whether localized or generalized, as follows:

Pathology	Causes
A. Inflammation	1. Acute appendicitis 2. Acute cholecystitis 3. Diverticulitis 4. Acute pancreatitis 5. Acute pyelitis/pyelonephritis 6. Salpingo-oophoritis 7. Acute regional ileitis 8. Peritonitis (acute primary pneumococcal peritonitis)
B. Perforation	1. Perforated peptic ulcer 2. Perforated typhoid ulcer
C. Torsion	1. Volvulus of the sigmoid, cecum or small bowel 2. Twisted ovarian cyst 3. Torsion of Fallopian tube, fimbrial and broad ligament cysts
D. Abdominal Colic	1. Renal colic—Intestinal colic—Biliary colic 2. Dysmenorrhea
E. Bowel Obstruction	1. Intrinsic: Stricture, Crohn's disease, tumor, intussusception 2. Extrinsic: Adhesions (congenital, acquired), hernia (external, internal), neoplasms 3. Intraluminal: Bezoar, parasites, fecolith, gallstone, F.B
F. Ischemia	1. Mesenteric vascular occlusion (MVO) 2. Omental infarction

Contd...

Contd...

G. Internal Hemorrhage	1. Ruptured ectopic pregnancy 2. Ruptured graafian follicle 3. Traumatic rupture of spleen, liver, or mesenteric tear 4. Ruptured aortic aneurysm.
H. Extra-abdominal Lesions	1. Pulmonary: Basal pleurisy, pneumonia, empyema. 2. Cardiac: Coronary thrombosis (myocardial infarction). 3. Acute tonsillitis (in children). 4. Neurogenic: Spinal cord tumors, spinal nerve root compression 5. Psoas abscess (TB) and osteomyelitis of the iliac bone.
I. Medical Disease:	1. Acute gastroenteritis 2. Acute mesenteric lymphadenitis 3. Generalized medical diseases: • Diabetic ketoacidosis (DKA), uremia, porphyria • Rheumatic pain in the abdominal muscles • Tabes dorsalis (tabetic crisis) • Herpes zoster (HZ) • Abdominal migraine and epilepsy • Neurosis • Hysteria.

A. INFLAMMATION

Acute Appendicitis

- In a typical case, pain starts around the umbilicus then shifts to the right iliac fossa (*shifting pain*).
- Temperature is slightly elevated (rarely exceeds 38°C). Pulse is correspondingly rapid.
- There is tenderness and rigidity at *McBurney's point* and rebound tenderness in the right iliac fossa.
- Pressure on the left iliac fossa leads to pain in the right iliac fossa (*Rovsing sign*).
- Blood count shows polymorphonuclear leukocytosis.

Acute Cholecystitis

- Pain starts in the epigastrium and right hypochondrium and refers to the right shoulder and scapular region. It is increased by movement and respiration.
- There is tenderness and rigidity in the right hypochondrium. The gallbladder may or may not be felt.
- If the patient is asked to take a deep inspiration while the doctor's hand exerts pressure below the right costal margin, a catch in breath due to pain occurs before full inspiration is completed (*Murphy's sign*).
- Temperature (reaches >40°C in acute obstructive cholecystitis) and pulse are elevated. Rigors and sweating.

Diverticulitis

- The *classic picture* is of left lower abdominal pain, low-grade fever, leukocytosis, nausea with occasional vomiting and mild abdominal distention. Rectal bleeding or occult blood in stools (50% of cases).
- A *palpable mass* may be detected rectally or bimanually.
- *Urinary symptoms*, usually burning and urgency, due to involvement in the inflammatory response.
- **Meckel's diverticulitis**: There is a midline hypogastric pain. A palpable fusiform mass is felt below the umbilicus, or increased pain on moving the navel upwards.

Acute Pancreatitis

- Shock, cyanosis and acute pain in the upper abdomen and back are constant features. Pain decreases on sitting.
- There may be ileus causing abdominal distention. Vomiting is early and profuse.
- There is deep upper abdominal tenderness but characteristically no rigidity (*not* in contact with the anterior abdominal wall).
- Discoloration of skin (*necrotizing pancreatitis*) at the loin (*Grey-Turner sign*) or umbilicus (*Cullen's sign*).

- Mydriasis on installation of adrenaline into the conjunctiva (normally there is no response) (*Lewis test*).
- Serum amylase should be estimated within 24 hours of onset of attack (it reaches > 1,000 SU).
- CT scan is currently the most sensitive non-invasive method for confirmation of diagnosis.

Acute Pyelitis/Pyelonephritis

- There is high fever, rigors, vomiting, frequency of micturition, and pain in the right loin.
- Tenderness in the right costovertebral angle. Urine analysis shows pyuria.

Pelvic Inflammatory Diseases (e.g. Pyosalpinx and Acute Salpingitis)

- History of previous attacks. Dysmenorrhea and menstrual irregularities. Burning micturition. Pain is characteristically one inch above the midpoint of inguinal ligament.
- Vaginal discharge + cervical swab (shows organism). PV examination reveals enlarged tubes and tender cervix (*diagnostic*).
- A pyosalpinx may be found to be mobile and smooth resembling an appendicular abscess.

Acute Regional Ileitis (Crohn's Disease)

- It is a rare condition that resembles acute appendicitis except that it is associated with *diarrhea* and a *mass* (ileal thickening) may occasionally be felt, being firm, mobile and slightly tender (*never hard or fixed*)
- The patient may present with features of acute on top of chronic intestinal obstruction.
- Other stigmata of Crohn's disease may be present, as well as weight loss, nutritional deficits and anemia.

Acute Pneumococcal Peritonitis (Primary)

- Occurs exclusively in girls under the age of 10 years, the infection spreading from the genital tract.
- Sudden onset, high fever, vomiting and diarrhea. Gradual lower abdominal distention is a constant feature.
- Unlike other types of peritonitis, tenderness and rigidity are not so marked.
- Revealing pneumococci in the vaginal discharge is diagnostic.

B. PERFORATION

Perforated Peptic Ulcer (PPU)

- Perforation occurs in the duodenal ulcer > gastric ulcer (10:1).
- Severe abdominal pain, marked tenderness, board-like rigidity (generalized but more marked in the right upper abdomen) and shock. The relation of the onset of the attack to a meal is significant.
- Air escapes leading to obliteration of liver dullness and is shown on X-ray as air under diaphragm **(Figure 5.2).**
- At first, temperature drops, but soon peritonitis leads to rise in temperature and pulse.

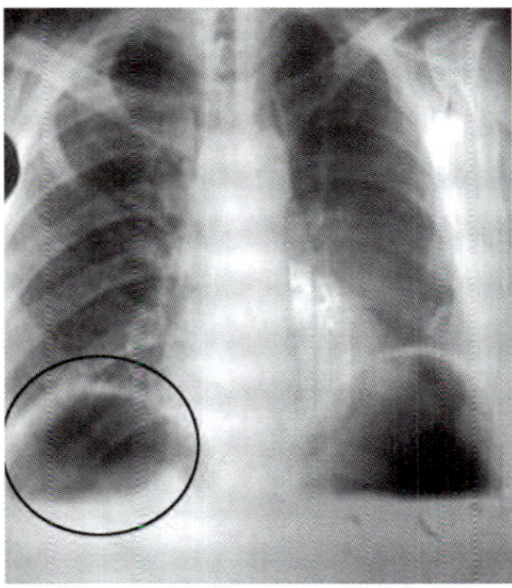

Fig. 5.2: Plain X-ray showing free air under right copula of the diaphragm

Perforated Typhoid Ulcer

- History of fever for at least 2 weeks before the onset of severe acute pain due to the perforation.
- Peritonitis is generalized due to poor power of localization and the fluid nature of the contents of the small bowel. There is shifting dullness in addition to tenderness and rigidity.
- Palpation of the enlarged spleen is difficult.

C. TORSION/VOLVULUS

Volvulus of the Sigmoid

- History of sudden attacks of vomiting, colicky pain, distention and constipation, followed by self-cure, with passage of large amounts of flatus and stools.
- Acute attacks present with features of colonic obstruction with acute tenderness on the left side of the abdomen. An abdominal mass may be felt. PR may reveal blood and mucus.
- Plain X-ray shows distended loop of bowel without haustrations often assuming a *kidney-bean* appearance **(Figure 5.3)**.

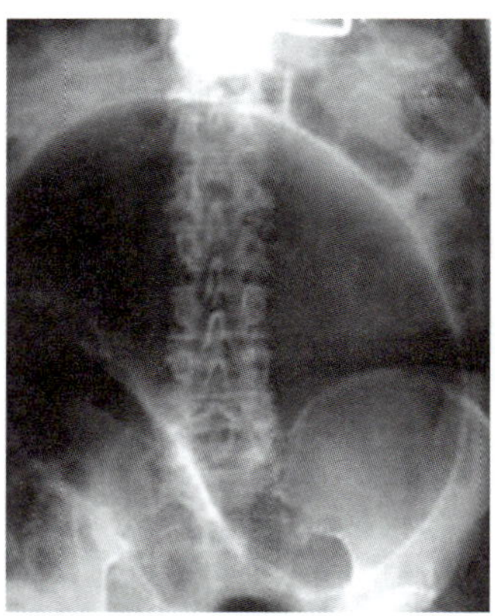

Fig. 5.3: Plain X-ray showing volvulus of the sigmoid colon

- Barium enema reveals the exact site of obstruction with a characteristic funnel narrowing (*Bird's peak*).

Volvulus of the Cecum

- It is better called "volvulus of the ileocolic or ileo-cecal region". The patient presents with acute intestinal obstruction. The volvulus may be palpable as a tender tympanic swelling in the right iliac fossa.
- Plain X-ray shows severe cecal distention and evidence of small bowel obstruction.
- Barium enema is done in chronic but not in acute cases. It shows cut-off of the barium at the transverse colon or right flexure, beyond which is seen the gas-filled right colon.

Volvulus of the Intestine

- Rotation of a segment of the intestine on an axis formed by its mesentery.
- It results in acute intestinal obstruction (pain, vomiting, constipation and distention), with a palpable swelling in the center of the abdomen. It may cause circulatory impairment of the bowel.

Twisted Ovarian Cyst

- Severe pain, which may be referred to the loin. Severe vomiting may be present. Tachycardia, but temperature is normal.
- With torsion, a smooth, tender and mobile swelling is felt by PV examination soon after the sudden onset of the attack (the most diagnostic).

Torsion of Fallopian Tube, Fimbrial and Broad Ligament Cysts

These are indistinguishable from pelvic appendicitis except by bimanual examination under anesthesia.

D. ABDOMINAL COLIC

Renal (Ureteric) Colic

- Pain is colicky, intermittent, less localized and radiates to the inner sides of the thighs (and right testicle or labium). Tender renal angles. Usually there is dysuria and urine frequency.
- Urine analysis, plain X-ray and IVU are the usual tests to be performed.
- Plain X-ray may show a stone **(Figure 5.4)**.
- It responds to antispasmodics.

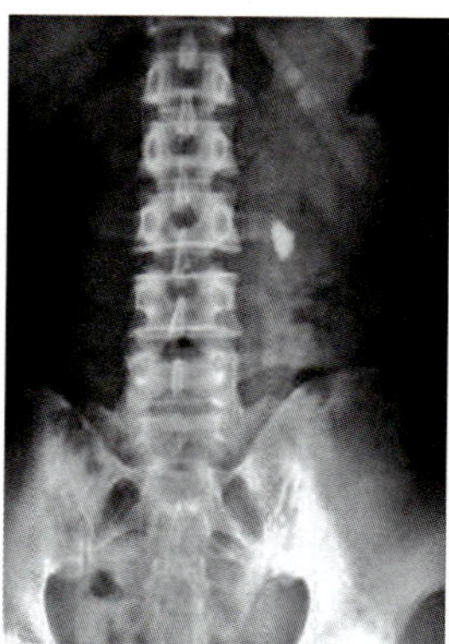

Fig. 5.4: Left ureteric stone

Intestinal Colic

- It starts around the umbilicus and is followed by diarrhea or the passage of loose stools.
- Temperature and pulse are normal. Palpation shows no tenderness, no rigidity, and no rebound tenderness.
- The condition should ameliorate within a few hours.

Biliary Colic

- It starts in the epigastrium and right hypochondrium and refers to the right shoulder and scapula.

- If it is followed by jaundice it must be due to a stone that migrated to the CBD. However, if a mucocele appears a few days later, the stone must have become impacted in the cystic duct.
- If the t° increased followed by tenderness and rigidity and palpable GB, the case is acute obstructive cholecystitis.

Dysmenorrhea

- Pain precedes and accompanies menstrual period.
- Pain lies in the lower abdomen and refers to the sacral region.
- History of previous similar attacks may be present.
- Pulse and temperature are normal.

E. INTESTINAL OBSTRUCTION

Main Features

- There is abdominal colic, vomiting, absolute constipation and abdominal distention.
- There may be shock when dehydration develops.
- Percussion shows resonance and auscultation reveals loud peristaltic movements.
- *Plain X-ray*, in the standing position, shows multiple fluid levels **(Figure 5.5)**.
- In *high gut obstruction*, vomiting is early with rapid dehydration and demineralization, while constipation is late.
- In *mid-gut obstruction*, colic and distension are central.
- In *low gut obstruction*, absolute constipation is early, vomiting is late or even absent, and distention occurs mainly in the flanks.

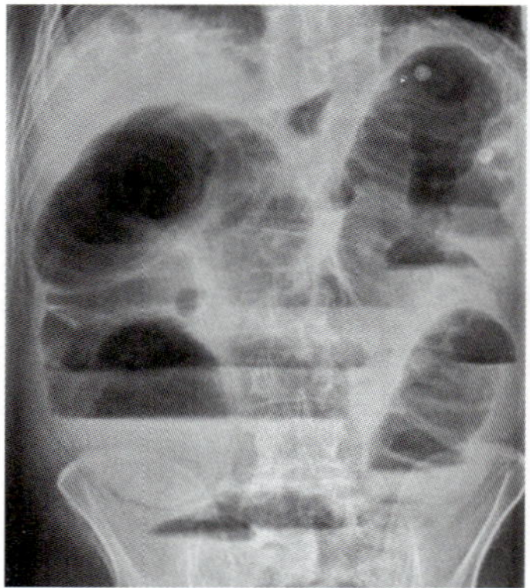

Fig. 5.5: Multiple fluid levels

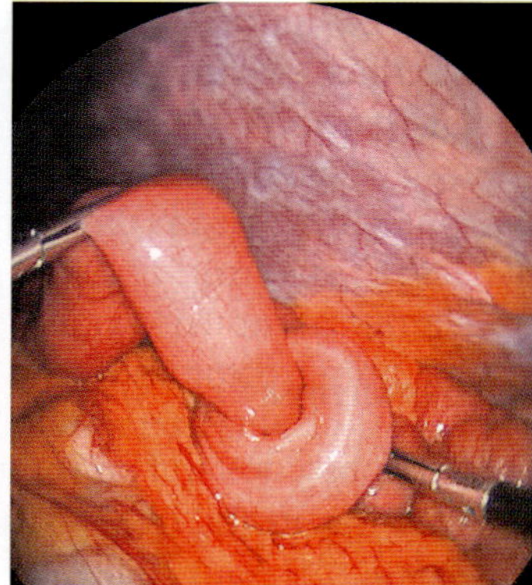

Fig. 5.6: Intussusception of small bowel

Intussusception (Intrinsic Cause) (Figure 5.6)

- Sudden onset of acute abdominal pain.
- The baby (< 2 years) cries and draws his legs to abdomen in attacks of about one minute.
- There is vomiting and constipation, but in 10% there is diarrhea.
- Passage of blood and mucus (*red currant jelly*) per anus.
- The apex may be felt by PR exam.
- Diagnosis is established by finding a curved sausage-shaped, firm, *mass* in the line of the colon with its concavity directed towards the umbilicus.
- Sensation of an empty right iliac fossa (*Sign de Dance*).
- Barium enema shows a cup-shaped filling defect at the apex (*Cobrahead or spring coil appearance*).
- The barium may reduce the intussusception.
- Ileocecal intussusception may be mistaken as acute appendicitis if there is no mass, or blood in stools.
- It may occur also in adults (secondary type).

Hernia (Extrinsic Cause)

- *External hernia*: Most hernias producing intestinal obstruction are external, usually inguinal, femoral or umbilical. Diagnosis may be difficult in very obese patients or in those with Richter's hernia. There is history of a reducible mass (the hernia), which now persists. Signs of inflammation or discoloration in the skin overlying the irreducible mass suggest non-viability of the hernial contents.
- *Internal hernia*: Bowel obstruction and strangulation may occur due to the presence of hernial apertures inside the abdomen. It is distinguishable in its early stages by the severe and obstructive picture, with lack of abdominal rigidity. In its later phases, with established peritonitis and a mass, diagnosis is difficult.

Gallstone Ileus (Intraluminal Cause)

- Symptoms of intestinal obstruction, mostly in old female, with a history of right hypochondrial pain.
- Examination reveals signs of obstruction and tenderness in the right hypochondrium. Rarely the stone is palpated. The stone is usually impacted 2 feet from the ileocecal valve (narrowest part of small bowel).
- X-ray shows multiple fluid levels, may be the stone (if radioopaque) and gas in the biliary tree.

F. ISCHEMIA

Mesenteric Vascular Occlusion (MVO)

- MVO results from mesenteric *embolism or thrombosis* and is ∴ seen in patients with valvular heart disease or atherosclerosis.
- The condition is diagnosed by constant severe central pain, copious vomiting, hematemesis or melena, associated

with a tender and rigid abdomen, as well as the presence of shock.

- Laboratory tests show leukocytosis (up to 40,000/mm^3 or more), increased serum amylase and hemoconcentration.
- X-ray shows air-fluid levels, distended loops, and intramural gas.

Omental Infarction

- It results from interference with blood supply of the omentum due to its torsion or strangulation in a hernial orifice or by extensive bands.
- Pain is central and severe. A tender mass in the abdomen may be felt.

G. INTERNAL HEMORRHAGE

Ruptured Ectopic Pregnancy

- Hemoperitoneum from leakage or rupture of tubal pregnancy causing pain due to irritation of peritoneum.
- Shock and shoulder tip pain on elevation of the foot of the bed are inconstant.
- Pain starts and stays on the right side with *no* shift.
- Missed period, soft and tender cervix (PV exam.) and vaginal bleeding. There may be other signs of pregnancy such as increased pigmentation of the nipple and areola and the linea alba.

Rupture of "Ovarian Follicle" (Mittelschmerz Pain)

- History of similar attacks of lower abdominal pain, on the 14th-16th day of the menstrual cycle, usually in a young female.
- Tenderness and rigidity are rare.
- No fever, no leukocytosis, no missed period and cervix is not soft.

- Sometimes bleeding is excessive giving rise to a picture similar to internal hemorrhage.

Traumatic Rupture (of Spleen, Liver, or Mesenteric Tear)

- History of trauma causing abdominal pain, pallor, thirst, tachycardia and may be fainting.
- Pain may be felt in the left shoulder in case of ruptured spleen (Balance's sign).
- The temperature becomes subnormal due to shock and as bleeding continues the patient becomes restless.
- Examination shows tenderness and rigidity over the bleeding organ + shifting dullness.

Ruptured Aortic Aneurysm

- *Pain* is usually mid-abdominal or paravertebral. With growing hematoma pain occurs in the flanks.
- Cardiovascular collapse and *shock* without warning (sweating, nausea, hypotension).
- The abdomen will usually reveal a pulsatile tender mass with mild abdominal fullness often extending toward the left flank.
- Ecchymosis may be present in the flanks, perineum, scrotum, or periumbilical area (Cullen's sign).

H. EXTRA-ABDOMINAL DISEASE

Pleurisy and Pneumonia

- Basal right-sided pleurisy and right lower lobe pneumonia may lead to pain and rigidity in the right side of the abdomen that is often mistaken for cholecystitis or appendicitis. Rigidity is more pronounced in the upper than in the lower quadrant. Rapid respiration and pleural rub heard on auscultation.
- There is usually dyspnea, cyanosis and working alae nasi. No bowel complaints.
- PXR confirms the condition **(Figure 5.7).**

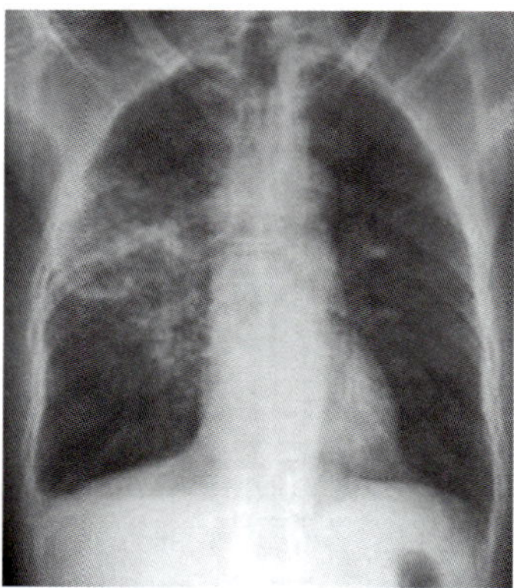

Fig. 5.7: Pneumonia of right lung

Coronary Thrombosis

- It causes reflex epigastric pain, but soon pain radiates to the sternum and left arm.
- The lower abdomen is free.

I. MEDICAL CAUSES

Acute Gastroenteritis

- The colic of acute gastroenteritis classically precedes the vomiting, this order being reversed in appendicitis.
- Tenderness is less sharply localized and is maximal around the umbilicus.
- It is usually associated with diarrhea.

Acute Mesenteric Lymphadenitis

- The patient is usually a child with history of upper respiratory tract infection.
- The child is usually free between attacks.
- Fever reaches 40°C.

- Diarrhea is common and shifting tenderness is characteristic (i.e. shifting on lying on the left side due to mobility of the mesentery).
- Abdominal or inguinal lymph nodes may be felt, but the abdominal signs are not of a sufficient degree.

Generalized Medical Diseases

- *Diabetic ketoacidosis* (DKA).
- *Uremia*: In advanced uremia (renal failure), abdominal distention, hiccup and intense vomiting are common. There is uriniferous odor of the breath. The kidneys may be enlarged. Blood urea is raised and urine shows much albumin.
- *Rheumatic pain in the abdominal muscles*: Pain is aggravated by contracting the affected muscle, which is tender on palpation. No bowel symptoms.
- *Tabes dorsalis (Tabetic crisis)*: Lightening-like pains that shoot for seconds along the distribution of a nerve. Abdominal examination reveals no abnormality. the clue to diagnosis is the discovery of absent knee jerk or ankle reflex, Argyll Robertson pupil, and rombergism.
- *Herpes zoster (HZ):* Severe pain referred to the umbilicus and RIF with herpetic eruption.
- *Abdominal migraine and epilepsy*: Tenderness and rigidity are absent and the patient may have normal bowel action in spite of the abdominal complaint.
- *Neurosis/Hysteria*: The patient is psychologically disturbed, with bizarre complaints. Abdominal examination reveals no organic abnormality.

Key Points — Acute Abdominal Pain

- *Acute appendicitis* is the commonest surgical cause of acute abdomen.
- In inflammatory conditions such as *acute appendicitis*, pressure at the site of pain increases the pain or there may even be cutaneous hyperesthesia so that the patient cannot tolerate his own hand. On the contrary, in colicky conditions such as *renal colic*, the patient is in agony, doubled-up or bent and usually dipping his hand into the side of the colic as this gives him some relief.
- Conditions requiring *urgent laparotomy* include:
  1. Inflammatory Diseases:
     Acute appendicitis, failure to localize (cholecystitis, diverticulitis), perforation (peptic ulcer, typhoid ulcer).
  2. Internal Hemorrhage:
     Ruptured ectopic pregnancy, ruptured aortic aneurysm, bleeding ulcer.
  3. Trauma:
     Damage to viscus such as liver, spleen, kidney, intestine, or gallbladder.
  4. Obstruction with or without strangulation:
     Dynamic, e.g. by peritoneal band, or adynamic, e.g. MVO.
  5. Pelvic causes such as:
     Twisted ovarian cyst or twisted uterine fibroid

4. EPIGASTRIC PAIN

I. SUDDEN SEVERE EPIGASTRIC PAIN

Etiology

Severe sudden epigastric pain may result from: 1. Perforated gastric or duodenal ulcer. 2. Gangrenous appendix. 3. Acute cholecystitis. 4. Acute pancreatitis.	→	The pain in such cases is attended by severe shock and signs of collapse. These conditions require immediate surgical treatment except when diagnosis of acute hemorrhagic pancreatitis is sure. This is achieved by finding Grey Turner's sign of blue discoloration, usually in the flanks, and the presence of raised serum amylase. Intraoperatively, fat necrosis confirms the diagnosis, but the majority of surgeons are opposed to operating.

It may also result from:

1. *Acute intestinal obstruction*: The pain in acute intestinal obstruction may be referred to the epigastrium. Vomiting is usually a prominent symptom in such a case.
2. *Coronary thrombosis*: The pain may be felt in the epigastrium and simulate an abdominal emergency.
3. *Acute pericarditis*: It may cause epigastric pain especially in children.
4. *Bornholm disease (epidemic myalgia)*: Although more usually thoracic, pain may be epigastric and sufficiently severe to encourage laparotomy.
5. *Acute porphyria*: It also often causes such acute abdominal pain that laparotomy is contemplated.

II. CHRONIC OR RECURRENT EPIGASTRIC PAIN

Extra-abdominal Causes

Extra-abdominal causes of chronic or recurrent epigastric pain must not be forgotten:

1. *Spinal caries* (specially in children) and other causes of spinal root irritation, e.g. spinal tumor.
2. *Pleurisy.*

3. *Small epigastric hernia*: They are usually in the linea alba and detected only by careful palpation.
4. *Vascular or circulatory causes,* e.g. angina.
5. *Affection of abdominal muscles*: Straining from coughing may also cause epigastric pain.

Abdominal Causes

When extra-abdominal causes are excluded, the cause of pain should be looked for in the following organs:

A. Stomach

1. *Gastric Carcinoma:*
   The pain in carcinoma is usually more or less continuous and may be aggravated by food. A tumor may be felt. Anorexia and nausea are usually present. Gastric contents in most cases show absence of free HCl and altered blood. X-ray examination if not conclusive is usually helpful. Endoscopy and biopsy confirm diagnosis.
2. *Benign Gastric Ulcer:*
   Pain usually occurs at a definite time after meals, and is generally temporarily relieved by eating, though it may be aggravated by meals. The pain often wakes the patient at 1-2 in the morning. Vomiting, with or without hematemesis, is a variable feature. There may be localized deep tenderness and rigidity on one side. X-ray examination usually reveals the ulcer and endoscopy with biopsy differentiates it from a malignant gastric ulcer.
3. *Hiatus Hernia:*
   Esophageal reflux associated with hiatal hernia may produce epigastric or retrosternal pain typically related to bending over or lying down.
4. *Pyloric Stenosis:*
   There is a history of projectile vomiting, the vomitus containing considerable undigested food. There is also a gastric splash 3 or 4 hours after the last meal. Visible

peristalsis and even a palpably distended stomach may be present in advanced cases. X-ray is diagnostic.

B. Duodenum

1. Duodenal Ulcer:
   The characteristic 'hunger pain" of a duodenal ulcer is often referred to the epigastrium.
2. Duodenal Diverticulum:
   It is usually symptomless unless very large or inflammation arises when food accumulates within. Symptoms resemble those of a duodenal ulcer but there is no regular food relationship (although a coexistent ulcer may be present). Patients as a rule are over the age of 50 years and the diverticulum is always on the inner (pancreatic) side of the duodenum.

C. Liver and Gallbladder

1. Hepatic Congestion:
   Epigastric pain may be produced by congestion of the liver, either active (hepatitis) or passive, as in mitral disease.
2. Hepatic Abscess and Carcinoma:
   These may also cause pain in the epigastrium.
3. Gallstones:
   They sometimes cause epigastric pain, which may be related to meals or a particular type of food; the pain however is less "punctual" than that of peptic ulcer. Pressure over the gallbladder often elicits tenderness and catch of breath. An X-ray of both the stomach and gallbladder will be of great help. Indeed these two common conditions often co-exist.

D. Pancreas

1. Pancreatic Calculi.
2. Chronic Pancreatitis.
3. Pancreatic Tumor.

They all may cause epigastric and high lumbar pain. An accurate diagnosis of all these conditions without laparotomy may be difficult, but other signs of disturbed function of the pancreas may be present such as fatty diarrhea (steatorrhea). A tumor (mass) may be felt. Glycosuria may be present, but is not invariable. In cases of chronic pancreatitis, there is usually a history of gallstones, and transient periods of jaundice.

E. Abdominal Aorta

1. Abdominal Aneurysm:
   It may cause pain in the epigastrium, but pain is more severe in the back. A pulsating expansile mass may be felt on deep palpation. The X-rays may confirm the diagnosis, though an aneurysm may exist without radiographic abnormality.
2. Abdominal Angina:
   It occurs in elderly patients as a result of progressive atheromatous narrowing of the superior mesenteric artery. Colicky attacks of central abdominal pain occur after meals and this is followed by diarrhea. Complete occlusion with infarction of the intestine is often preceded by attacks of this nature.

F. Colon

Enterospasm:
Spasmodic contraction of the intestine may be a cause of epigastric pain, which may simulate gastric pain by being induced by food intake. Such pain, however, tends to be relieved by pressure, and the passage of gas per anum. Obstinate constipation is usually a feature, and there are often mucus and shreds of membrane in the motions (mucomembranous colic). A similar pain may be due to *plumbism*.

5. PAIN IN THE UMBILICAL REGION

Pain felt by the patient at or near the umbilicus may arise in the umbilicus itself, or may be referred to that region from some distant lesion.

I. PAIN ARISING IN THE UMBILICUS

If pain is due to some causes in the umbilicus itself, it will be localized, movements of the abdominal wall will be restricted, and the umbilicus will be tender to palpation.

Umbilical Hernia and Paraumbilical Hernia (PUH) (Figure 5.8)

- In children, umbilical hernia is usually a small spherical swelling easily reducible and usually symptomless. It should not be considered as the cause of umbilical pain unless other more likely causes such as acute appendicitis have been eliminated.
- In middle-aged adults, the hernia usually lies just above the umbilicus, giving impulse on cough but rarely completely reducible. Pain may arise from inflammation of the overlying skin with no abdominal colic, or from obstruction or strangulation of the hernial contents where pain becomes deeper. If strangulated, the hernia becomes tender, tense, irreducible and with no impulse on cough.

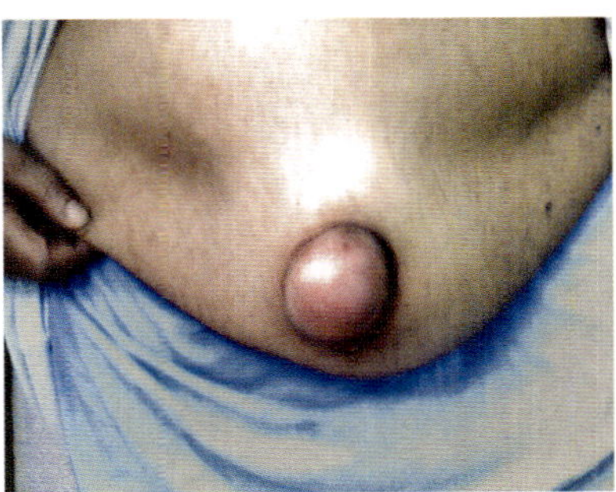

Fig. 5.8: Irreducible PUH

Eczema and Suppuration of the Umbilical Scar

- Due to fat or an umbilical hernia, the scar is deepened and leads to a retention of secretions.
- The diagnosis is obvious.

Extension of Abdominal Lesions to the Umbilicus

- *Chronic abdominal infections,* such as TB and pneumococcal peritonitis, and *tumors,* particularly those of the stomach, may reach the umbilicus.
- The discovery of an abscess or a nodule in this situation may give the clue to some obscure abdominal pain, but the lump itself is usually painless.

II. PAIN REFERRED TO THE UMBILICUS

A. Pain Arising in the Area Supplied by Visceral Nerves

The *"visceral level"* of the umbilicus is that part of the alimentary tract supplied by the superior mesenteric artery, i.e. from the 2nd part of the duodenum to the middle of the transverse colon; the segmental level is the 10th dorsal nerve and its corresponding cord segment. Visceral pain is usually colicky, referred to a diffuse and indefinite area, usually accompanied at first by nausea or vomiting.

a. The Commonest and Most Important Causes

The commonest and by far the most important variety of pain in the umbilical region is a colic accompanied by nausea and vomiting. This could be caused by the following three conditions have a similar clinical picture in the early stages.

1. Appendicitis
2. Intestinal obstruction.
3. Intestinal colic.

The following Table shows the main points of differentiation:

	Appendicitis	Intestinal Obstruction	Colic due to Irritants
History	Possibly previous attacks	Herniae, previous operation or history of peritonitis. Swallowed FB in child or gallstone in adult	Doubtful food. Others in family affected
Pain	Shifts from colic at the umbilicus to steady pain in the RIF	Remains colicky and increased in severity	Remains colicky, but decreases by vomiting or diarrhea
Vomiting	Soon ceases, but may return with extensive peritonitis	Increases in frequency. Vomitus becomes intestinal	Maximal at the beginning and then decreases
Bowels	Constipated, but enema produces action	Constipation, becomes absolute after bowel distal to obstruction is evacuated	Diarrhea soon appears unless forestalled by enemas
Temperature and Pulse	Low-grade fever, pulse raised moderately	Temperature normal or subnormal. Pulse mounting steadily	Temperature normal or subnormal. Pulse in ordinary case soon returns to normal
Abdominal Wall	First slight tenderness over appendix, later more marked with guarding and rebound	Usually no tenderness. Distention and peristalsis may be seen	No visible or palpable abnormality
Auscultation	Silence round cecum: normal sounds elsewhere	Increased peristaltic sounds	Increased peristaltic sounds
PR Exam	Feces. may be tender	No feces. No tenderness	Feces. No tenderness

b. Other Visceral Pain Referred to the Umbilicus

1. *Gall Stone Colic or Acute Pancreatitis*:
   Pain may be referred to the umbilicus but is usually higher.
2. *Renal Colic*:
   Pain may exceptionally center on the umbilicus.

B. Pain Arising in the Spinal Nerves and Spinal Cord

Pain arising in spinal nerves is accurately localized, burning or aching, and often associated with muscular guarding or rigidity, and with hyperesthesia in the skin of the part concerned.

Chest Conditions

An early pleurisy may be characterized by sharp umbilical pain. The high temperature, rapid breathing, and working of the alae nasi will usually suggest that the lesion is above the diaphragm.

Spinal Caries

In children, umbilical pain may be the 1st symptom of TB (*Pott's disease*). The peculiar trunk rigidity and unwillingness to bend should call attention to the spine. There will be localized tenderness over one of the vertebrae and deformity. An X-ray will confirm the diagnosis. Pain may also be referred from other spinal disorders such as *crush fractures, neoplastic deposits, or ankylosing spondylitis*.

Tabes Dorsalis

Abdominal pain, often referred to the umbilicus, may be the only complaint. The typical gastric crisis may be replaced by a much more diffuse pain. CNS examination should be made in all cases.

Lead Poisoning

Severe attacks of cramp-like abdominal pains referred to the umbilicus may be the chief or only complaint. Diagnosis is suggested by the patient's occupation (*plumber*) and confirmed by seeing a blue line on the gums during examination. Other manifestations may be present such as constipation, various paralyses, particularly wrist-drop, optic neuritis, and in late stages, arterial and chronic renal disease.

Tumors of the Spinal Cord and Compression Myelitis

Though a less common source of error, these must be borne in mind. The pain is usually of a *girdle* character, and some evidence of motor or sensory deficits in the lower limb can be found.

6. CHRONIC BACK PAIN

Pain in the back is one of the commonest complaints in general and specialist practice. The differential diagnosis, therefore, covers most of medicine. The first important subdivision is acute and chronic back pain. Causes may be in the back or organs other than the back.

ACUTE BACK PAIN

Acute back pain may occur in any *febrile disorder* such as dengue or "break-bone" fever. It may also result from injury particularly in sportsmen, gardeners, and horse-riders. Such injuries usually rapidly settle when the cause is removed or the injured tissue heals.

CHRONIC BACK PAIN

In any backache lasting >2-3 weeks the conditions listed in the Table below should be considered. *The commonest causes are the first four mentioned.* In eliciting the cause, a good history is essential, as well as examination of the way the patient moves, walks, sits or lies, and how he rises from sitting and lying positions. Spinal range of movement should be measured. *Details are beyond the scope of this book.*

Chronic Back Pain—Etiology

1. Traumatic, mechanical or degenerative
2. Metabolic
3. Unknown causes
4. Infective conditions of bone, joint and theca of spine
5. Neoplastic: Benign or malignant (primary or secondary)
6. Cardiac and vascular
7. Gynecological conditions
8. Gastrointestinal conditions
8. Renal and genitourinary causes
10. Blood disorders
11. Drugs
12. Psychogenic

Traumatic, Mechanical or Degenerative

1. Low-back strain: fatigue, obesity, and pregnancy.
2. Injuries of bone, joint or ligament.
3. Degenerative diseases of the bone (osteoarthrosis).
4. Intervertebral disc lesions.
5. Lumbar instability syndromes, e.g. spondylolisthesis.
6. Scoliosis: Primary and secondary.

Metabolic

1. Osteoporosis
2. Osteomalacia
3. Hyperparathyroidism
4. Ochronosis
5. Fluorosis
6. Hyperphosphatemic rickets.

Unknown Causes

1. Inflammatory arthropathies of the spine (ankylosing spondylitis, spondylitis of Reiter's = Brodies disease)
2. Psoriasis
3. Inflammatory bowel disease (ulcerative colitis, Crohn's disease)
4. Whipple's disease
5. Rarely:
   - Polymyositis and polymyalgia rheumatica
   - Paget's disease of the bone
   - Epiphysitis (Scheuermann's disease).

Infective Conditions of Bone, Joint and Theca of Spine

1. Osteomyelitis
2. Tuberculosis (TB)
3. Typhoid and paratyphoid
4. Syphilis.

5. Yaws
6. Very rarely:
   - Weil's disease (leptospirosis icterohemorrhagica)
   - Spinal pachmeningitis
   - Chronic meningitis
   - Subarachnoid or spinal abscess.

Neoplastic: Benign or Malignant (Primary or Secondary)

1. Osteoid osteoma.
2. Eosinophilic granuloma.
3. Metastatic (usually from breast, bronchus, kidney, suprarenal, prostate, thyroid and GIT).
4. Bronchial carcinoma.
5. Esophageal carcinoma.
6. Sarcoma.
7. Multiple myeloma.
8. Primary and secondary tumors of the spinal canal and nerve roots:
   - Ependymoma
   - Neurofibroma
   - Glioma
   - Angioma (Hemangioma)
   - Meningioma
   - Lipoma
   - Chordoma (rarely).
9. Hodgkin disease.

Cardiac and Vascular

1. Subarachnoid or spinal hemorrhage.
2. Dissecting aortic aneurysm. Ischemic pain from aortic or iliac arteries occlusion.
3. Grossly enlarged left atrium in mitral valve disease.
4. Rarely, myocardial infarction.

Gynecological Conditions

1. Tuberculosis.
2. Prolapse, or retroversion of the uterus.
3. Dysmenorrhea.
4. Chronic salpingitis.
5. Pelvic abscess.
6. Chronic cervicitis.
7. Tumors.

Gastrointestinal Conditions

1. Peptic ulcer.
2. Hiatus hernia.
3. Cholelisthiasis.
4. Cholecystitis.
5. Pancreatitis (very important).
6. Rarely:
   - Appendicitis
   - Tumors of intraabdominal viscus (stomach, colon, pancreas)
   - Tumors of retroperitoneal structures.

Renal and Genitourinary Causes

1. Renal carcinoma.
2. Calculus (renal or ureteric).
3. Hypernephrosis.
4. Polycystic kidney.
5. Pyelitis and pyelonephritis.
6. Perinephric abscess.
7. Seminal vesiculitis.
8. Prostatic infections or tumors.

Blood Disorders

1. Sickle-cell crisis.
2. Acute hemolytic states.

Drugs

1. Corticosteroids (osteoporosis).
2. Methysergide (retroperitoneal fibrosis).

Psychogenic

1. Anxiety.
2. Depression.
3. Hysteria.
4. Compensation neurosis.
5. Malingering.
   - In this case, no organic cause for low back pain could be found. The patient usually suffers from anxiety or depression.
   - Two tests can detect such condition:
     - Aird's Test:
       The patient is asked to flex forwards to touch his toes in the standing position with his knees straight. He usually fails and complains of pain. He is now asked to sit down and to touch his toes by flexing his spine. He is usually able to do so as there is no organic lesion in the spine.
     - Magnuson's Test:
       The patient is asked to point the most painful area of the spine, and this is marked out. The patient's attention is now diverted by examining other organs and then he is asked to point out again the most painful spot on his back. He points out to another spot.

7. PAIN IN THE PERINEUM

The complaint of perineal pain *per se* does not convey much information to the clinician, and is practically never present as the only symptom in a case.

It may be a manifestation of an anxiety state.

Aching in the perineum is frequently present in diseases of the following

Organ	Diseases
Prostate	Prostatitis (acute, subacute, or chronic) Prostatic abscess, or TB Calculus Adenomatous enlargement Carcinoma
Seminal Vesicles	Acute inflammation, TB
Testicle	Congenital misplacement (ectopic) in the perineum
Urinary Bladder	Cystitis, TB, Calculus, carcinoma
Urethra	Gonorrhea, injury and rupture, stricture with extravasation or urethral abscess, fistula, calculus impacted in the bulbo-prostatic portion
Anal Area	Anal fissure (acute or chronic) Follicular abscess, carbuncle Anal Crohn's disease Anal fistula Cancer of the anus, or ulcerated anal tumor Prolapsed hemorrhoids
Rectum	Ulcerative proctitis Cancer of the rectum Solitary rectal ulcer syndrome Descending perineum syndrome
Vagina	Acute inflammation Inflammation or abscess of Bartholin's glands Cystocele Epithelioma

Contd...

Contd...

Skin Disease	Intertrigo, diabetic inflammation, condylomata
Bone	Bone tumor, retrosacral tumor, coccygeal arthritis
Nerves	Spinal tumor, peripheral nerve compression
Idiopathic	Chronic idiopathic anal or perineal pain

ANAL AND PERIANAL CONDITIONS

Anal Fissure

- *Inspection*: A tightly closed anus, with a sentinel tag in chronic cases, but the fissure itself can be seen on gentle separation of the anal margin. The circular fibers of the internal sphincter are seen at the base of the ulcer.
- *Palpation*: An acute fissure is impalpable, but a chronic fissure is felt like a button-hole with a firm edge.
- A complicating abscess or fistula should be looked for.
- *PR examination*: For chronic cases only because of severe pain in acute fissures. It reveals induration of the lateral edges of the fissure ± hypertrophic papillae.
- *Avoid proctoscopy,* because it causes severe pain.
- *Sigmoidoscopy (may be delayed or done under anesthesia)* should be performed to R/O IBD or carcinoma.

Perianal Hematoma

- *Inspection*: A small bluish swelling is seen to one side of the anus and extending into the anal canal. It is spherical in shape and covered by skin. It may rupture spontaneously through ulceration of the skin.
- *Palpation*: It is tender and firm or tense cystic in consistency. The emainder of the anal skin and anal canal is usually normal but there may be a palpable cord running up the anal canal from the hematoma. This is probably caused by thrombosis in the vein that has ruptured. Inguinal LNs should *not* be enlarged.

Perianal Abscess

- Early in the disease, when the abscess is small and confined to the inter-sphincteric space, the only finding may be a hot, tender, indurated area in the posterior or lateral anal canal. Fluctuation should never be waited for.
- If the abscess has been present for a time and expanded downwards, swelling and erythema of the anal verge occur.
- If on the other hand, the abscess has extended laterally into the ischiorectal fossa, tenderness over the buttocks will be present and a bulge may be felt adjacent to the rectum by PR.

Complicated Piles

- *Inspection*: The hemorrhoids are seen prolapsing **(Figure 5.9)**, congested, and edematous. They are purplish black in color and the mucous membrane looks unhealthy. Sloughing, ulceration and infection may follow.
- *Palpation*: They are tense and tender.

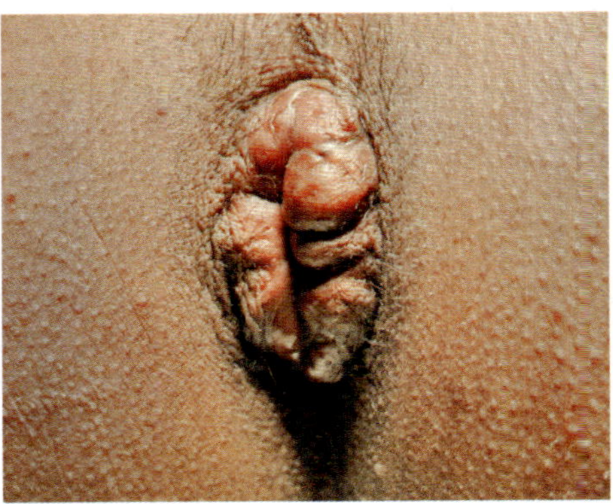

Fig. 5.9: Prolapsed hemorrhoids

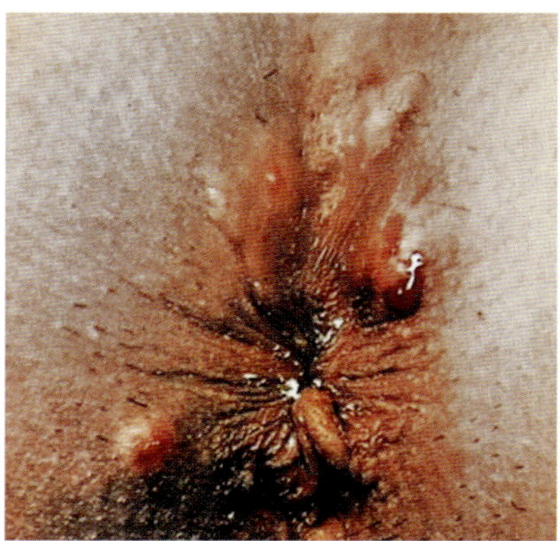

Fig. 5.10: Multiple perianal fistulae

Perianal Fistula

- *Inspection*: The following should be defined regarding the external opening: number, site (anterior or posterior), distance from the anal canal (the nearer the external opening from the anus, the lower is the fistula) and discharge **(Figure 5.10).**
- *Palpation*: The fistulous tract is felt and its relation to the ARMR is determined.
- *PR Exam*: The internal opening may be felt and other pathologies excluded, e.g. cancer.
- *Probe Test*: Not done because, it is painful, unreliable and may lead to the formation of a "false passage".
- *Good-Sall's Rule:* Fistulae with their external opening in the anterior 1/2 of the anus have their internal opening opposite the external one, while those with the external opening in the posterior half, have their internal opening in the midline, i.e. have curved or horseshoe tracks.
- *Proctoscopy and Sigmoidoscopy*: To show the internal opening and exclude underlying disease such as cancer, Crohn's disease, ulcerative colitis or TB.

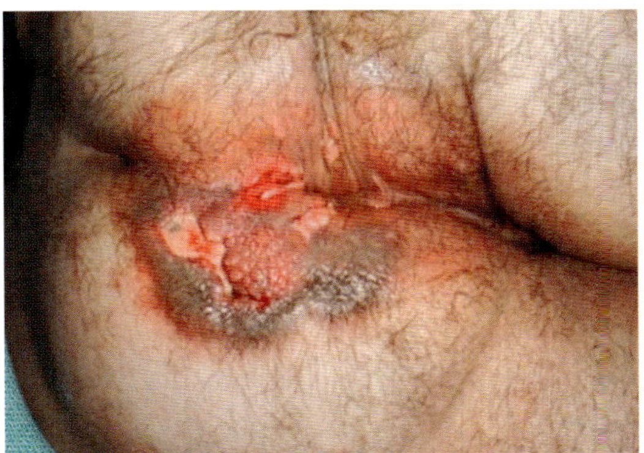

Fig. 5.11: Anal carcinoma (SCC)

Anal Carcinoma

- It shows as an ulcer with everted edges and indurated base **(Figure 5.11)**.
- It bleeds easily on touch.
- Superadded infection is common and causes a foul smell.
- Inguinal lymph nodes should be palpated for the presence of metastases.
- Carcinoma should be suspected if a fissure is not in its typical position and is persistent to treatment. Pain is due to infiltration of somatic sensory nerves supplying the anal verge.

Proctalgia Fugax

- It is a rare condition that causes severe episodic pain due to segmental spasm in the pubococcygeus muscle in young patients with anxiety and stress. Pain usually disappears spontaneously and suddenly.
- No abnormal signs are detected.

Pruritis Ani

- It means intractable itching around the anus due to irritation of the perianal skin and the skin lining the lower part of the anal canal, which causes the patient to scratch. This results in excoriation of the skin and possibly infection.

- Local examination is important to exclude fissures, fistulae, piles and thread worms.
- Scratch markings are usually evident. Perianal skin may be thrown into whitish, sodden, hyperkeratotic skin.
- Localized zone of dermatitis is seen where the skin of the buttocks appears to have rubbed together.
- The whole perianal skin may be red and blistered.

Key Points — Perineal Pain

- Pain in the perineum occurs with numerous lesions; other symptoms are almost well marked in every case.
- *Anal lesions* that cause perineal pain, include anal fissure, perianal abscess, perianal hematoma, prolapsed hemorrhoids, and proctalgia fugax.
- In *prostatic disease*, perineal pain is an indication of inflammation rather than of enlargement.
- In *prolapsed hemorrhoids*, pain may be referred to as heaviness or discomfort.
- When the presenting symptom is *only pain*, surgical correction must be viewed with the greatest caution.
- The diagnosis of *chronic idiopathic anal or perineal pain* is based upon a whole spectrum of arguments:
  1. Most patients are women, usually above the age of 50 years.
  2. The type and distribution of pain are unclear.
  3. Pain and its radiation do not follow the usual distribution of nerve segments.
  4. Pain has often been present for a long time, with many doctors have been consulted.
  5. Standard treatments are ineffective.
  6. It coexists with a special psychological profile, i.e. with a marked anxious or depressive connotation.
  7. There are no other causes.

8. PAIN IN THE TESTICLE

Pain in the testicle may be present in many conditions, which may be discussed under separate headings as follows:

- Diseases of the body of the testis or epididymis.
- Affections of the coverings of the testicle.
- Affections of the spermatic cord.
- A retained or misplaced testicle.
- Pain from lesions remote from the testis.

I. DISEASES OF BODY OF TESTIS OR EPIDIDYMIS

A. Inflammatory Lesions

Inflammatory lesions may attack the testis proper, or, as is more common, may begin in the epididymis.

Causes of Acute Epididymitis	Causes of Chronic Epididymitis	Causes of Acute Orchitis	Causes of Chronic Orchitis
1. Causes of urethral origin: gonorrheal urethritis, septic urethritis, passage of catheters, instru-mentation, infection behind a stricture 2. Ulceration about an impacted stone or a prostatic stone	1. Tuberculosis 2. Resolving acute epididymitis	1. Fevers: • Parotitis (mumps). • Typhoid. • Brucellosis. • Leptospirosis • Chicken-pox • Scarlet fever 2. Injury	1. Tuberculosis 2. Syphilis: • Diffuse interstitial orchitis. • Gummatus orchitis

Contd...

Contd...

3. Injections into posterior urethra 4. After operations on the prostate 5. Urinary infections 6. Non-specific epididymitis			

1. Acute Epididymitis

- It arises most commonly by spread of infection from the urethra via the vas deferens or by the lymphatics accompanying the vas. When any inflammation has reached the prostatic portion of the urethra, the orifices of the vasa deferentia may become infected, and inflammation spreads along the duct to the epididymis.
- Acute epididymitis begins as a painful thickening of the epididymis associated with febrile symptoms and pyuria, dysuria, frequency ± urethral discharge. The epididymis swells and a secondary effusion of exudate into the tunica vaginalis occurs (secondary hydrocele). The whole organ thus becomes enlarged, painful and tender. Pain is relieved by elevating and supporting the testis.
- Diagnosis is confirmed by history and finding gonococci in the discharge collected after prostatic massage. The prostate is firm and tender. Pressure on it may bring turbid prostatic fluid from the external urethral meatus.
- Acute epididymo-orchitis should be differentiated from *torsion of the cord* (*refer back*).

2. *Acute Orchitis*

- It usually occurs in eruptive fevers such as *mumps*, especially when it occurs in adolescents or adults. The testis becomes uniformly enlarged, extremely painful and tender. Acute hydrocele may be present. Both testes may be affected. Suppuration is unusual, but atrophy of the testis is rather more common.

- Much less often the testis may be affected in *typhoid, scarlet fever or influenza.*
- Less frequently, testicular inflammation may occur after a direct injury to the organ, such as a *blow or squeeze* !!

3. Tuberculous Epididymo-orchitis

- One or more nodule in the epididymis (behind the testis). They are hard, nodular and slightly tender. At first, the nodules are painless, but as they enlarge they cause dull ache. The cord is thickened, and vas beaded. A lax secondary hydrocele is present.
- If untreated, the skin of the *back* of the scrotum may become adherent and an ulcer is formed *posteriorly.*
- Rectal examination reveals a thickened, irregular, indurated seminal vesicle on the same side.

4. Syphilitic Disease of the Testis

- It causes very little testicular pain, but there is often a sense of dragging or heaviness. The outstanding feature is that it affects the body of the testis rather than the epididymis, thus differing greatly from TB.
- *Interstitial orchitis*: There is thickening of the intertubular connective tissue, with fibrous tissue infiltration, which may subsequently cause atrophy of the testis. The epididymis *rarely* shows nodularity.
- *Gumma of the testis*: Syphilis is now a rare condition. It presents as a painless lump in the testis or an enlargement of the whole testis. It is hard, and usually associated with slight tenderness on palpation or loss of testicular

sensation and secondary hydrocele. It may ulcerate through the skin of the scrotum *anteriorly*. The epididymis and cord are normal. A previous history of exposure to venereal disease followed by hard chancre and rash may be obtained.

B. Malignant Tumors of the Testis

- Malignant tumors of the testis may cause pain in the organ, but as a rule pain is experienced only in the *later stages*, as testicular sensation is completely lost.
- They affect young and adult men. The commonest types are **seminoma** (30–50 years) and **teratoma** (20–30 years).
- The usual presentation is a *painless* swelling or sense of heaviness of the testicle. Rarely, it is painful simulating epididymo-orchitis. The patient may present with symptoms of metastases, e.g. abdominal pain or swelling (para-aortic lymph nodes), cough, dyspnea and hemoptysis (lung secondaries), or bone aches (bone metastases).
- Examination reveals:
    1. A purely scrotal swelling, usually not tender. It is firm to hard, and smooth or irregular.
    2. Loss of testicular sensation.
    3. There may be secondary hydrocele.
    4. Para-aortic lymph nodes may be enlarged. Inguinal lymph nodes are involved only when skin is affected.
    5. There may be gynecomastia in patients with teratoma.
    6. In many teratomata and some seminomata, the anterior hypophyseal sex hormone (Prolan A) is present in the urine in sufficient quantities to give a +ve Aschheim-Zondek test (-ve finding being of little value).
- For differences between *mumps, syphilis and tumor of the testis refer back.*

C. Torsion of the Testis

- Testicular torsion on its vascular pedicle may occur in a testis that has a mesorchium or in an ectopic one.
- It occurs most commonly soon after puberty or in infants.
- There may be history of repeated attacks that may have even involved the other testis.
- At the moment of torsion, there is severe pain, which may be felt at first in the abdomen but is quickly localized to the testis.
- There is usually nausea and sometimes vomiting (it may mimic acute appendicitis). The testis forms a tense tender swelling in the upper part of the scrotum or at the external abdominal ring, and the scrotum below is empty (this sign helps to differentiate it from strangulated hernia or inflamed lymph node). For differentiation from acute epididymo-orchitis *refer back.*

D. Cysts of the Testis

- They occur most frequently in connection with epididymis, very rarely with body of testis.
- It is called "spermatocele" although all do not contain spermatozoa (term better avoided).
- The cysts may be multiple and/or bilateral, causing scrotal swelling and usually ache in the testis (by pressure upon, or stretching of epididymis), groin or lumbar region. They are usually placed above and to the outer side of the testis, occasionally behind it. They move with movement of the testis and can be distinguished from it by translucency. Their increase in size is very slow.
- They can be distinguished from hydrocele by their position relative to the testis and their colorless or slightly opalescent (contain *spermatozoa*) fluid, in distinction from the straw-colored clear fluid of hydrocele.

II. DISEASES OF COVERINGS OF THE TESTIS

Hydrocele

- *Primary vaginal hydrocele*: It usually arises slowly. The patient is well complaining of a lump or the *drag* it causes. The swelling is usually large, heavy, ovoid, tense and elastic rather than fluctuating. Neither the testis nor the epididymis can be felt apart from the swelling. It can be transilluminated. The testicular shadow will be felt at one edge of the swelling, usually behind.
- *Secondary hydrocele*: It follows disease of the testis or epididymis such as acute epididymo-orchitis, syphilitic orchitis, TB epididymitis, and new growths of the testis. The amount of fluid is usually small, and the swelling lax, so that the finger can touch the testis. The complaint is of the causative disease rather than of the hydrocele. Transillumination confirms the presence of fluid.
- A hydrocele must be distinguished from a *scrotal hernia, hematocele, cyst of the epididymis and tumor*.

Hematocele

- It has the physical characters of a hydrocele except that it is not translucent (i.e. opaque).
- Hematocele is due to tapping of hydrocele, trauma, torsion, or tumor of the testis, and its discovery is therefore the indication for exploration unless the history of trauma is recent and definite.
- Tapping may be required for diagnosis.
- If it becomes *chronic*, the blood will clot and will become hard simulating tumor or gumma.

Pyocele

- It is merely part of a suppurative process arising in the testis or the epididymis such as epididymo-orchitis.

- In addition to the enlarged, tender epididymis and testis, a cystic, tender swelling exists in front of and on the testis. It is *painful,* hot, red, tender, and the overlying skin is edematous.

III. DISEASES OF THE SPERMATIC CORD

- Tumors of the cord, lipomata, sarcomata (very rare), and hydroceles of the cord, cause no pain in the testis.
- Affections of the spermatic cord causing testicular pain include the following:
    1. *An inflammatory affection of the cord*:
       It is usually secondary to urethral infection (not uncommon).
    2. *TB infection of the cord*:
       It is practically never present without corresponding infection of the epididymis.
    3. *Varicocele*:
       A varicocele, especially if large, in a pendulous scrotum, causes dull aching pain in the testicle. It is most commonly left-sided. the characteristic feel of enlarged veins in the erect position, and the slight impulse and thrill on coughing, will readily point to the correct diagnosis.

IV. RETAINED OR MISPLACED (ECTOPIC) TESTIS

- An undescended or ectopic testicle **(Figure 5.12)** may suffer from diseases that affect the normally placed testis and thus cause pain. In addition, owing to the effect of recurrent muscular strains and the comparative immobility of the testis when retained in the inguinal canal, it is more liable to attacks of ***inflammation***.
- In the intra-abdominal position it remains protected from the muscular injury.

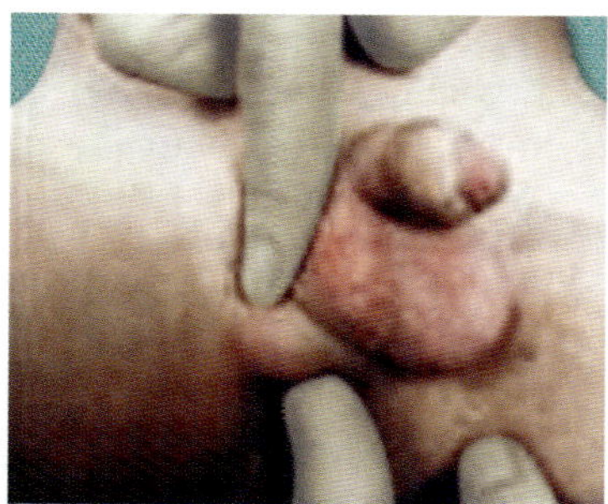

Fig. 5.12: Right ectopic testis

- In ectopic sites, it has a wider range of mobility and is thus more liable to torsion. A misplaced testis is liable to be the seat of ***malignant disease.***
- Inflammation of an undescended testis may be so acute as to cause *gangrene,* with or without torsion. Pain may be complained of first when the testes begin to enlarge at puberty (it may simulate appendicitis).
- The diagnosis of misplaced testis rests upon the fact that one side of the scrotum is empty, feeling the testis (if it lies in a palpable position), testicular sensation upon pressure and the recurrent attacks of pain.

V. TESTICULAR PAIN FROM EXTRA-TESTICULAR LESIONS

Pain may be felt in the testicle in the following situations:

1. A ***calculus*** is present in the renal pelvis or upper ureter.
2. Stimulation of the peripheral nerves by ***secondary deposits in the bodies of the lumbar vertebrae.***
3. Pressure from an ***extra-medullary intraspinal*** tumor such as neurofibroma, meningioma, or ependymoma, or the pressure of an ***aneurysm*** in this situation.
4. ***Appendiceal inflammation*** when the appendix turns down into the pelvis.
5. ***Neuralgia testis***, i.e. aching pain with no obvious cause, usually in patients with a neurotic tendency.

9. PAIN IN THE PENIS

Pain in the penis is a symptom, which occurs not only in association with lesions of the penis or urethra, but also as a referred pain from disease of the prostate, bladder, or kidney. Penile pain may be present either during or immediately after micturition, or may be entirely independent of the act. If pain is felt only during micturition there is probably some inflammatory lesions of the urethra or prostate; if it occurs *immediately after the flow of the urine* it suggests some lesions in the urinary bladder; pain present quite apart from micturition may be due to various diseases of the penis, bladder, ureter, or kidney.

I. CAUSES OF PAIN IN THE PENIS DURING MICTURITION

Diseases of Urethra

- Acute inflammation (gonorrheal or other).
- The passage or impaction of a calculus.
- Stricture of the urethra.
- Injury of the urethra.
- Foreign body in the urethra.

Diseases of the Prostate

- Acute prostatitis
- Prostatic abscess
- Prostatic carcinoma
- Prostatic calculus.

Diseases of the Bladder

- Acute cystitis
- Vesical calculus
- Papilloma
- Pedunculated carcinoma.

II. PENILE PAIN FOLLOWING MICTURITION

1. **Vesical**: Calculus, bilharziasis, TB, tumor (carcinoma, papilloma), acute cystitis.
2. **Ureteric**: Calculus in the lower end, descending ureteritis, descending TB.
3. **Prostate**: Acute inflammation, abscess, carcinoma, calculus.
4. **Vesicular**: Acute seminal-vesiculitis.
5. **Rectal**: Carcinoma.
6. **Anal**: Fissure or ulcer, inflamed hemorrhoids.

PAIN IN THE PENIS APART FROM MICTURITION

A. Local Lesions of the Penis and Urethra

1. *Balanitis.*
2. *Phimosis and Para-phimosis.*
3. *Lymphangitis of the penis* due to a septic sore or abrasion of the skin or mucous membrane.
4. *Herpes* of the skin of the prepuce or penile skin.
5. *Cordee*: Infiltration of the cavernous tissue of the penis causes pain during erection (as in urethritis).
6. *Chronic indurative cavernositis* (= Chronic form of Peyronie's disease): A condition of unknown etiology but similar to, and sometimes associated with, Dupuytren's contracture and retroperitoneal fibrosis. It causes pain during erection as well as lateral deviation of the organ.
7. A similar condition arises from *organized hematoma* in the cavernous tissues from a *local injury*, or spontaneously in blood disease, especially *lymphatic or myeloid leukemia.*
8. *Epithelioma of the penis*: On rare occasions, it gives pain in the organ.

B. Pain Referred from Disease Elsewhere

1. *Renal colic*:
   Renal colic accompanying the passage of a stone, blood clot or debris of caseous material may cause aching pain in the penis apart from the increase desire to pass urine. Penile pain in this condition is minimal compared to renal or ureteric pain.
2. *Acute appendicitis*:
   Few cases reported. All were pelvic in position.
3. *Anxiety state* or mental cause.

10. PAIN IN THE LOWER LIMBS

I. SCIATICA

The term "sciatica" is applied to pain radiating from the buttock, down the back of the thigh, and along the posterior or lateral aspect of the calf to the foot. Causes of sciatic pain include:

Affections of Nerve-Roots, Lumbosacral Plexus and Sciatic Nerve

1. Cauda Equina:

Neurofibroma (or other tumor), backward protrusion of intervertebral disk, irritation of the meninges by hemorrhage, infection and intrathecal injections, hydatid cyst, postherpetic neuralgia.

2. Lumbar Vertebrae

Disk lesions, spondylosis, Pott's disease, osteomyelitis, tumors, fracture-dislocations, spondylolisthiasis.

3. Lumbosacral Plexus

Cysts and tumors of the pelvic adnexa and rectum, the uterus during labor (due to pressure of the fetal head upon the lumbosacral trunk as it crosses the pelvic brim), pelvic inflammation (very rare).

4. Sciatic Nerve

Neurofibroma (other evidence of von Recklinghausen's disease, i.e. neurofibromatosis is suggestive), penetrating injuries.

Extraneural Causes

1. Sacroiliac Joints

Subluxation, tuberculous and non-tuberculous arthritis (pyogenic or osteoarhtritic), ankylosing spondylitis and other spondyloarthropathies.

2. Sacrum and Pelvic Bones

Primary and secondary neoplasms.

3. Soft Tissues

Cellulitis, gluteal bursitis, fat herniation (through the deep fascia and becomes strangulated may occasionally cause referred sciatica).

Key Points — Sciatica

- Commonest causes of sciatica are intervertebral discs (L4/5, L5/S 1), spondylosis, or sacroiliac disease.
- It is important to distinguish between sciatica due to implication of the *nerve or its roots* on one hand, and sciatic pain referred from extra-neural lesions on the other, as follows:
  1. Complaints of paresthesia, tingling or numbness always indicate involvement of the sensory pathways, but paresthesia may be absent. It never occurs in "referred" pain.
  2. Aggravation of pain and paresthesia by flexion of the hip (which stretches the cauda equina) indicates a root lesion.
  3. Pain down the leg on coughing occurs in root lesions, but occurs also in acute extra-neural disease of the spine, pelvis and sacroiliac joints; its value is therefore slight.
  4. Pain induced by straight-leg raising (Lasegue's sign) is more likely to be present in neural lesions than in others, but it is unreliable.
  5. Muscular weakness, sensory loss, and depression or loss of ankle-jerk, indicate a neural lesion.
     Wasting of muscles usually has the same significance, but may occur from disuse or pain from extra-neural disease.
- X-ray and lumbar puncture are desirable in every case.

II. PAIN IN THE FRONT AND SIDES OF THE THIGH

A. Pain Down the Front of the Thigh to the Knee

- It may be referred from the (1) hip as in TB and osteoarthrosis of the joint, (2) upper part of the iliac bone, or (3) the 2nd or 3rd lumbar vertebra.

- In such cases there may be wasting of the quadriceps, but there is no weakness, sensory loss, or interference with the patellar reflex. The presence of these neurological signs means that the pain is due to a lesion implicating the 2nd or 3rd lumbar roots or the femoral nerve itself.
- Most cases are due to spondylosis of upper lumbar vertebrae with protrusion of the upper lumbar disks. Some are due to diabetes and few are due to Pott's disease of the meninges and cauda equina.
- As with sciatica, X-ray and lumbar puncture are desirable in every case.

B. Obturator Pain

- Obturator pain, down the inner aspect of the thigh, results from:
  1. Disease of the hip joint (most common).
  2. Obturator hernia (rare).
  3. Gross neoplastic or inflammatory disease within the pelvis (rare).

C. Meralgia Paresthetica

- It means numbness and pain over the lateral aspect of the thigh due to entrapment of the lateral cutaneous nerve of the thigh as it passes from the pelvis under the lateral aspect of the inguinal ligament.
- Pain develops on exertion causing intermittent claudication, resembling ischemia.
- Sensory loss may be demonstrated over a variable area on the lateral aspect of thigh.

III. PAIN IN THE FOOT

Pain in the foot is usually due to a *local disease* or abnormality and *rarely* occurs as a *referred pain* from elsewhere, radicular or nonradicular.

A. Local Disease or Abnormality

1. Causes to be remembered include gout, rheumatoid arthritis, TB, bunions, plantar warts, calcanodynia from Reiter's disease or from a calcaneal spur, flat foot, metatarsalgia, and march fracture (pied force).
2. Raynaud's disease may cause severe pain in the toes. It is usually present in the fingers as well. Relationship of symptoms to cold makes diagnosis easy.
3. Erythromelalgia: Pain is burning and may be severe. It may be continuous or intermittent, and is aggravated by heat, dependency and walking. Hyperhidrosis of the foot is common. Pain is soon followed by the appearance of cutaneous flushing, going on to cyanosis and there is increased pulsation of the vessels. Tenderness is extreme and in long-standing cases, there is some edema of the affected part.

B. Referred Pain

1. Radicular (Root pain): Cases are occasionally encountered in which a sharp pain in the side of the foot, the big toe, the lateral border of the foot or ankle, has been the first manifestation of nerve root pain, but root pains usually spare the foot and favor the upper part of the limb.
2. Non-radicular: Painful feet are a feature of the polyneuritis caused by alcohol and arsenic, and are a conspicuous symptom in the neuropathy, which occurs in starvation.

IV. TABES DORSALIS

- The lightning pains of tabes dorsalis are, unlike the neuralgias, usually bilateral and not referred to the distribution of any particular peripheral nerve. The area in which a paroxysm of pain occurs is never much larger than the palm of a hand and it often remains hypersensitive for hours after the paroxysm has passed.

- The following points should be investigated carefully to reach a diagnosis: a history of syphilis, pupils not reacting to light but reacting to convergence, absent knee- and anklejerks, loss of sensation to pain below the knees and over the trunk and inner arms, lymphocytosis in the CSF, +ve TPI and VDRL tests in the blood and CSF (though they may be -ve).

V. VASCULAR CAUSES

Acute Ischemia

- Acute interruption of the blood supply usually results from embolism, thrombosis or trauma.
- The sequence of events is as follows: loss of sense of position, followed by loss of pressure sensation + anesthesia and intense pain. Motor loss then follows.

Chronic Ischemia

- Gradual diminution of the blood supply to the organ due to gradual occlusion of the lumen of the artery giving time for progressive opening of the collaterals.
- It results from atherosclerosis (most common cause) with or without thrombosis, Buerger's disease, spastic arterial diseases (e.g. Raynaud's disease), aneurysms and rarely syphilitic arteritis.

  It is aggravated by anemia.
- *Risk factors* include old age, males > females, smoking, diabetes mellitus, hypercholesterolemia and hypertension.
- *Clinical Presentation:*
  1. Intermittent Claudication:

     It means cramp-like pain or dull aching pain in a group of muscles after a certain amount of exercise that usually disappears by rest and reappears by an equal amount of exercise. The pain is due to "accumulation of metabolites" during exercise that stimulates the sensory nerve endings. They are gradually washed away during "rest". It usually occurs distal to the level of arterial obstruction, but because calf muscles do most of the work during walking and have the greatest metabolic needs, pain usually occurs in the calf regardless of the site of obstruction. About 50% of patients have associated severe coronary artery disease (the commonest cause of death is myocardial infarction).

2. Rest Pain:
   It is a late symptom indicating advanced ischemia and severe tissue starvation. It typically occurs in *the toes and forefoot* during the night, which awakens the patient from sleep. Temporary relief is obtained by dangling the limb over the side of the bed or getting up and walking (i.e. it improves with dependency or gravity). Pain increases by elevation and warmth. It is not affected by analgesics.
3. Muscle Cramps:
   Sudden nocturnal painful contractions of calf muscles that last for a few minutes only.
4. Ischemic (Arterial) Ulceration:
   A typical arterial punched out ulcer that usually occurs on the toes, heel, dorsum of foot or lower 1/3 of leg, after trivial trauma.

Deep Vein Thrombosis

- *High Risk Patients*: Old age (> 40 years), obesity, trauma (injury, burns, parturition), postoperative (3-7 days), prolonged or complex procedures, immobility (leg immobilization or paralysis), history of prior "phlebitis,

DVT, or PE", central venous catheter, malignancy (visceral carcinoma), congestive heart failure, and acute myocardial infarction.

- *Clinical Picture*: DVT can be completely *asymptomatic* in about 1/3 of cases. *Early manifestations* include aching pain and heaviness on moving the calf or thigh, frog-leg position of the involved leg, tenderness on pressure on the instep of the sole of the foot, and tenderness along the affected veins.
- *Obstructive Manifestations* include swelling, cyanosis, warmth, and varicose veins (late sign).

Key Points — Leg Pain

Vascular Causes
- Atherosclerosis
- Buerger's disease
- Abdominal coarctation
- Popliteal entrapment syndrome
- Chronic compartment syndrome
- Venous claudication
- Deep vein thrombosis (DVT)

Degenerative and Neurological Causes
- Peripheral neuropathies and neurospinal disorders (sciatica due to prolapsed disc) (precipitated by heavy weight and straining, not by walking).

Orthopedic Causes
- Osteoarthritis (X-ray picture, absence of local manifestations of chronic ischemia, restricted joint movements).

Trauma
- Fractures
- Dislocations
- Ligament rupture.

Infection
- Cellulitis
- Osteomyelitis.

Tumors
- Primary (osteogenic sarcoma)
- Secondaries.

11. PAIN IN THE UPPER LIMBS

I. LOCAL CAUSES

Trauma

- Fractures.
- Dislocation.
- Ligament tears.

Inflammation

- Cellulitis.
- Osteomyelitis.

Bone Tumors

- Primary (osteogenic sarcoma).
- Secondaries.

Vascular Causes

- Atherosclerosis.
- Buerger's disease.
- Thrombosis, etc.

Orthopedic Causes

- Osteoarthritis.

II. REFERRED PAIN

Pain referred to the upper limb from the lower cervical area and the region of the brachial plexus may result from the following:

Lesions in the Cervical Spine and Cord

- Disc lesions.
- Spondylosis.

- Syringomyelia.
- Fracture-dislocations.
- Tumors of the spinal cord.
- Post-herpetic neuralgia.
- Tumors of the spine.
- Paralytic radiculitis.
- Pachymeningitis cervicalis.
- Pott's disease.
- Tumors of the meninges and roots.

Lesions of the Brachial Plexus

- Cervical ribs.
- Malignant and inflammatory infiltration from the apex of the lung.
- Costoclavicular compression.
- Pressure of subclavian aneurysm.
- Scalenus anterior syndrome.

Pain Referred from Viscera

- Angina pectoris and coronary thrombosis.
- Syphilitic aortitis.

Pain Referred from Extraneural Lesions

- Periarthritis of the shoulder joint.
- Tendonitis of the long head of the biceps.
- Tendonitis of the supraspinatus tendon.

CHAPTER

6

Differential Diagnosis of Dyspepsia

DYSPEPSIA

Patients with dyspepsia suffer from such complaints as pain or discomfort or vaguely unpleasant sensation in the abdomen, vomiting, flatulence, alteration of appetite, heartburn, or acidity. The subject of dyspepsia involves those causes in which the alimentary tract is free from abnormality, those in which the digestive organs are diseased (organic dyspepsia), and those in which they are structurally intact but functionally disturbed (functional dyspepsia).

I. SIMULATION OF SYMPTOMS OF DYSPEPSIA BY OTHER CONDITIONS

The Vomiting of Pregnancy

Pregnancy should always be thought of when a young woman complains of vomiting and vague indigestion. In some cases, the woman herself may be unaware of her pregnant state.

Cerebral Vomiting

In children particularly, meningitis or tumor may cause vomiting that may be mistaken for dyspepsia. Signs of cerebral irritation (photophobia, squint, irritability, headache, Kernig's sign, etc.) point to meningitis, while paralyses, headache and optic neuritis point to tumor. CSF examination may be required.

Uremia

It may cause loss of appetite and vomiting (*uremic gastritis*). The uremic odor in breath, mental blurring, high arterial tension, proteinuria and high blood urea confirm the diagnosis.

Pulmonary TB

It is associated with loss of appetite, and nausea, with or without vomiting. Careful clinical and radiological examination of the chest as well as sputum should not be omitted to reach diagnosis.

Gastric Crises of Tabes (Syphilis)

Paroxysmal marked vomiting with severe abdominal pain is the usual form patients assume that may even simulate gastric perforation. Absent knee jerks and non-reactive pupils to light make diagnosis easy if they are present. Serological tests of the blood and CSF may determine the diagnosis.

Chronic Intestinal Obstruction (Cancer Colon)

There is abdominal pain and vomiting. Examination reveals abdominal distention often with visible peristalsis and a history of gradually increasing constipation. X-ray and endoscopy will reveal the diagnosis.

Cholecystitis

When a patient, particularly a middle-aged woman, complains of abdominal spasms and nausea, the possibility of cholecystitis should be considered. Examination reveals tenderness in the right hypochondrium or +ve Murphy's sign. An ultrasound will confirm or dispute the clinical diagnosis.

Recurrent Appendicitis

The pain may have the character of typical "*hunger pain*" and relieved by alkalis, thus pointing to the stomach rather than the appendix. It should be always thought of especially in children.

Angina Pectoris

In one of its forms it may be accompanied by *flatulence*. Presence of symptoms on exertion, radiation of pain to left arm, presence of hypertension, and relief by vasodilators point to the right diagnosis.

Chronic Bronchitis

Dyspneic patients may experience discomfort in the upper abdomen and flatulence.

Migraine

The chief diagnostic point is the occurrence of severe headache and visual disturbance with or before the gastric symptoms, and the periodicity of the attacks.

Acute Glaucoma

Vomiting is generally an accompaniment.

Extra-abdominal Causes of Pain

These are often attributed by patients to indigestion such as *pleurisy, tumor of the spine, and aortic aneurysm.*

Nervous or Hysterical Vomiting

Diagnosis must be made largely by the method of exclusion. The patient is usually a woman, and other signs of hysteria will be present.

Eructio Nervosa

It is due to swallowing of air (*aerophagy*). It is also described as dyspepsia.

Porphyria

It may cause acute abdominal pains described by the patient as acute indigestion.

II. ORGANIC VERSUS FUNCTIONAL DYSPEPSIA

- If *loss of weight and/or severe pain* are prominent symptoms, the disease is probably **organic**.
- If these are absent, and the affection has persisted for some time, it is more likely to be a **functional** disorder.
- *Functional pain* tends to be present continuously, day in and day out, year after year, compared to periodicity of *organic pain*.

III. CAUSES OF ORGANIC DYSPEPSIA

The chief organic diseases of the **stomach,** which have to be thought of, are the following:

Carcinoma

- *Age and sex:* Usually above 50 years. Men are more affected than women (3:1).
- *Mechanical effects:* Large tumor in the *antrum* → pyloric obstruction (**Figure 6.1**), large tumor in the *cardia* → dysphagia, in the *middle* of stomach → filling dyspepsia (**Figure 6.2**).

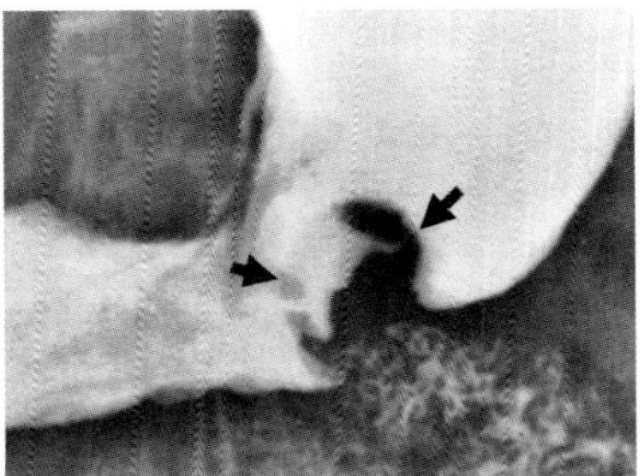

Fig. 6.1: Gastric carcinoma – pyloric region

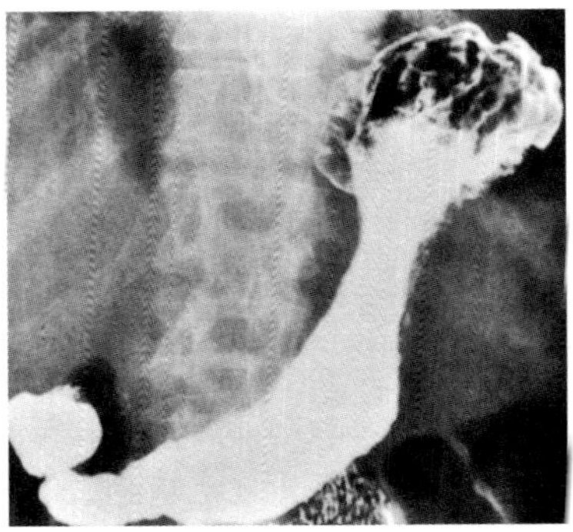

Fig. 6.2: Gastric carcinoma – body of the stomach

- *Ulcerative type* → dyspeptic manifestations similar to gastric ulcer. It can be differentiated from chronic PU by older age, anorexia, shorter duration with persistent symptoms (not periodic), continuous pain which ↑ by food and *not* relieved by vomiting or alkalis, and by foul coffee ground material due to altered blood.
- A tumor of the body of the stomach causes *no* early interference with gastric function. ***It is characterized by 3A***: **A**norexia (→ loss of weight), **A**thenia (→ weakness), and **A**nemia (→ pallor). H*emorrhage* (hematemesis/melena) and *perforation* may occur.

- *Latent (Silent) type:* Remains symptomless until signs of dissemination appear such as jaundice, ascites, Krukenberg tumor, and Virchow's lymph nodes (*Troisier's sign*).
- The patient may present with a *mass* in the epigastrium, or below the left costal margin.
- *Investigations:* Laboratory (anemia, occult blood in stools), radiological, endoscopy and biopsy.

Gastric Ulcer

- Characteristically, pain comes after food and decreased by vomiting. It occurs in "attacks of a few weeks" duration separated by free intervals. Hematemesis is confirmatory but is absent in the majority.
- Radiology (**Figure 6.3**) and endoscopy should be done.

Gastritis

- There is loss of appetite and fullness with a sense of oppressive weight in the epigastrium. Pain is not a feature but nausea is common and vomiting may occur.

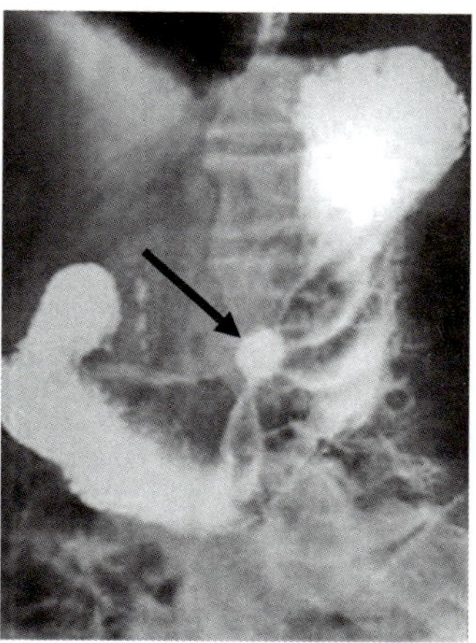

Fig. 6.3: Gastric ulcer at the lesser curvature

- Diagnosis is made with certainty by endoscopy and biopsy.

Gastric Dilatation

- There is enlargement of the stomach and stagnation of the contents.
- A gastric splash is present, and peristalsis may be visible. There is history of projectile vomiting containing undigested food.
- Radiology shows delayed gastric emptying (**Figure 6.4**).
- It has to be differentiated from "*hour-glass stomach*", which is more common in women than in men and is diagnosed by X-ray examination, which shows the division of the stomach into 2 pouches. There usually is a history of chronic peptic ulcer that caused cicatrization.

Hiatal Hernia

- There is flatulence and retrosternal pain which by standing or lying on the back, or the left side or on wearing tight belts or corset.

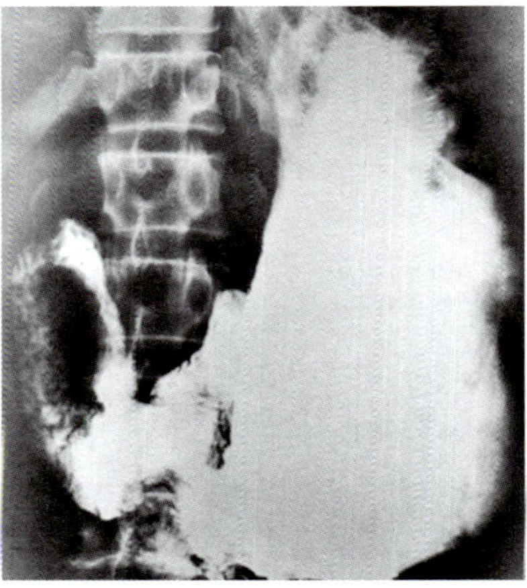

Fig. 6.4: Acute gastric dilatation

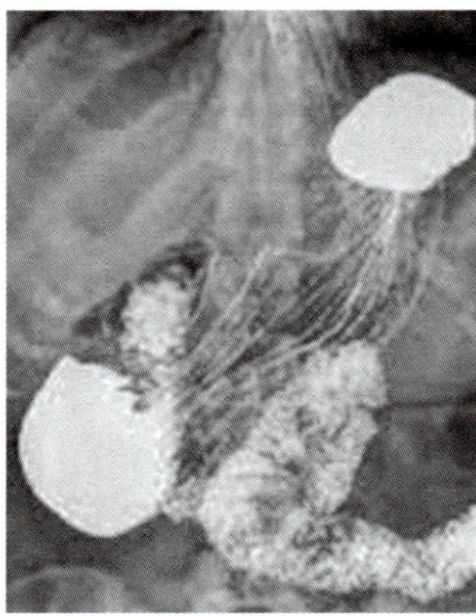

Fig. 6.5: Hiatal hernia

- Barium meal, in the Trendelenburg position shows either part of the fundus rolled up in the chest (*rolling type*) or the upper part of the stomach has sledded into the chest (*sliding type*) (**Figure 6.5**) with loss of the gastroesophageal angle and regurgitation of acid into the esophagus, which is confirmed by *endoscopy*.

IV. CAUSES OF FUNCTIONAL DYSPEPSIA

Dietetic Causes

These include unsuitable badly cooked unpalatable food, hasty meals, overeating, underfeeding, abuse of alcohol, tea, tobacco or drugs.

Physical Causes and Bad Habits

These include imperfect chewing, defective teeth, oral sepsis, deficient exercise, general and local infective disease such as pulmonary TB and severe anemia.

Mental Causes

Overwork, especially extending into the periods of eating and digestion can cause dyspepsia.

Emotional Causes

Emotional causes include shock, love affairs, and in general, a faulty mental or nervous adjustment, which will include worry and anxiety, states, hysteria and hypochondriasis.

CHAPTER

7

Differential Diagnosis of Dysphagia

DYSPHAGIA

Dysphagia means painless difficulty in swallowing while *odynophagia* means painful difficulty in swallowing.

FUNCTIONAL GRADES OF DYSPHAGIA

Grade I	Requires liquids with meals.
Grade II	Able to take semi-solids, but not solids.
Grade III	Able to take liquids only.
Grade IV	Unable to take liquids, but able to swallow saliva.
Grade V	Unable to swallow saliva.

CAUSES OF DYSPHAGIA

Causes at the Oral Level (Mouth and Tongue)

1. **Inflammation:** Stomatitis, glossitis, tonsillitis.
2. **Ulcers:** E.g. Tuberculous or malignant ulcers of the tongue.
3. **Cleft palate**.
4. **Palatal paralysis** (due to diphtheria in children, or bulbar in adults).

Causes at the Pharyngeal Level (Larynx and Pharynx)

In the Lumen	In the Wall	Outside the Wall
Foreign bodies (impaction)	1. Inflammatory: • Acute pharyngitis • Laryngitis • TB 2. Malignancy • Spasm • Hysterical 3. Plummer-Vinson syndrome 4. Bulbar paralysis	1. Retropharyngeal abscess 2. Cervical lymph nodes 3. Malignant tumors

Causes at the Esophageal Level

Congenital

1. Atresia (with or without TE fistula).
2. Stenosis.
3. Short esophagus.
4. Hiatal hernia.
5. Dysphagia lusoria.

Acquired

In the Lumen	In the Wall	Outside the Wall
Foreign bodies, including food	1. Stricture (traumatic, corrosive, reflux) 2. Carcinoma 3. Benign tumors 4. Motility disorders (e.g. achalasia, scleroderma) 5. PVS 6. Schatzki's ring (circumferential web at cardia) 7. Tetanus	1. Pharyngeal pouch 2. Retrosternal goiter 3. Mediastinal lymph nodes and tumors 4. Periesophagitis 5. Paraesophageal hiatal hernia (HH) 6. Tight esophageal hiatal repair 7. Aortic aneurysm

Contd...

Contd...

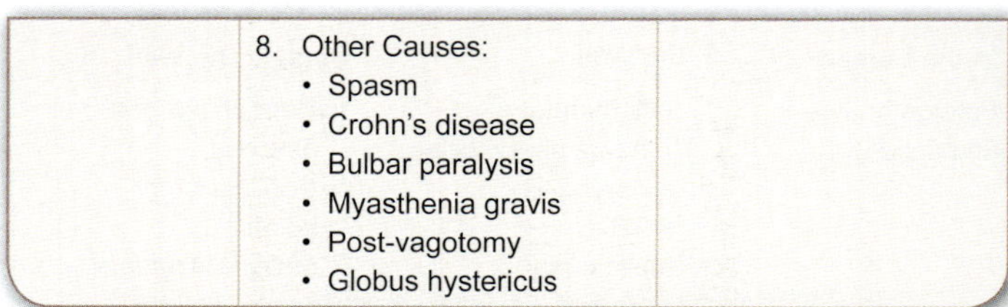

	8. Other Causes: • Spasm • Crohn's disease • Bulbar paralysis • Myasthenia gravis • Post-vagotomy • Globus hystericus	

NB Most common causes of dysphagia:

1. Achalasia
2. Hiatal Hernia
3. Esophageal cancer
4. Reflux stricture.

DIFFERENTIAL DIAGNOSIS

For differential diagnosis, dysphagia is considered to result from (I) mechanical obstruction to the esophagus, (II) nervous causes without obstruction, (III) mechanical defects of the mouth or pharynx, and (IV) pain, which causes the patient to refrain from swallowing despite absence of mechanical obstruction.

I. MECHANICAL OBSTRUCTION TO THE ESOPHAGUS

Carcinoma of the Esophagus

- The patient is usually, an elderly man with inability to swallow, at first solids and then liquids, of recent onset and slow progressive course. The patient gradually loses weight and becomes dehydrated and emaciated.
- *Barium swallow* shows the typical "rat tail appearance" (**Figure 7.1**) and *esophagoscopy* shows the malignant lesion.

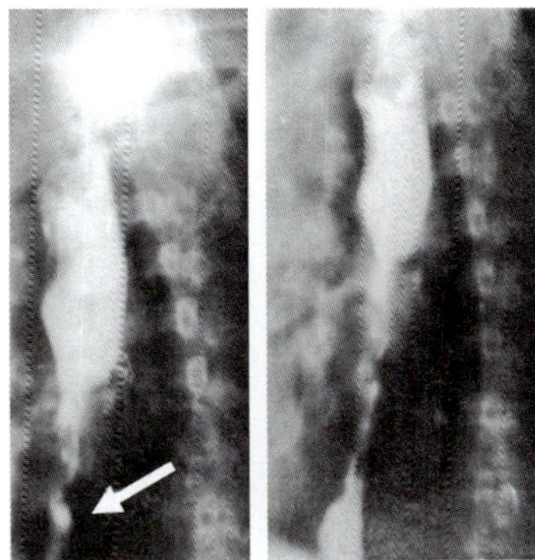

Fig. 7.1: Cancer esophagus (rat tail appearance)

- The differentiation between carcinoma of the lower esophagus (*squamous cell carcinoma*) and infiltration of the esophagus by a carcinoma starting at the cardiac end of the stomach (*adenocarcinoma*) is very difficult, and may be reached only by *biopsy* (endoscopic).

Corrosive Stricture

- The patient, usually a child, complains of dysphagia after a history of drinking a corrosive material, usually *accidental*. Intake in adults may be *suicidal*.
- The barium swallow shows narrowing of a long segment (stricture) (**Figure 7.2**), or more than one segment.

Congenital Stricture of Esophagus

- It is suspected if a newborn exhibits respiratory distress immediately on being fed.
- Passage of a soft rubber catheter revealed obstruction, which will be confirmed by the installation of a few drops of lipiodol and X-ray examination.

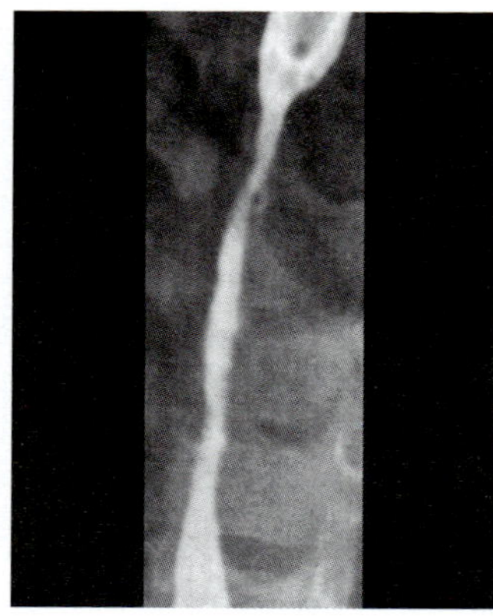

Fig. 7.2: Corrosive stricture 3 months after caustic injury

- Usually there is a fistulous communication between the lower esophageal segment and the trachea (Tracheo-esophageal fistula).

Hiatal Hernia (Causing Peptic Esophagitis)

- It usually becomes manifest in late middle life.
- The patient complains of:
  1. Dysphagia
  2. Retrosternal pain
  3. Regurgitation
  4. May be hematemesis.
- There is a typical history of heartburn and reflux on lying down and bending over.
- Barium meal in the Trendelenburg's position shows part of the stomach in the chest.

Aortic Aneurysm (*Compressing the Esophagus*)

- The aneurysm most likely to compress the esophagus from outside is the one affecting the *descending thoracic aorta,* behind the heart, where it can be neither felt nor heard, and in a situation unlikely to cause the conventional physical signs, i.e. inequality of the pulses, inequality of the pupils (from interference with the cervical sympathetic), paralysis of a vocal cord (from interference with left RLN), tracheal tugging, or pain down either arm.

- The only effects besides esophageal obstruction to be due to an aneurysm in this position are: (1) pain in the dorsal region of the spine, possibly radiating along the course of one of the intercostal nerves towards the left and simulating neuralgia, and perhaps (2) obstruction to the lower part of the root of the left lung, causing impairment of note, of air-entry, or of voice-sounds, with or without some crackling rales over the left lower lobe behind.
- *Chest X-ray* is essential preferably an oblique view (the best to show lesions in the posterior mediastinum), to avoid obscuring the aneurysm by the heart shadow in front of it.
- A history of syphilis and evidence of syphilitic aortic regurgitation, especially in a man between the ages of 40 and 50 years, would render the diagnosis of aneurysm likely.
- When an aortic aneurysm can be excluded, information as to the nature of esophageal obstruction can be obtained by *esophagoscopy*.

Pharyngeal Pouch (Diverticulum)

- The patient, usually an old man, complains of dysphagia with the appearance of a swelling in the neck, which is resonant and compressible (yielding undigested food or causing irritative cough).
- The pouch does not obstruct the esophagus until it becomes much distended by the gradual accumulation

of swallowed food in it; relief occurring when the greatly distended sac empties itself back into the esophagus.
- Barium fills the diverticulum.

Carcinoma of the Thyroid Gland

- The patient complains of dysphagia, usually associated with dyspnea and hoarseness of voice, together with a swelling in the lower part of the neck.
- The swelling takes the shape of the thyroid gland (may be irregular), compressing or most likely involving the esophagus. Mobility with deglutition may be restricted due to malignant infiltration.

Dysphagia Lusuria

- A very rare condition due to esophageal compression by an aberrant right subclavian artery, which arises from the aorta beyond the left subclavian and passes to the right side, in front of or behind the esophagus.
- Diagnosis is difficult and may be suspected only if there are other congenital anomalies, e.g. transposition of viscera. It may manifest itself as chronic superior mediastinal compression.

Impacted Foreign Bodies

- Esophageal obstruction may occur after swallowing a foreign body e.g. a tooth-plate, a large piece of bone, or a coin.
- Diagnosis is easy by history taking, X-ray and esophagoscopy, which at the same time, is therapeutic.

II. DYSPHAGIA DUE TO NERVOUS CAUSES

Achalasia of the Cardia

The patient, usually a young or middle-aged female, complains of repeated attacks of dysphagia, more to liquids than to

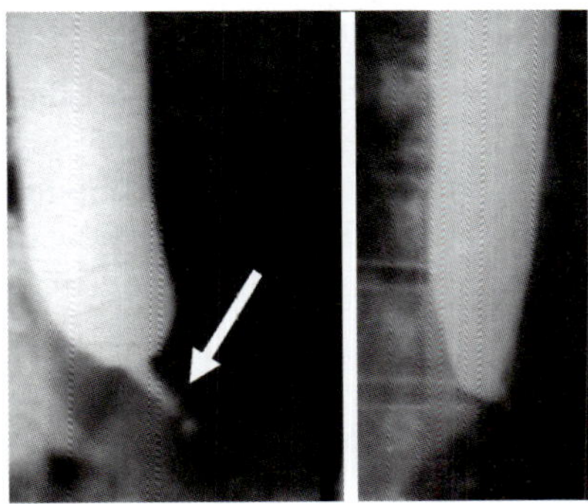

Fig. 7.3: Achalasia of the cardia (smooth pencil)

solids. In spite of the long history (years), the patient is relatively in good health with little wasting or dehydration. At times the patient *cannot* swallow though a mercury-*bougie* passes perfectly well. Whatever the pathology, the esophagus becomes more dilated and hypertrophied from the cardia upwards. *Barium swallow* shows a smooth tapering lower end of esophagus (*smooth pencil*) with marked dilatation above, and absence of the fundic gas bubble (**Figure 7.3**). *Esophagoscopy* reveals non-relaxation of the cardiac end, but can be passed by the esophagoscope (opposite to cancer esophagus).

Plummer-Vinson Syndrome

The patient, almost always a *woman*, middle-aged, with marked iron deficiency *anemia* complains of dysphagia; the food being arrested at the level of the cricoid cartilage due to spasm of the circular muscle fibers of the pharyngo-esopahgeal sphincter. It is associated with the formation of webs. Glazing of the tongue, spooning of the nails and enlargement of the spleen are also present.

Post-diphtheritic Dysphagia

It is characterized by regurgitation of food *through the nose* due to paralysis of the soft palate. There may be history of sore throat and *Klebs-Loeffler bacilli* may still be found is a swab from the throat. There may be paralysis of the ciliary muscles of the eyes or other signs of peripheral neuritis.

Globus Hystericus

Spasm of the muscular coat of the esophagus and pharynx is probably the cause of dysphagia in globus hystericus. Diagnosis is not difficult if the patient is a young woman who has suffered from other functional nervous affections such as *hysterical* aphonia.

Bulbar Paralysis

There is progressive disability in the use of the lips, tongue, pharynx, and larynx which points at once to the diagnosis.

Syphilitic Degeneration

Syphilitic degeneration of the medullary centers may be differentiated from *bulbar paralysis* by the simultaneous affection of other cranial nerves, particularly those of the eyeball. There may be also +ve history of syphilis, with or without a +ve serological reaction in the blood of CSF.

Lead Poisoning and Alcoholism

These may also be responsible for degenerative lesions, which affect the nerves concerned in the process of swallowing.

Rabies

Spasticity may occur in *hydrophobia* in which any effort to swallow liquids produces the symptom in a severe degree. History of *dog-bite* is the chief point in arriving at diagnosis.

Tetanus

Similar spasm occurs in case of tetanus and causes dysphagia.

Acute Encephalitis Lethargica

Acute dysphagia may precede coma, and the patient being in a state of delirium at the same time. A lesser degree of the condition may occur in Parkinson's disease.

Botulism (*Poisoning by the Bacillus botulinus*)

The patient feels nauseated 6–24 hours after ingesting the infected preserved food, vomits and has difficulty in swallowing even water, the tongue feels stiff, the muscles of deglutition become ineffective, the voice becomes husky and weakens until there is complete aphonia and aphagia. The t° is often raised and the pulse rate is raised. The eyes exhibit asymmetrical ptosis or strabismus. Vomiting may persist with headache and abdominal cramps, drowsiness supervenes, deepens to coma, and the patient dies of respiratory failure within a few days of the onset of the illness.

Myasthenia Gravis

The muscles of the neck, eye, larynx and mouth become fatigued rapidly and are involved early. Difficulty in swallowing occurs after the first few mouthfuls. The *myasthenic electrical reaction* serves to distinguish these cases from those due to bulbar paralysis. The therapeutic test by *neostigmine* is diagnostic.

III. MECHANICAL DEFECTS OF MOUTH AND PHARYNX

- This group of cases includes patients suffering from such conditions as *wide cleft palate, syphilitic stenosis of the pharynx, inability to use the tongue,* either because it is acutely swollen from glossitis, bee-sting, or Ludwig's angina, or because it is fixed from carcinomatous inflammation and so forth.

- *Mumps, quinsy, tuberculous caries of the cervical spine, retropharyngeal abscess, and carcinoma of the hypopharynx* belong to the same group (the latter causes more dyspnea than dysphagia and being confined to early childhood).

IV. PAIN - BUT NO MECHANICAL OBSTRUCTION

Inflammatory Affections of the Mouth or Tongue

- *Stomatitis:* All types of stomatitis cause pain that causes the patient to refrain from swallowing.
- *Pemphigus or erythema bullosum of buccal cavity,* evidenced by similar skin eruption.
- *Ulcers of the tongue,* whether malignant, gummatous, tuberculous, actinomycotic, leprous or due to chronic streptococcal glossitis, or due to erosion by a carious tooth.

Laryngeal Diseases

- *Sore throat* of various kinds.
- *Laryngitis*: *Acute laryngitis, TB laryngitis, syphilis, carcinomatous ulceration* of the larynx.

CHAPTER

8

Differential Diagnosis of Constipation

CONSTIPATION

DEFINITION

The symptom of constipation has different meaning for different individuals. It has an objective component that can be measured and a subjective component, which is experiential.

Objectively

It may be defined in terms of:

1. Weight: < 35 gm (normal = 35-225 gm).
2. Frequency: < 5 times/week when eating high residue diet (normal = > 5 times/week) or < 3 times/week, if on regular diet.

Subjectively

It may be defined in terms of:

1. Infrequency of bowel motion.
2. Hard consistency of stools.
3. Difficult expulsion of stools, straining during defecation, sensation of anal blockage.
4. Feeling of incomplete evacuation after defecation.

COMMON COMPLICATIONS OF CONSTIPATION

- Abdominal pain and aggravation of cancer pain in patients with abdominal or retroperitoneal malignancy.
- Abdominal distension and discomfort.
- Nausea and vomiting.
- Overflow diarrhea.
- Hemorrhoids and anal fissures.
- Bowel pseudo-obstruction.
- Urinary retention.

PATHOPHYSIOLOGY

Abnormalities of Colonic Motility

Constipation of colonic origin may be caused by:

1. Excessive smooth muscle activity as in distal spasticity, which prevents effective propulsion.
2. Atonicity of colonic musculature.

From radio-opaque marker studies, patients with constipation are divided into 3 categories:

1. *Colonic inertia:* The marker stagnates along the entire colon.
2. *Hindgut dysfunction:* Transit time is normal in the ascending colon only.
3. *Outlet obstruction*: Delayed passage through the rectoanal structures.

Colonic Absorption

- Excessive absorption of water in the large bowel contributes to constipation.
- It results from delayed transit and prolonged storage.

ETIOLOGY

Drug-induced Constipation

Some medications can cause constipation. These include:

- Analgesics and narcotics.
- Antacids (Ca and Al compounds).
- Anticholinergics, anticonvulsants, antidepressants, antiparkinson drugs, and antihypertensives (Calcium channel blockers).
- Barium sulfate, bisthmus compounds, diuretics and hematenics (iron compounds).

Metabolic and Endocrine Disorders

- *Metabolic:* DM (diabetic ketoacidosis, neuropathy), porphyria, uremia, hypokalemia.
- *Endocrine:* Panhypopituitarism, hypo- or hyperthyroidism, hypercalcemia (due to hyperparathyroidism, milk-alkali syndrome, or carcinomatosis), pheochromocytoma, glucagonoma.

Systemic Disorders

- Amyloidosis
- Systemic lupus erythematosis (SLE)
- Scleroderma.

Neurogenic Constipation

Peripheral

- Aganglionosis (Hirschsprung's disease).
- Ganglioneuromatosis: Primary, Von-Recklinghausen's, MEN type IIB.
- Autonomic neuropathy: Paraneoplastic, pseudo-obstruction.
- Chaga's disease.

Central

- *Spinal cord*: Cauda equina lesion, meningocele, tabes dorsalis, multiple sclerosis.
- *Brain*: Parkinsonism, tumors, cerebrovascular accidents.

Constipation due to Bowel Disorders

1. Colonic Disorders

Mechanical Disorders

- *Extraluminal:* Tumors, chronic volvulus, hernias, rectal prolapse.
- *Luminal:* Tumors, strictures, chronic diverticulitis, chronic amebiasis, ischemic colitis, LGI, syphilis, TB, corrosive enema, surgery.

Functional Disorders

- *Mucosal*: Ulcerative colitis.
- *Muscular*: Diverticular disease, irritable bowel syndrome, myotonic dystrophy, systemic sclerosis, dermatomyositis.

2. Rectal Disorders

Rectocele.

3. Anal Disorders

Mechanical Disorders

- Stenosis.

Functional Disorders:

- Anal fissure, mucosal prolapse, puborectalis syndrome.

EVALUATION OF PATIENTS WITH SEVERE CHRONIC CONSTIPATION

1. *Onset of constipation:* Most of congenital types as Hirschsprung's disease present since "birth". Some others present at any time during the first decade.

2. *Search for the cause:* Constipation is NOT a disease. It is a symptom of many diseases or disorders, or it may be drug-induced.
3. *Physical examination:*
   a. Digital examination of the rectum and vagina is mandatory:
      - Anal lesions (chronic fissure) and cancer of pelvic organs are often easily detected.
      - Presence of large masses of feces (fecal impaction).
      - Absent anal and perianal sensation indicates a neurological lesion.
      - Excessive perineal descent on straining suggests a mechanical obstruction.

   b. Abdominal examination for:
      - Tenderness.
      - Masses.
      - Gaseous or fluid distension.
4. *Radiological and endoscopic studies (sigmoidoscopy or colonoscopy)* of the large bowel: Endoscopy and barium enema should be carried out without delay to rule out an inflammatory or neoplastic lesion of the colon if:
   a. The constipation is severe and of recent onset.
   b. The bowel disturbance is accompanied by weight loss.
   c. Loss of blood or mucus has occurred.
   d. The patient is febrile or has general malaise.
5. *Proctoscopy*: It identifies fissures, hemorrhoids, and ulceration or redness of the anterior rectal wall, suggesting solitary rectal ulcer or anterior mucosal prolapse.
6. *Studies of colonic transit time*: By following the progression of radio-opaque markers along the colon by daily abdominal films, the segmental colonic transit time can be evaluated.
7. *Ano-rectal manometry* for:
   a. Diagnosis of outlet obstruction induced by hypertonic or hypotonic rectum.

   b. Diagnosis of anal achalasia.
   c. Evaluation of the anorectal inhibitory reflex.
8. *Biopsy:*
   a. Rectal suction biopsy in infants, 15 mm above the dentate line → diagnosis of Hirschsprung's disease (25 mm above the distal edge of the internal sphincter).
   b. Biopsy can also aid in the diagnosis of autonomic neuropathy in adults with severe constipation as a paraneoplastic manifestation.
9. *Dietary trial:* To evaluate patients whose constipation is due to low-residue diet: A diet containing 30 g/d of dietary fiber is given and the patient should carefully note the number of stools and consistency. A man should normally pass > 5 motions/week and a woman > 3 motions/week.
10. *Psychiatric evaluation:* This is resorted to when the cause of constipation remains unknown in spite of extensive investigation.

PERTINENT QUESTIONS THAT MAY AID IN DIAGNOSIS OF CONSTIPATION

- Most people do not need extensive testing and can be treated with changes in diet and exercise. For example, in young people with mild symptoms, a medical history and physical examination may be all the doctor needs to suggest successful treatment. The tests the doctor performs depend on the duration and severity of the constipation, the person's age, and whether blood in stools, recent changes in bowel movements, or weight loss has occurred.
- The doctor may need to ask a patient to describe his or her constipation in details. The following are pertinent questions, which may aid in the diagnosis of constipation:

Question	Possible Diagnosis/ Comments
Does the patient seldom feel like going to the toilet?	Colonic inertia or megacolon
Does the patient feel like going to the toilet, but has considerable difficulty in evacuating the stool?	Obstructed defecation
Does the patient have a frequent desire to defecate, strain or pass a few small pellets, and leave the toilet feeling that stool is still present in the rectum?	Irritable bowel syndrome
After straining for some time, does the stool come half way through a bulging anal outlet?	Hemorrhoids – a common cause of obstructed defecation
After passing one stool, does the patient still feel and intense desire to defecate, but is unable to pass anything but a little blood or mucus?	Anterior rectal prolapse or solitary rectal ulcer syndrome
Does the patient insert a finger into the vagina to assist defecation?	Rectocele
Does the patient insert a finger and push up on the pelvic floor behind the anus?	Weak levators
Does the patient find that defecation is facilitated by inserting a finger in the rectum to push away a flap?	Solitary rectal ulcer syndrome
Is the patient taking adequate amounts of dietary fiber or fluid?	
Is the patient dieting to lose weight?	Little in, little out!
Is the patient taking any drugs that cause constipation?	Drug-induced constipation
Has there been any change in life style?	
Does the patient allow sufficient time to defecate?	
Does the patient have the urge to defecate only when he/she is on a crowded train or on the way to work?	
Does the patient take as much exercise as used to?	
Have the patient's occupation or personal relationships become more demanding?	
Does the patient's bowel habit vary with her menstrual cycle?	
Did the constipation come on only after childbirth, or after hysterectomy?	Hysterectomy may damage the delicate autonomic nerve fibers
Is there history of spine injury? Is micturition normal?	Neurogenic constipation

INDIVIDUAL CAUSES OF CONSTIPATION

Conditions that most commonly present as constipation are described below:

Not Enough Fiber in the Diet

- The most common cause of constipation is a diet *low* in fiber found in vegetables, fruits, and whole grain and *high* in fats found in cheese, eggs, and meats.
- People who eat plenty of high-fiber foods are less likely to become constipated.

Not Enough Liquids

- Liquids like water and juice add fluid to the colon and bulk to stools, making bowel movements softer and easier to pass. People who have the problem of constipation should drink enough of these fluids each day, about 8-ounce glasses.
- Liquids that contain caffeine, like coffee and cola drinks, and alcohol have a dehydrating effect.

Lack of Exercise

- Lack of exercise can lead to constipation, although doctors do not know precisely why.
- For example, constipation often occurs after an accident or during an illness when one must stay in bed and cannot exercise.

Irritable Bowel Syndrome (IBS)

- Constipation is a common feature of the IBS (also known as *spastic colon*). It is often associated with abdominal pain and bloating, and can alternate with diarrhea.

- Constipation in IBS may be related to the presence of small pellet-like stools that are difficult to evacuate from an abnormally sensitive rectum.

Medications

- Drug-induced constipation.

Change in Life or Routine

- During *pregnancy,* women may be constipated because of hormonal changes or because the heavy uterus compresses the intestine.
- *Aging* may also affect bowel regularity because a slower metabolism results in less intestinal activity and muscle tone.
- In addition, people often become constipated when *traveling* because their normal diet and daily routine are disrupted.

Abuse of Laxatives

- *Laxatives* are not necessary and can be habit forming. The colon begins to rely on laxatives to bring on bowel movements. Over time, laxatives can damage nerve cells in the colon and interfere with the colon's natural ability to contract.
- For the same reason, regular use of *enemas* can also lead to loss of normal bowel function.

Ignoring the Urge to have a Bowel Movement

- People who ignore the urge to have a bowel movement may eventually stop feeling the urge, which can lead to constipation.

- People ignore the urge because of emotional stress or being busy or outside home.

Hirschsprung's Disease

- Hirschsprung's disease, in which there is spasticity and amotility of the distal colon caused by the absence of neurons, accounts for 15–25% of cases of intestinal obstruction in the neonate.
- Short-segment Hirschsprung's disease, causing failure of internal anal sphincter relaxation, may present later in life with progressive constipation.
- Diagnosis can be established by:
  1. Manometry: It shows failure of the anal sphincter to relax when the rectum is distended with a balloon.
  2. A thick rectal biopsy, taken at least 2 cm from the dentate line: It shows the absence of ganglion cells.

Mechanical Causes

1. ***Descending perineum and anterior mucosal prolapse:*** Excessive stretching or trauma to the pelvic floor during child birth or prolonged straining may cause the perineum to descend to an abnormal degree when the patient attempts to defecate. This leads to neuropathic weakness of the external anal sphincter due to stretching of the pudendal nerve below the ischial spine. Obstructed defecation may result from tightening of the puborectalis sling around the anorectal angle as the pelvic floor descends and from herniation of redundant anterior rectal mucosa into the weakened anal canal.
2. ***Hypertrophied anal cushion or first-degree hemorrhoids:*** Although it is a common condition, it is often overlooked

as a cause of constipation. The patient may complain of the stool appearing to stick to the anal canal, where it can be felt protruding from a "ballooning" anal margin.

3. ***Rectocele:*** The presence of a rectocele may misdirect the force of defecation forward into the vagina; a posterior vaginal repair often fails to relieve the constipation.

Fecal Impaction

- It most commonly affects the very young and the very old.
- Most patients may have impaired anal and rectal sensation, and may be unable to perceive the presence of feces in the rectum until the mass becomes too large to pass.
- Incontinence of mucus or liquefied feces is common.
- It is uncertain as to whether fecal impaction is the result of a primary neurological disturbance or is secondary to chronic fecal retention.
- *Contributory causes* of fecal impaction in the elderly include immobility, confusion, depression, admission to hospital, and administration of constipating drugs.

Ten most commonly missed causes of constipation

- Hypothyroidism
- Drugs
- Hypercalcemia
- Spinal disease or injury
- Cerebral tumors
- Cerebrovascular disturbances
- Ulcerative colitis
- Pneumatosis coli
- Hemorrhoids
- Anterior mucosal prolapse.

Points to Remember

- Constipation affects almost everyone at one time or another.
- Many people think they are constipated when, in fact, their bowel movements are regular.
- Constipation is not a disease. It is a symptom of many diseases or disorders, or it may be drug-induced.
- The most common causes of constipation are poor diet and lack of exercise.
- Additional causes of constipation include medications, irritable bowel syndrome, abuse of laxatives, and specific diseases.
- A medical history and physical examination may be the only diagnostic tests needed before a doctor suggests treatment.
- In most cases, following these simple tips will help relieve symptoms and prevent recurrence of constipation.
  - Eat a well-balanced, high-fiber diet that includes beans, bran, whole grains, fresh fruits, and vegetables.
  - Drink plenty of liquids.
  - Exercise regularly.
  - Set aside time after breakfast or dinner for undisturbed visits to the toilet.
  - Do not ignore the urge to have a bowel movement.
  - Understand that normal bowel habits vary.
  - Whenever significant or prolonged change in bowel habits occur, check with doctor
- Most people with mild constipation do not need laxatives. However, doctors may recommend laxatives for a limited time for people with chronic constipation.

CHAPTER

9

Differential Diagnosis of Jaundice

JAUNDICE

Jaundice means yellow staining of the body tissues and fluids (except brain, CSF, tears, saliva and milk) produced by an excess of "circulating bilirubin". It is most evident in tissues, which have a high elastic tissue content (skin, sclera and blood vessels) (Normal serum bilirubin = 0.2–0.8 mg/dL, in latent jaundice = 0.8–2 mg/dL, in clinical jaundice > 2 mg/dL).

Jaundice may be classified according to the predominance of either unconjugated or conjugated bilirubin in the blood	Unconjugated hyperbilirubinemia	1. Pre-Hepatic (Hemolytic) 2. Hepatic
	Conjugated hyperbilirubinemia	1. Hepatic • Acute damage • Chronic damage • Cholestasis 2. Post-hepatic

I. UNCONJUGATED HYPERBILIRUBINEMIA— PREHEPATIC (HEMOLYTIC)

Increased hemolysis is the most common cause resulting in increased production of bilirubin, that the liver cannot deal with it, leading to accumulation of unconjugated bilirubin in blood, i.e. ***increased bilirubin load.***

Etiology

I. Congenital: Inborn defect of RBCs	A. Abnormal Shape ....Spherocytosis, elliptocytosis. B. Abnormal Hb .... Thalassemia, sickle cell anemia. C. Enzymopathy ....G-6-P-D deficiency, pyruvate kinase deficiency.
II. Acquired	A. Immune Hemolytic Anemia: • Drugs ....Methyl dopa, aspirin, tagamet, tetracycline • Collagen vascular.....SLE, rheumatoid arthritis. • Tumors ....Lymphoma, leukemia. • Infections.................Mycoplasmosis, malaria, syphilis. B. Non-immune Hemolytic Anemia: • Septicemia, severe burns. • Heavy metal poisoning, snake venom. • Sequestrated blood (big hematoma, hemothorax and hemoperitoneum).

Diagnosis

- Clinical examination reveals a ***triad*** of:
  1. Anemia.
  2. Jaundice (usually not severe).
  3. Splenomegaly.
- No bile salts in serum (*no* itching) and urine.
- No conjugated bilirubin in urine.
- Bilirubin is not found in urine and stools are of normal color.
- Positive indirect VDR.
- Peripheral blood shows increased reticulocytosis, a sign of increased bone marrow activity.
- Examination of the bone marrow shows hyperplasia of erythropoietic cells.
- Hemolysis can be confirmed by and its extent documented by measurement of RBC half-life using cells labeled with radioactive chromium (^{51}Cr).
- LFTs are normal.

II. UNCONJUGATED HYPERBILIRUBINEMIA—HEPATIC

Etiology

- Any condition which interferes with the passage of bilirubin into the hepatic cell, or with the process of conjugation, will result in jaundice, i.e. ↓ ***uptake or conjugation of bilirubin***.
- The consequent serum level of unconjugated bilirubin may be detected by the diazo reaction of Van den Bergh as the "indirect" form.

Failure to Transport into Hepatocyte

1. Gilbert's syndrome
2. Male fern extract (flavaspidic acid).

Impaired Conjugation

1. Absent: Crigler-Najjar (Type I)
2. Low: Crigler-Najjar (Type II), neonates
3. Inhibited: 3,20-pregnanediol, Lucey-Driscoll syndrome.

III. CONJUGATED HYPERBILIRUBINEMIA—HEPATIC

Jaundice due to Acute Hepatocellular Damage

This type of jaundice may be caused by:

1. Infections
2. Poisons
3. Drugs.

The depth of jaundice is variable, serum transaminases always ↑ highly, while alkaline phosphatase ↑ only moderately and may be normal.

Infections	1. Viral hepatitis, infectious mononucleosis (IMN), yellow fever, others (Coxsackie B virus, Herpes simplex, cytomegalovirus "CMV", rubella).	
	2. Portal pyemia, septicemia (causes severe hepatic destruction).	
	3. Leptospirosis (Weil's disease caused by Leptospira icterohemorrhagiae), relapsing fever, syphilis "$" (congenital or rarely diffuse hepatitis in 2^{ry} $), tuberculosis (TB) (granulomatous hepatitis), other bacterial infections (*Klebsiella pneumoniae*, *Salmonella typhi*, bacteroids).	
	4. Protozoal: Congenital toxoplasmosis (neonatal), hepatic amebiasis.	
Poisons	• Carbon tetrachloride:	Inhaled during drycleaning or handling fire extinguishers.
	• Dicophane (DDT)	Used as an insecticide.
	• Benzene derivatives	A rare cause of hepatotoxicity.
	• Tannic acid	Absorbed when put on burnt areas of skin.
	• Muscarine	Follows ingestion of Amanita mushrooms.
	• Aflatoxin	Derived from Aspergillus flavus (fungal infection of ground nuts).
	• Phosphorus (yellow form)	Taken by accident or with suicidal intent.
	• Physical agents	Fever, severe burns, liver irradiation (cause liver damage).
Drugs	• Hydrazine and related drugs	MAO inhibitors and anti-TB drugs.
	• Halothane	Anesthetic agent.
	• Cytotoxic drugs	Methotrexate, 6-MP.
	• Tetracyclines (IV, large dose)	In late pregnancy or in the malnorished.
	• Paracetamol	Overdose.
	• Obsolete drugs	Withdrawn from the market, e.g. ibufenac

Jaundice due to Chronic Hepatocellular Damage

Etiology

Chronic liver disease may cause failure due to ***infection, degeneration, infiltration or malignancy.***

Cirrhosis	Cryptogenic, viral, alcoholic, cardiac failure, Budd-Chiari syndrome, chronic active hepatitis (CAH), cholestasis and primary biliary cirrhosis (PBC), hepatolenticular degeneration (Wilson's disease), hemochromatosis, fibrocystic disease (mucoviscidosis), galactosemia, congenital $, schistosomiasis, glycogen-storage diseases.
Amyloidosis	Primary amyloidosis or secondary to chronic infection, myelomatosis, or rheumatoid arthritis.
Tumors	• Primary tumors: Carcinoma (hepatoma), sarcoma, malignant hemangioendothelioma. • Secondary tumors: The liver is the most frequent site of blood-borne metastases. • Reticuloendothelial disease: Hodgkin's disease.

Jaundice due to Intrahepatic Cholestasis

Etiology

- Drug-induced cholestasis: E.g. chlorpromazine, methyltestosterone.
- Primary biliary cirrhosis: Usually in women (35–70 years) - no known cause for cholestasis.
- Pregnancy (last trimester): Some women develop cholestasis due to sensitivity to sex hormones.
- Hemolytic disease of newborn: Probably due to liver-cell damage (inspissated bile syndrome).
- Congenital biliary atresia: It causes jaundice apparent a few days after birth.
- Virus hepatitis: It may present with a cholestatic picture.
- Cirrhosis: Alcoholic and post-necrotic cirrhosis may be complicated by cholestasis.

- Sclerosing cholangitis: Primary or secondary to prolonged extrahepatic biliary obstruction (with infection).
- Cholangiocarcinoma: Carcinoma of intrahepatic bile ducts is a rare cause of cholestasis.
- Dubin-Johnson syndrome: Rare, benign, intermittent condition, diagnosis made by bromsulphthalein test.
- Rotor syndrome: It differs from Dubin-Johnson by absence of brown pigment in the liver.

General Picture

- Characteristics of obstructive jaundice (intrahepatic), itching, pale stools and dark urine.
- Predominance of conjugated bilirubin in blood.
- LFTs are disturbed. Serum alkaline phophatase (AP) level >30 KAU/dL.
- It is necessary to distinguish this situation from extra-hepatic obstruction to avoid unnecessary surgery:
  1. A history of drug-ingestion should be sought.
  2. The liver is often enlarged, but pain and fever are normally absent.
  3. Liver biopsy, PTC, and response to prednisone may provide further information. In *extrahepatic* obstruction, PTC reveals dilated bile ducts within the liver and a block below. In *intrahepatic* cholestasis, the bile ducts are not dilated and no obstruction is seen. Recently, magnetic resonance cholangiopancreatography (MRCP) can be used (non-invasive but expensive and requires experience).

Differences between Intrahepatic and Extrahepatic Obstruction

Criteria	Intra-hepatic Obstruction	Extra-hepatic Obstruction
History Onset Course Obstruction	PBC, Alcoholic Cirrhosis or VH, Drugs Usually rapid Usually fluctuating Incomplete	Biliary colic, dyspepsia, ulcer cancer. Insidious Rarely fluctuating Complete
Liver Spleen GB	Normal or enlarged Palpable Not felt.	Always enlarged Not palpable May be felt
LFTs	Early disturbance, ↑↑ SGPT	Late disturbance, ↑↑ AP
Treatment	Medical	Surgical

IV. CONJUGATED HYPERBILIRUBINEMIA—POSTHEPATIC

SURGICAL JAUNDICE

Etiology

Congenital	Acquired		
	Inside the Duct	In the Duct Wall	Outside the Duct
1. Biliary atresia 2. Choledochal cyst 3. Sclerosing cholangitis 4. Congenital stricture	1. Stone 2. F.B. 3. Parasites: Clonorchis sinensis, Ascaris lumbricoides	1. Traumatic stricture 2. Sclerosing cholangitis 3. Radiotherapy 4. Malignant stricture (cholangio-carcinoma).	1. Cancer head of pancreas 2. Periampullary carcinoma 3. Porta hepatis secondaries (lymph nodes) 4. Liver secondaries

Contd...

Contd...

5. Annular pancreas			5. Hydatid or retroperitoneal cyst 6. Pancreatitis and chronic DU 7. Duodenal diverticulum 8. Hepatic artery aneurysm

Clinical Picture

1. Sclera → deep yellowish green.
2. Stools → clay-colored (no pigment).
3. Urine → liquorice (due to urochrome and conjugated bilirubin).
4. Serum bilirubin → ↑ conjugated (early) and ↑ conjugated and non-conjugated (late due to ↓ LFTs).
5. VDB reaction → direct (violet ring), but later becomes biphasic.
6. Urobilinogen → Absent in urine and stools (not formed).
7. Bile salts → absent from the intestine leading to (a) impaired fat absorption and bulky offensive stools (↑ fat in stools), and (b) lack of absorption of fat-soluble vitamins especially vitamin K → hypoprothrombinemia and prolonged prothrombin time → bleeding tendency.
8. Bile salts → escape into the systemic circulation resulting in:
   - SAN inhibition (bradycardia).
   - Itching.
   - Excretion of bile salts in urine.
9. LFTs → disturbed (deteriorated) in prolonged obstruction.

The main causes that should be distinguished from each other are:
1. *Stones* in the CBD (Calcular or benign obstructive jaundice).
2. *Carcinoma* of the head of pancreas or periampullary carcinoma (Malignant obstructive jaundice).

CALCULAR OBSTRUCTIVE JAUNDICE

It usually results from impaction of a ***gallstone*** in the CBD and rarely in the hepatic ducts. Sometimes, pigment stones are formed *primarily* in the ***CBD*** (not migrating from the GB). ***Sites of impaction*** in order of frequency are as follows: Supraduodenal part of CBD, retroduodenal part of CBD, ampulla (only 10%), and CHD (rare).

Clinical Picture

- CBD stones may be *asymptomatic*, but in most cases, they produce the symptoms of **Charcot's triad** (associated with *ascending cholangitis*), which is characterized by:
  1. *Recurrent biliary pain*: Usually colicky and epigastric or in the right hypochondrium.
  2. *Intermittent fever* with rigors.
  3. *Fluctuating jaundice* of the obstructive type
- In addition to Charcot's triad, the presence of *hypotension and mental confusion* is called **Reynold's pentad**. The patient has acute suppurative cholangitis (pus under pressure), which is a surgical emergency.
- Other manifestations include loss of weight, muddy complexion (due to toxic absorption and liver insufficiency), and the liver is often palpably enlarged and tender, but the GB is usually not palpable.

Courvoisier's Law

In a jaundiced patient, if the gallbladder is palpably enlarged, it is probably *not* due to stones in the CBD, because in such case the previous cholecystitis has already made the GB fibrotic. In malignant obstruction, the GB is usually enlarged, as it was previously normal and the pressure rises gradually and progressively (not intermittently).

Exceptions of Courvoisier's Law

A. *In calcular obstructive jaundice, the GB may be palpably enlarged due to:*
   1. Stone in CBD causing jaundice + stone in cystic duct causing mucocele or empyema (enlarged GB).
   2. A large stone in "Hartmann's pouch" obstructing both, the cystic duct (causing enlargement of the gall bladder) and the CBD (causing obstructive jaundice). This is known as **Mirrizi syndrome**.

B. *In malignant obstructive jaundice, the GB may NOT be felt due to:*
   1. Cancer + chronic fibrotic GB.
   2. Cancer of the CHD.
   3. Obstruction at the porta hepatis (secondaries).
   4. GB hidden under the lower border of the liver, and therefore, not felt.

Investigations:

1. *Laboratory:* blood - stools - urine.
2. *Radiological:* PXR - ERCP - MRCP - US - CT - PTC.
3. *Liver biopsy:* If parenchymatous liver disease is suspected.
4. *Laparoscopy or laparotomy.*

MALIGNANT OBSTRUCTIVE JAUNDICE

Etiology

1. Carcinoma of head of pancreas (**Figure 9.1**).
2. Ampullary carcinoma (carcinoma of the ampulla of Vater or duodenal papilla).

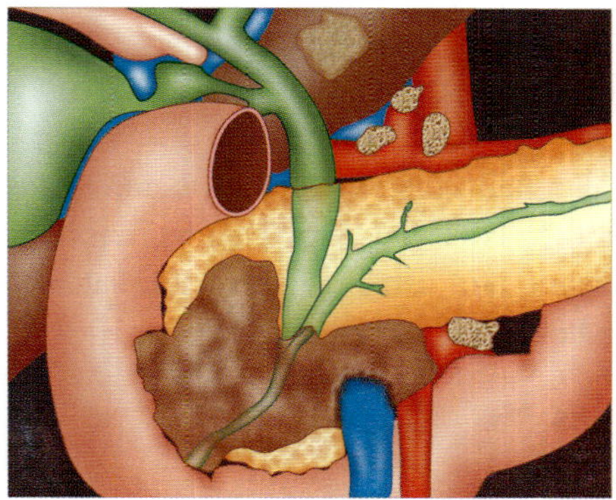

Fig. 9.1: Cancer head of pancreas causing CBD obstruction

3. Carcinoma of the bile or hepatic ducts.
4. Malignant lymph nodes in the porta-hepatis compressing or invading the CBD.
5. Malignant liver, compressing the intrahepatic ductules.

Clinical Picture

Symptoms

1. The most important point is history of *painless progressive jaundice* for few weeks.
2. In carcinoma of the head of pancreas, there may be boring epigastric pain radiating to the back. Vomiting is late except with duodenal involvement.
3. Jaundice is exceptionally "intermittent" with tumor necrosis or ulceration into the duodenum.
4. Rapid loss of weight, malignant cachexia, and marked itching.
5. Ulcerating ampullary carcinoma (into the duodenum) may cause melena.

Examination

1. *Generally:* Deep jaundice, scratch marks on the skin, no fever, and Virchow's lymph nodes in advanced cases
2. Locally: Palpable distended GB (usually), the liver may be smoothly enlarged ± epigastric mass (cancer body of pancreas), and ascites and peritoneal secondaries in advanced cases.

Investigations

1. *Laboratory Tests:*
   - Blood examination: LFTs, CBC.
   - Urine analysis.
   - Stool analysis (occult blood in carcinoma of ampulla or carcinoma of the CBD).
2. *Radiological Investigations:*
   - Plain X-Ray.
   - Barium meal or hypotonic duodenography (widening of the C-curve of the duodenum in cases of cancer head of pancreas or inverted "3" in ampullary carcinoma).
   - Ultrasonography (US).
   - Computerized tomography (CT).
   - Percutaneous transhepatic cholangiography (PTC).
   - Endoscopic retrograde cholangiopancreatography (ERCP).
   - Magnetic resonance cholangiopancreatography (MRCP).
3. *Laparotomy.*

Differences between Calcular and Malignant Obstructive Jaundice

Criteria	Calcular Obstructive Jaundice	Malignant Obstructive Jaundice
Age	Usually about 40 years	Usually > 60 years
Sex	Females > males.	Males > females.
Charcot's Triad		
1. Pain	Colicky and intermittent.	Constant and dull aching (±)
2. Fever	Intermittent	Absent
3. Jaundice	Intermittent	Progressive
Itching	±	Evident
General Condition	Good or moderate	Moderate to bad
GB	Not felt	Enlarged
Abdominal Mass	-	± (epigastric)
Ascites	-	+ (in late cases)
Occult Blood in Stools	Usually -ve	Usually +ve
Barium Meal	Normal duodenum (±)	Wide C-shaped duodenum
Plain X-ray	May show stone	No stones
Treatment	Curable	Radical or Palliative

What does Surgical Jaundice mean?

It means "jaundice that can be corrected by surgery". It includes the following:

1. *Posthepatic jaundice*: All causes are included.
2. *Hepatic jaundice*: Hepatic tumors - hepatic cysts.
3. *Prehepatic jaundice*: Corrected by splenectomy, e.g. hereditary spherocytosis.

Differences between Different Types of Jaundice

Criteria	Hemolytic Jaundice	Hepatic Jaundice	Obstructive Jaundice
Etiology	↑ hemolysis	Hepatic insult	Obstruction
Sclera Urine Stools	Yellowish ↑ urobilinogen, Deep amber color	Yellowish green Deep More or less normal	Greenish Liquorice Clay color
Serum bilirubin VDB Reaction LFTs	↑ ↑ unconjugated Indirect Normal	↑ Both Biphasic Impaired	Mostly conjugated Direct Impaired later
Other Features	Anemia, reticulocytosis and enlarged spleen	Hepatomegaly, enlarged tender spleen	Itching, bradycardia, fat malabsorption and steatorrhea
Liver Biopsy	Normal, ↑ pigment	Liver damage	Dilatation of bile canaliculi

Diagnosis of Jaundice

The following questions should be answered: Presence of jaundice? Degree of jaundice? Type of jaundice (Unconjugated-conjugated)? Site of obstruction (Intra-hepatic; extrahepatic)? or Whether CHD or CBD?, Cause of obstruction (Calcular, inflammatory stricture, malignancy)?

To reach the answers to these questions, the following algorithm should be considered:

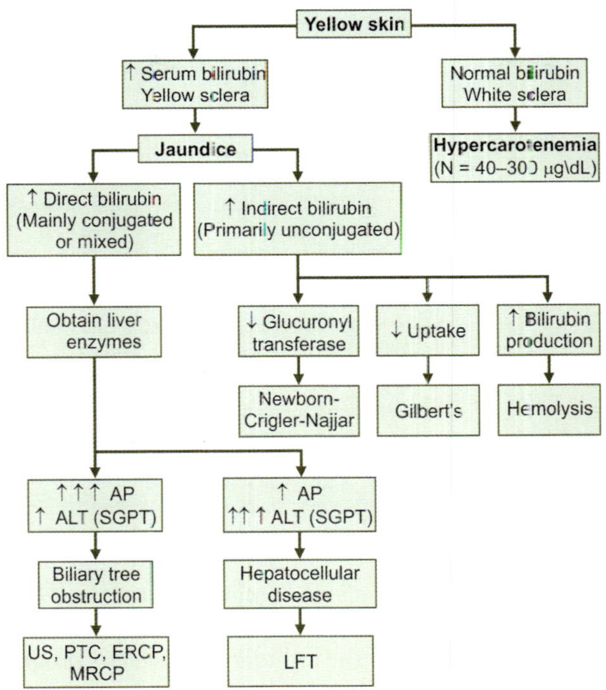

POSTOPERATIVE JAUNDICE

Definition

It means jaundice that occurs, *for the first time,* in the post-operative period.

Etiology

Unconjugated Hyperbilirubinemia	a. Massive blood Transfusion b. Hemolysis (e.g. mismatched blood transfusion) c. Resorption of residual hematomas or bilomas d. Others (drugs, e.g. antihypertensive drugs, sepsis, and hypoxia)
Hepatocellular Damage	1. Hepatocellular necrosis due to: • Adverse Drug Reaction: e.g. Tylenol (Acetaminophen). • Sepsis from leaking anastomosis, abscess, septicemia. • Hypoxia by decreasing O_2 delivery to the liver. • Hypotension by decreasing hepatic blood flow. • Anesthetic Agents: e.g. Halothane. • Virus hepatitis e.g. HBV, HCV, and CMV. 2. Activation of pre-existing liver disease. 3. Extensive hepatic resection.
Extrahepatic Obstruction	1. Primary biliary pathology: Residual stones - trauma-missed tumors of biliary tract. 2. Bile duct injury (refer back). 3. Postoperative pancreatitis.

Clinical Picture

Jaundice may be *mild, slowly progressive and self-limited.* This signifies benign postoperative cholestasis or conjugated hyperbilirubinemia. On the other hand, *severe progressive jaundice* usually indicates biliary tract problem, significant liver disease or severe sepsis.

Investigations

- *Laboratory:* LFTs (Serum bilirubin, AST, ALT, AP, blood culture), urine (bile pigments and bile salts).
- *Radiological:* US (To differentiate between cholestatic and hepatocellular jaundice), ERCP and PTC (in case of extra-hepatic cholestasis), CT scanning (for intra-abdominal suppuration).
- *Biopsy:* Liver biopsy for diagnosis of hepatocellular disease, or drug-induced jaundice.

Algorithm for Diagnosis

After full clinical examination and estimation of LFTs, the following should be performed in sequential order:

Determination of the Nature of Jaundice by LFTs, Urine and US

- Unconjugated hyperbilirubinemia: Normal conjugated bilirubin + no bile pigment or bile salts in urine.
- Hepatocellular affection: Both conjugated and unconjugated hyperbilirubinemia + ↑ AST and ALT + US shows no intrahepatic biliary dilatation.
- Cholestatic jaundice: Conjugated hyperbilirubinemia + bile salts and pigments in urine + ↑ AP + Us shows intrahepatic biliary dilatation and may even show the pathology in the liver.

If Unconjugated Hyperbilirubinemia

The most possible causes include:

- Massive blood transfusion...... history of transfusion.
- Incompatible blood transfusion .... history of transfusion + systemic manifestations.
- Hemolytic reaction.................. +ve Coomb's test.
- Absorption of large hematoma................................discovered by US, or CT scan.

If Hepatocellular

- Hepatitis.......................... +ve HBsAg.
- Halothane hepatitis........ anesthesia.
- Drug-induced.......................improvement with drug withdrawal.
- Sepsis.................................. S/S of anastomotic leak, sepsis and +ve blood culture.
- Liver biopsy..................... for undiagnosed cases.

CHAPTER

10

Differential Diagnosis of Bleeding

1. HEMATEMESIS

Bleeding in the upper GIT results in **hematemesis** (vomiting of blood), **melena** (passage of black tarry stools), **occult blood in stools**, or **anemia**.

- **Hematemesis** almost always infers the site of bleeding to be from the *oro-pharynx to proximal to the ligament of Treitz.*
- **True melena** usually follows bleeding *proximal to the jejunum.* As little as 50 ml of blood from the upper GIT can cause clinically obvious melena. With a bleeding of 1000 ml, melena can persist for 5 days and stool can remain hemo-occult positive for 3 weeks !

CAUSES OF HEMATEMESIS

Swallowed Blood	1. Epistaxis. 2. Hemoptysis. 3. Bleeding from the mouth and throat. 4. Malingering.
Diseases of Esophagus	1. Rupture esophageal varices. 2. Reflux esophagitis (associated with *hiatal hernia*). 3. Simple ulcer. 4. Epithelioma. 5. Mallory-Weiss syndrome. 6. Aortic aneurysm rupturing into the esophagus. 7. Mediastinal tumor perforating the esophagus and aorta. 8. Foreign body perforating the esophagus and aorta.

Contd...

Contd...

Diseases of Stomach	1. Gastric ulcer (peptic ulcer). 2. Gastritis (acute, chronic, drug-induced). 3. Hemorrhagic erosions. 4. Tumors: Carcinoma, leiomyosarcoma, hemangioma. 5. Gastric varices. 6. Mallory-Weiss syndrome. 7. Telangiectasia (Osler-Rendu-Weber).
Diseases of Duodenum	1. Duodenal ulcer. 2. Carcinoma (Primary or invasion from the pancreas). 3. Duodenal diverticula. 4. Gallstone ulcerating into the duodenum.
Portal Obstruction	1. Cirrhosis of the liver (including **SHF**). 2. Portal vein thrombosis or obstruction (compression).
Blood Diseases	1. Purpura. 2. Scurvy. 3. Polycythemia. 4. Hemophilia and allied disorders. 5. Leukemia. 6. Aplastic anemia with thrombocytopenia. 7. Malarial cachexia. 8. von Willebrand's disease. 9. Ehlor-Danlos syndrome. 10. A-V malformations.
Acute Febrile Diseases	1. Malignant variola. 2. Malignant scarlet fever. 3. Malignant measles (black measles). 4. Anthrax. 5. Malaria. 6. Black water fever, yellow fever and dengue fever. 7. Cholera. 8. Bacterial endocarditis. 9. Weil's disease (leptospirosis).
Miscellaneous Causes	1. Abdominal aneurysm opening into the stomach. 2. Chronic nephritis or uremia. 3. Anticoagulant therapy. 4. Following abdominal operations, trauma and burns (Curling's ulcer). 5. Prolonged jaundice. 6. Polyarteritis nodosa. 7. Abdominal injury. 8. Malignant hypertension. 9. Amyloidosis. 10. Sarcoidosis.

The four common causes of profuse hematemesis are:
1. Esophageal varices.
2. Erosive gastritis.
3. Gastric ulcer.
4. Duodenal ulcer.

SWALLOWED BLOOD

Epistaxis

- It is obvious when bleeding from the nose is followed by hematemesis.

Hemoptysis

- Blood coming from the lungs may be swallowed, especially when hemorrhage occurs during sleep.
- The following Table shows the distinguishing features between hemoptysis and hematemesis.

	Suggesting Hemoptysis	Suggesting Hematemesis
Previous History:	**Respiratory symptoms**	**Dyspepsia**
Immediately Before the Episode	1. Tickle or gurgle in the throat. 2. Cough.	1. Faintness. 2. Abdominal pain. 3. Nausea.
Characteristics of the Episode	• Blood produced by repeated cough. • May be mixed with sputum. • Usually bright red • May be frothy. • Reaction on alkaline side.	• Blood produced by acts of vomiting. • May be mixed with food debris. • Usually dark in color. • May resemble coffee-grounds. • Usually acid in reaction.
After the Episode	• Blood-stained sputum for several days. • Stools normal, may contain occult blood (rarely after severe hemoptysis).	• Stools often dark and tarry (melena). • Always give positive test for occult blood.

Bleeding from the Mouth and Throat

- The gums, tongue and fauces should be examined carefully to exclude causes of bleeding from the mouth and throat.

Malingering

- The possibility of malingering with the intent to deceive must be considered in some cases.
- Nasogastric aspirate will not contain blood.
- No melena.

DISEASES OF THE ESOPHAGUS

Esophageal Varices

- *History* of bilharziasis, previous attacks of hepatitis or jaundice.
- On *examination*, spleen is enlarged and liver is firm, with irregular surface.
- Ascites may be present. *Esophagoscopy* may determine the site of bleeding.
- Multiple filling defects on *barium swallow* (honey-comb appearance) (**Figure 10.1**).

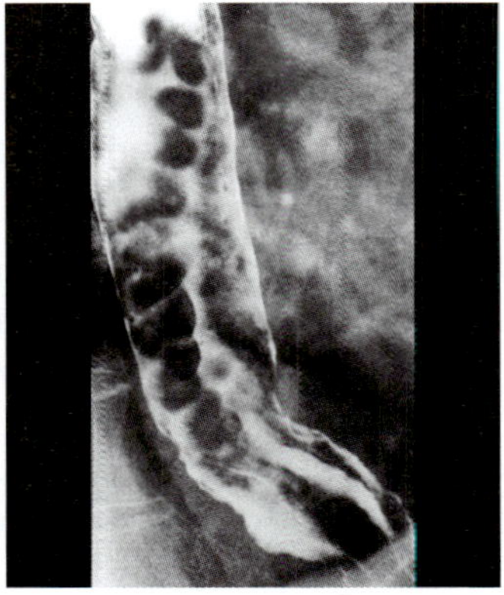

Fig. 10.1: Esophageal varices

Reflux Esophagitis (Hiatal Hernia)—Esophageal Ulcer

- An esophageal ulcer is comparatively rare, usually existing as ulceration in a peptic-lined esophagus.
- Bleeding is more likely to be from reflux esophagitis associated with hiatus hernia, which becomes evident in late middle life and is responsible for dysphagia, painful dyspepsia and hematemesis.
- There is history of heartburn and reflux on lying down.

Esophageal Carcinoma (Epithelioma)

- The commonest form is an annular stricture, which causes dysphagia as the earliest symptom.
- However, hemorrhage may occur from erosion of small blood vessels as the result of ulceration, the amount of blood being small.
- When the ulceration is deep and extensive a larger vessel, even the aorta, may be opened, causing sudden, profuse and rapidly fatal hemorrhage.

An Aneurysm of the Thoracic Aorta

- An aneurysm of the thoracic aorta compressing the esophagus may finally erode and open into it, with profuse and fatal hematemesis.

Rupture or Laceration of the Esophageal Wall (Mallory-Weiss Syndrome)

- Massive, painless hematemesis results from lacerations that traverse the gastroesophageal junction from forced vomiting or from severe coughing bouts, usually in alcoholics.
- The lacerations extend into the submucosa but do not rupture through the entire thickness of the wall.

Mediastinal Tumor Perforating the Esophagus and Aorta

- It is most likely to be mistaken for aneurysm or epithelioma of the esophagus.
- Cyanosis and dilated superficial veins are generally characteristic and serves to distinguish it from aneurysm in which severe venous obstruction is much rarer.

Foreign Body Perforating the Esophagus and Aorta

- A history of such a foreign body (pin, fish-bone, toothplate) being swallowed, followed by a feeling of discomfort in the esophagus, would suggest such a condition.
- It may be confirmed by the use of *X-rays* or the *esophagoscope*.

DISEASES OF THE STOMACH

Gastric Ulcer

- *History* of dyspepsia, abdominal pain after meals, relieved by vomiting or alkalis, melena or previous attacks of hematemesis.
- There may be also history of receiving medical treatment or having *radiographs* done for the stomach and duodenum.
- *Examination* reveals tenderness behind the upper part of the right rectus muscles, or deeply seated pain in the back.
- In severe bleeding, the patient develops manifestations of hemorrhagic shock (pallor, rapid pulse, sweating, etc).
- The ulcer can usually be seen through the *gastroscope*.

Acute Gastritis

- *Causes* include irritant food, alcohol, or corrosive or irritant poisons.
- The mucosa becomes congested and small hemorrhages and erosions are seen by the *endoscope*.

- Usually blood occurs in the form of streaks mixed with mucus in the vomit.
- The main *symptoms* are:
  1. Discomfort and tenderness in the epigastrium.
  2. Nausea, eructation and vomiting.
  3. Constipation or in children diarrhea.

Chronic Gastritis

- It may follow acute gastritis but is most frequently *caused* by continued excessive intake of alcohol, tobacco, or irritating food.
- The main *symptoms* are:
  1. Epigastric tenderness.
  2. Nausea, vomiting, flatulence and foul breath.
  3. Constipation.
- The *gastroscope* shows thickened, congested mucosa with scattered hemorrhagic erosions. It may show the typical appearance of atrophic gastritis.

Drug-induced Gastritis

- There is *history* of intake of strong acids or alkalis, or poisoning with arsenic or phosphorus, or of drug-intake such as indomethacin or phenylbutazone.
- Cortisone is not a gastric irritant but may activate a quiescent ulcer.
- Iron-containing tablets such as ferrous sulfate or carbonate may produce gastric erosion in children and in some adults.
- Chief *symptoms* include:
  1. Epigastric pain and tenderness.
  2. Nausea and vomiting.
  3. Dysphagia.
  4. There may be diarrhea, faintness and depression (arsenic poisoning).

Hemorrhagic Erosions

- They are virtually minute ulcers.
- They are usually caused by:
  1. Specific fevers of malignant severity.
  2. Purpura.
  3. Infective endocarditis.
  4. Septic states.
  5. Yellow fever.
  6. Anthrax
- Hematemesis may be as severe as that of ordinary gastric ulcer.

Gastric Carcinoma

- Frank hematemesis is rare and is usually of coffee-grounds rather than bright red
- Most patients are between 40 and 60 years.
- The chief *manifestations* are:
  1. Epigastric pain, nausea, vomiting, anorexia, loss of weight and strength.
  2. Pyrexia.
  3. Anemia and cachexia.
  4. Abdominal mass.
- The tumor may be silent and the patient presents with vague illness or just loss of weight.
- If the tumor is not obstructing the cardia or pylorus the patient may present with only dyspepsia simulating gastritis; while with diffuse carcinoma of the stomach (leather-bottle) there is no vomiting or bleeding or palpable tumor and diagnosis is reached by *barium meal.*
- A growth in the stomach may be seen and *biopsied* by the *gastroscope.*
- *Troisier's sign* (enlargement of left supraclavicular lymph node) may be positive in some patients.

Leiomyosarcoma

- It is rare.
- Together with leiomyoma, it has a high propensity to ulcerate and bleed.

Hemangioma

- It may also bleed and cause hematemesis.

Injuries

- Hematemesis may follow blows, stabs or gunshot wounds in the epigastric region.

Abdominal Aneurysm Opening into the Stomach

- Rupture of the sac may lead to a sudden, profuse and fatal attack of hematemesis.
- The condition may have been previously known by the presence of an epigastric swelling with distinct expansile pulsation, and severe pain, both in the abdomen and back, in a male atherosclerotic patient (abdominal aneurysm in a woman is very rare).

DISEASES OF THE DUODENUM

Duodenal Ulcer

- It is most common in men.
- Pain usually occurs 2–3 hours after food intake and is generally deep-seated in the upper part of the abdomen.
- Vomiting may occur but may be entirely absent.
- The ulcer is shown by *barium meal* (trifoliate deformity) and is seen by *endoscopy*.

Duodenal Diverticulum

- It is always on the inner (pancreatic) side of the duodenum and is asymptomatic unless very large or become inflamed from accumulation of food.

- Symptoms resemble those of a duodenal ulcer but with no regular food relationship.
- Patients as a rule are over the age of 50 years.
- A co-existent ulcer may be present and responsible for the symptoms including hematemesis.

Duodenal Carcinoma

- It is very rare.
- In most cases it proves to arise in the ampulla of Vater and thus is apt to cause obstructive jaundice and pale or "silver" stools.

Gallstones Ulcerating through the Gallbladder into the Duodenum

- They rarely cause hematemesis and melena and may be mistaken for a gastric or duodenal ulcer.
- Colicky pain, tenderness below the tip of the 9th right rib with jaundice, should put the diagnosis of gallstones in mind.
- Diagnosis may be confirmed by radiology, passage of stone in stools or intestinal obstruction if a large stone gets impacted.

PORTAL OBSTRUCTION

Liver Cirrhosis

- It causes portal hypertension and the development of varices that cause severe hematemesis.
- The spleen is enlarged and the liver is firm.
- Jaundice, ascites and cholemia may supervene.

Portal Vein Thrombosis or Compression

- It also causes portal hypertension and gives rise to sudden and profuse hematemesis.
- It is usually associated with ascites and jaundice.

BLOOD DISEASES

Purpura Hemorrhagica

- Hematemesis may occur from swallowed blood (from nose or mouth) or from small gastric erosions.
- There will be other hemorrhages, i.e. epistaxis, oral and rectal bleeding, hematuria, vaginal or uterine bleeding.
- Blood examination is necessary for diagnosis.

Scurvy

- Hematemesis occurs in severe cases.
- The swollen, spongy gums, anemia, cutaneous hemorrhages and SC indurations, in a patient who has vitamin C deficiency, would point to scurvy.
- Confirmation is accorded by response to administration of ascorbic acid.

Hemophilia and Allied Disorders

- The patient is a male with a positive family history.
- The patient suffers from excessive bleeding from slight cuts or after tooth extraction, in addition to bleeding from other sites particularly the joints.

Leukemia

- Hematemesis and enlarged spleen are not pathognomonic for leukemia as they may be present in other diseases such as chronic malaria and bilharziasis.
- Diagnosis is established by blood examination and bone marrow biopsy.

Hodgkin's Disease

- Hematemesis may rarely occur in the late stages of the disease.

- In addition, there may be bleeding from other sites such as epistaxis, bleeding from the mouth or cerebral hemorrhage.

Malarial Cachexia

- Anemia and splenic enlargement may follow repeated attacks of malaria.
- Severe hematemesis may occur.

ACUTE FEBRILE DISEASES

Malignant Variola

- Hematemesis occurs in about 1/3 of cases of hemorrhagic ***small pox***.
- It is associated with cutaneous, SC and submucous hemorrhages, hematuria, epistaxis and bleeding from the gums.

Malignant Scarlet Fever

- Hematemesis occurs very rarely; epistaxis, hematuria and cutaneous hemorrhages being more common.
- The sudden and severe onset, the very high fever, the rapid and feeble pulse, the headache and delirium, and the appearance of rash on the 2nd day would point to scarlet fever.

Malignant (Black) Measles

- Hematemesis is less prominent than is the generalized purpura.
- Diagnosis is indicated by the nature of the general epidemic.

Yellow Fever

- The onset is sudden with a chill, headache and severe pain in the back and limbs.

- The face is flushed and jaundice very soon appears.
- In addition to "black vomit", there may be cutaneous petechiae and bleeding from gums.
- It simulates malignant malaria and both may co-exist.

Cholera

- Hematemesis may occur.
- Sudden onset and rice-water stools in an epidemic point to diagnosis.

Acute Massive Liver Necrosis

- Hematemesis is the most common form of hemorrhage in this rare disorder.
- It may result from industrial chemicals, such as TNT, yellow phosphorus or benzole, and as a sequel of infective hepatitis.

Leptospirosis

- Severe hemorrhagic manifestations occur in very ill patients but some bleeding is present in 40% of all cases, hematemesis and hemoptysis being the most common.

MISCELLANEOUS DISEASES

Chronic Nephritis

- Hematemesis may occur.
- There is hypertension, cardiac hypertrophy, retinopathy, polyuria and urine of low specific gravity containing albumin and renal tube casts.

Following Abdominal Operations

- Hematemesis may follow abdominal operations independently of gastric or duodenal injury.

- It may follow other forms of ***stress*** such as severe burns (***Curling's ulcer***).

Prolonged Jaundice

- The importance of jaundice as a cause of almost any variety of bleeding by oozing, lies chiefly in the added danger attending operations in such cases.

Sea-Sickness - Airplane Sickness

- It may cause hematemesis from violent strain on the stomach from retching and vomiting.
- The amount of blood is usually not large.

Injury to the Epigastrium

- An injury caused by a kick, punch or steering-wheel in a motor-car accident, may be followed by hematemesis from direct injury to the stomach.

2. MELENA

DEFINITION

Melena is a term applied to the black motion (black tarry stools) resulting from hemorrhage that has occurred in the alimentary canal at a high enough level for chemical alteration to have taken place, usually proximal to the ligament of Treitz (middle of the 2nd portion of the duodenum) - or after the swallowing of blood derived from hemoptysis or epistaxis.

CAUSES (SOURCE)

Usually melena is due to bleeding from the **esophagus, stomach, or duodenum** and is associated with hematemesis. If melena occurs ***alone*** from these sources, it usually indicates that the rate of bleeding is relatively *slow*.

Lesions Lower Down (Distal to Duodenum)

Such lesions, as a rule, give rise to dark or bright red blood in stools rather than melena, but melena may occur in the relatively uncommon group of causes of **small intestinal** bleeding which include:

1. *Typhoid fever,* from an ulcerated Peyer's patch in the upper ileum or from an ulcer in the jejunum.
2. *Leiomyoma or hemangioma* of the upper jejunum.
3. *Mesenteric thrombosis or embolism.*
4. *Direct abdominal injury* causing contusion of the bowel.
5. *A peptic ulcer in a Meckel's diverticulum,* particularly in children.

Blood Dyscrasias

Any of these disorders may result in oozing from the mucosa in the GIT and the commonest cause of this today is anti-coagulant therapy.

OTHER CAUSES OF BLACK STOOLS

1. *Iron therapy* by mouth in large quantities (the iron being converted into the *sulfide*).
2. Ingestion of *charcoal* biscuits or much red wine.
3. *Certain foods,* such as bilberries or blackberries.

If there is doubt, the diagnosis can be confirmed by laboratory investigation of the stool.

3. BLEEDING PER RECTUM

DEFINITION

Hemorrhage *beyond the range of the gastroscope* has empirically been called "lower gastrointestinal bleeding". It has also been defined as blood loss *distal to ligament of Treitz*.

The passage of blood per anus may be

- *Obvious to the patient* because blood is still of its recognizable color (**frank red blood**).
- *Obvious to the doctor* but not the patient, when blood has become black (**melena**).
- *Recognizable only when lab tests for blood are applied to stools* (**occult blood in stools**).

Causes (Sources)

Frank Red Blood Per Rectum	
Anal Causes	• Piles, fissure, fistula. • Foreign body and trauma. • Tumors (anal carcinoma). • Primary syphilis, non-specific inflammation associated with pruritis. • Sensitivity to certain topically applied drugs, e.g. cinchocaine HCl.
Rectal Causes	• Tumors (carcinoma, lymphoma) – polyps. • Injury (e.g. by sigmoidoscope or enema nozzle) – foreign body. • Rectal invasion by carcinoma of the bladder, uterine carcinoma, pelvic sarcoma, pelvic abscess, actinomycosis, schistosomiasis. • Infective proctitis including lymphogranuloma venereum and primary syphilis. • Tuberculous ulceration - solitary rectal ulcer. • Non-specific proctitis.

Contd...

Contd...

Colonic Causes	• Carcinoma (from sigmoid to cecum) - polyps. • Intussusception. • Dysentery (amebic, bacillary, bilharzial). • Tuberculous ulceration of the colon. • Ulcerative colitis - granulomatous colitis (*Crohn's*). • Actinomycosis of the cecum. • Diverticular disease. • Colonic vascular occlusion of artery or vein by thrombus or embolus. • Injury - Irritant drugs (arsenic, phosphorus, calomel) - excessive purgation. • Acute summer diarrhea of infants - *Oxyuris vermicularis*.
Ileal Causes	• Intussusception. • Typhoid fever (typhoid ulcer) - Tuberculous ulcer - Dysentery. • Mesenteric vascular occlusion (MVC) by thrombosis or embolism. • Injury. • Diverticula - *Meckel's diverticulitis*. • After delivery, if the stump of the umbilical cord becomes infected. • Granulomatous ileitis (*Crohn's disease*). • *Tumors*: lymphoma, leiomyosarcoma, multiple polyposis (*Peutz-Jegher syndrome*), hemangioma.
Jejunal Causes	• Peptic ulcer. • After gastro-jejunostomy.
Blood Diseases	Leukemia - thrombocytopenic purpura - Henoch-Schonlein purpura - hereditary capillary fragility - von Willebrand's disease - hemophilia - hypoprothrombinemia.
MELENA	
Duodenal Causes	• Chronic duodenal ulcer. • Duodenal diverticulum. • Injury. • Carcinoma (rare). • Carcinoma of the ampulla of Vater.

Contd...

Contd...

Gastric Causes	• Gastric ulcer - erosive gastritis. • Drug-induced gastritis or ulcer (aspirin, phenylbutazone, cortisone). • Injury - *Mallorey-Weiss syndrome*. • Tumor: carcinoma - sarcoma. • Gastric varices (portal hypertension). • Hereditary telangiectasia, *Osler-Weber-Rendu disease*. • *Gronblad-Strandberg syndrome* (pseudoxanthoma elasticum).
Esophageal Causes	• Esophageal varices. • Hiatal hernia. • Carcinoma of the esophagus. • Trauma - *Mallorey-Weiss syndrome*. • Esophageal ulcers - esophagitis.
Swallowed Blood	• Epistaxis. • Hemoptysis. • Ruptured aneurysm. • Malingering.
General Infections	• Cholera. • Yellow fever - intermittent fever - relapsing fever. • Sprue. • Septicemia.
Occult Blood in Stools	
• The nature of blood passed in the stools depends on: 1. The quantity of the bleeding. 2. Its position in the GIT, high or low. 3. The rate of intestinal transit. • Thus, bleeding in the cecum may appear as bright red blood, melena, or be in such small quantities as to be undetectable to the naked eye (occult) and be detectable only by microscopy or biochemical tests. • Most of the conditions described above may sometimes lead to the passage of occult blood in stools.	

FRANK RED BLOOD PASSED PER ANUS

- When red blood is passed by anus and there is no general pyrexial illness (e.g. typhoid fever) or abdominal catastrophe (e.g. direct injury or MVO), ***the first point*** is to decide whether the blood originates from piles or any other anal lesion, or from a lesion higher up in the GIT.

- In case of **piles, fissure or fistula**, the blood is passed unmixed with feces, and as a rule, not associated with much mucus; with lesions of the **pelvic colon**, or of parts higher up, there may be no mucus. When mucus is passed as well as blood, or if blood is mixed with feces, the lesion is generally more serious than piles, although a rectal carcinoma or a polyp may lead to blood passing in drips or even in gushes quite separate from feces.
- One rule should therefore be considered ***"no case in which blood is passed per anum can be regarded as unimportant until careful examination - visual, digital and instrumental (proctoscopy or sigmoidoscopy) - has been made to exclude the more serious cases than piles such as rectal carcinoma".***

In adults, the chief lesions to diagnose or exclude are the following:

Malignant Disease of the Rectum and Colon

- By digital examination a *rectal carcinoma or polyp* is felt. A microscopic diagnosis is necessary.
- *Higher lesions* require further investigation by radiology or sigmoidoscopy. This will be indicated by the presence of additional symptoms such as spurious diarrhea, pain, constipation, loss of weight, anemia, or general ill-health. A swelling may be felt in the left iliac fossa.
- *Carcinoma of the upper parts of the colon* may be suspected by the passage of blood and mucus associated with increasing constipation and discomfort or pain. A mass may be palpable.

Polyps of the Rectum and Colon

Solitary Polyp

It may be felt digitally or seen by sigmoidoscopy. There may be no pain and no diarrhea and bleeding may be attributed to internal piles. Removal of the polyp should terminate bleeding.

Multiple Polyps

These cause constipation with passage of bloody mucus rather than profuse hemorrhage. They may be detected digitally or by sigmoidoscopy. Sometimes they are flat and sessile, and sometimes they are so numerous as to cause intestinal obstruction. They may turn malignant. Using endoscopy, not only may polyps be located and biopsied, but, providing they are not too large and sessile, they may also be removed using a diathermy snare.

Non-malignant Ulceration

Amebic Dysentery

There is diarrhea, abdominal pain, tenesmus and protracted diarrhea succeeded by the passage of blood-stained mucus or pure blood. It may be followed by an amebic abscess of the liver. Endoscopy, microscopical, and bacteriological examination of stool are necessary to reach diagnosis. Therapeutic test by emetine is helpful.

Bilharzial Dysentery

It affects males > females, especially young adults, due to more exposure. There is diarrhea, tenesmus, mucus and bleeding per rectum, abdominal pain, in addition to anemia and vitamin deficiency. In the diffuse form of colonic schistosomiasis, a mass may be felt in the left iliac fossa. Polyps may be felt by PR examination. Stools should be examined for bilharzial ova.

Bacillary Dysentery (Shigella)

Patients become severely ill with abdominal pain followed by severe diarrhea with passage of blood, pus and mucus many times a day.

Malarial Dysentery

This is usually only seen in acute *falciparum* malaria and is often associated with vomiting, jaundice and collapse. It responds to anti-malarial drugs.

Ulcerative Colitis

Bloody diarrhea and discharge ± tenesmus, abdominal pain, vomiting and loss of weight. Examination reveals dehydration, toxemia and emaciation + tenderness and rigidity on the affected segments. PR may reveal anal fissure, abscess or fistula. *Barium enema* reveals loss of haustrations, narrow contracted colon, undermining of mucosa, or pseudo-polyposis. *Endoscopy* shows mild granular proctitis or extensively ulcerated rectum. Ulcerative colitis may be associated with pyoderma gangrenosa, polyarthritis, iritis, portal hepatic cirrhosis, anal fissure and fistula, and later, the development of colonic carcinoma, which may be multifocal in origin.

Granulomatous Colitis (Crohn's Disease)

Manifestations include fever, malaise, loss of appetite and loss of weight. Middle and lower abdominal crampy pain and diarrhea (may be bloody). Nausea, vomiting, and bloating (obstructive symptoms) may also occur. Rectal bleeding is less common than in ulcerative colitis). Colonic perforation, sinuses, fistulas and strictures are characteristic in contrast to ulcerative colitis (but less frequent than in the terminal ileum). A fistula may involve the UB, causing urgency, dysuria, and pneumaturia. Extra-intestinal manifestations are common, with musculoskeletal abnormalities being the most frequent. *Perianal disease* is a frequent complication. *Colonoscopy* shows aphthous ulcers and *skip areas. Barium enema* shows skip areas, longitudinal ulcerations, transverse fissures, pseudodiverticula, narrowing, strictures, pseudopolypoid changes, a cobblestone pattern, internal fistulas, and sinus tracks.

Uremic Colitis

It is distinguishable by the picture of renal failure and high blood urea.

Syphilitic Proctitis

In primary syphilis where an anal ulcer (chancre) extends into the rectum (in homosexuals), or in tertiary syphilis, which is very rare but has to be distinguished from rectal carcinoma.

Tuberculous Ulceration

It is usually associated with active pulmonary TB and bacilli are found in swabbing from the lesions or feces. It has to be distinguished from carcinoma, $ and ulcerative colitis.

PASSAGE OF BLOOD PER ANUS IN A CHILD

Acute Intussusception

- Severe abdominal pain, passage of bloody mucus (red current jelly) in small amounts at intervals.
- Vomiting is usual.
- A sausage-shaped lump may be identified in the right hypochondrium, epigastrium or left side of the abdomen.

Prolapse of the Anal Mucosa

- It may cause passage of blood per anum.
- It is associated with constipation and straining at stool, but not necessarily with ill-health.

4. HEMATURIA

DEFINITIONS

- **Hematuria** .... Passage of blood in urine.
- **Frank Hematuria** .... Presence of blood on macroscopic examination.
- **Microscopic Hematuria** ..... RBCs are only seen on microscopy (***smoky urine***).
- **Hemoglobinuria** .... Presence of free hemoglobin (Hgb) in urine. Urine is dark brown from the presence of methemoglobin.

PATHOGENESIS OF HEMATURIA

Mechanism	Examples of Causes
1. Undue permeability of nephrons to RBCs (usually glomeruli).	• Bleeding disorders. • Some systemic diseases, e.g. SLE and PAN.
2. Parenchymal renal affection by:	• Anti-coagulants or nephritis. • Micro-infarcts, e g. SABE.
3. Ulcerated surface affecting the urinary tract from the renal pelvis to the urethra:	• External trauma. • Calculi and foreign bodies (internal trauma). • Inflammation (acute or chronic). • Neoplastic (e.g. cancer bladder).

OTHER CAUSES OF RED COLORATION OF URINE

These should be excluded first before attempting to diagnose the cause of hematuria:

Cause of Red Urine	Examples	Characteristic Features
1. *Drugs*	Pyridium, phenophthalin, senna	• History of intake. • Urine translucent not opaque • No RBCs under microscope.
2. *Dyes*	Aniline - coloring agents (juice)	Same as above.
3. *Diet*	Beet root (Beeturia)	Same as above.
4. *Hemoglobinuria:* Passage of oxy-Hb or met-Hb in urine due to hemolysis	• Inections: e.g. Typhoid • Toxins: Carbolic acid. • Incompatible blood Tn. • Some crush injuries.	• Urine is purple in color. • No clots. • No RBCs under microscope. • Distinguished by spectroscopy.
5. *Metabolic Disorders*	Hematoporphyrinuria (should be differentiated from urethral causes)	The patient complains also of dribbling of blood apart from micturition.

CAUSES OF HEMATURIA

Blood may appear in the urine as the result of *injury*, of *disease* in some part of the urinary system or of other organs involving the urinary apparatus, or of a few *general diseases*.

Hematuria from Affection of Some Part of the Urinary Tract (Figure 10.2)

Organ	Cause (Local)	Characteristic Features
Kidneys	Trauma	Mild to moderate trauma commonly causes renal bleeding; severe injuries may not bleed (avulsed kidney - complete disruption) - There is history of trauma - may be renal swelling - other injuries.
	Tumor	Bleeding may be profuse or intermittent: • *Renal cell carcinoma:* Associated mass, loin pain, clot colic or fever, occasional polycythemia, hypercalcemia and hypertension. • *Transitional cell carcinoma (TCC):* Painless, intermittent hematuria. • *Renal adenoma or angioma* at or near the apex of the renal papilla may cause profuse hematuria. • *Papilloma of renal pelvis:* Uncommon but may cause profuse intermittent hematuria.
	Stone	Severe loin/groin pain, gross or microscopic, associated infection, previous attacks or passage of small stones.
	Infection	• *Glomerulonephritis:* usually microscopic, associated systemic disease (e.g. SLE). • *Pyelonephritis* (rare). • *Renal TB:* Sterile pyuria, weight loss, anorexia, ↑ frequency day and night, IVU shows "moth-eaten appearance" (early) or irregular calyces or loss of function (late).
	Hydronephrosis	Hematuria is rarely copious + renal swelling. IVU (characteristic).
	Polycystic disease	Rare, palpable kidneys, hypertension, CRF, IVU (elongated calyces).
	Renal artery aneurysm	Rare, bruit may be heard, hypertension, PXR (shadow), aortography.
	Renal infarction	Very rare, caused by arterial embolus, painful tender kidney.
	Pyelonephritis	Fever, rigors, frequency + organisms, albumin and pus in urine.

Contd...

Contd...

Ureters	Stone	Severe loin/groin pain, gross or microscopic, associated infection.
	Carcinoma	TCC: characteristically painless, intermittent hematuria, ureterography shows filling defect.
	Papilloma	May cause hematuria even after removal of the primary disease in the renal pelvis by nephrectomy.
Bladder	Trauma or F.B.	Foreign bodies are shown by cystoscopy or radiography.
	Stone	Sudden cessation of micturition, pain in the perineum and tip of penis.
	Inflammation	• *Acute Cystitis:* Supra-pubic pain, dysuria, frequency and bacteriuria. • *Interstitial Cystitis (rare):* may be auto-immune, drug or radiation-induced, frequency and dysuria (common).
	Schistosomiasis	Terminal "hematuria and dysuria", burning and frequency of micturition.
	Tumors	*TCC* - characteristically painless, intermittent hematuria, history of work in rubber or dye industries.
Prostate	Hyperplasia	Painless hematuria, associated obstructive symptoms, recurrent UTI.
	Cancer prostate	Late hematuria, difficulty in micturition, heaviness in perineum, back pressure symptoms.
Urethra	Trauma	Blood at meatus, history of direct blow to perineum and retention.
	Stone	Acute penile pain, stone may be palpable or shown by X-ray or endoscopy.
	Urethritis	Rare, septic or gonnorheal, presence of discharge.
	Tumor	*Papillomata* may cause initial hematuria or not related to micturition. *Carcinoma and angioma* are rare.

HEMATURIA FROM NEIGHBORING VISCERA INVOLVING THE URINARY TRACT

Carcinoma of the Uterus, Vagina or Colon

Hematuria results from malignant infiltration of the bladder wall.

Acute Appendicitis

Hematuria may occur due to spread of inflammatory process to vesical wall (pelvic appendicitis or abscess).

Acute Salpingitis

Hematuria may occur due to spread of inflammatory process to vesical wall. It is rarer than in appendicitis.

Pelvic Abscess

Hematuria may occur due to spread of inflammatory process to vesical wall. It is also rarer than in appendicitis.

Dysenteric or TB Ulceration of the Intestine

Hematuria may occur due to adhesion of the bowel to the fundus of the urinary bladder.

Diverticulitis of the Colon

It often causes a pelvic abscess, which may ulcerate into the urinary bladder resulting in hematuria.

HEMATURIA IN GENERAL DISEASE

1. Renal infarction in subacute bacterial endocarditis.
2. Arteriosclerosis.
3. Leukemia.

4. Bleeding disorders:
   - Purpura
   - Scurvy
   - Hemophilia
   - Other bleeding diatheses including anticoagulant therapy
5. Acute fevers:
   - Malaria
   - Small pox
   - Yellow fever
   - Black water fever
6. Excessive exercise.
7. Sickle-cell trait or disease.

GENERAL CAUSES OF HEMATURIA

- Renal infarction (SABE).
- Atherosclerosis.
- Leukemia.
- Bleeding disorders.
- Acute fevers.
- Severe exercise
- Sickle cell disease

Diagnosis of Hematuria

The following points will often help in the differential diagnosis.

Color of Urine:

Bright red .... Hemorrhage is most likely to arise from UB or lower urinary tract.

Dark-colored .... Due to retention of blood in the UB for some time, or due to large amount of blood present in urine.

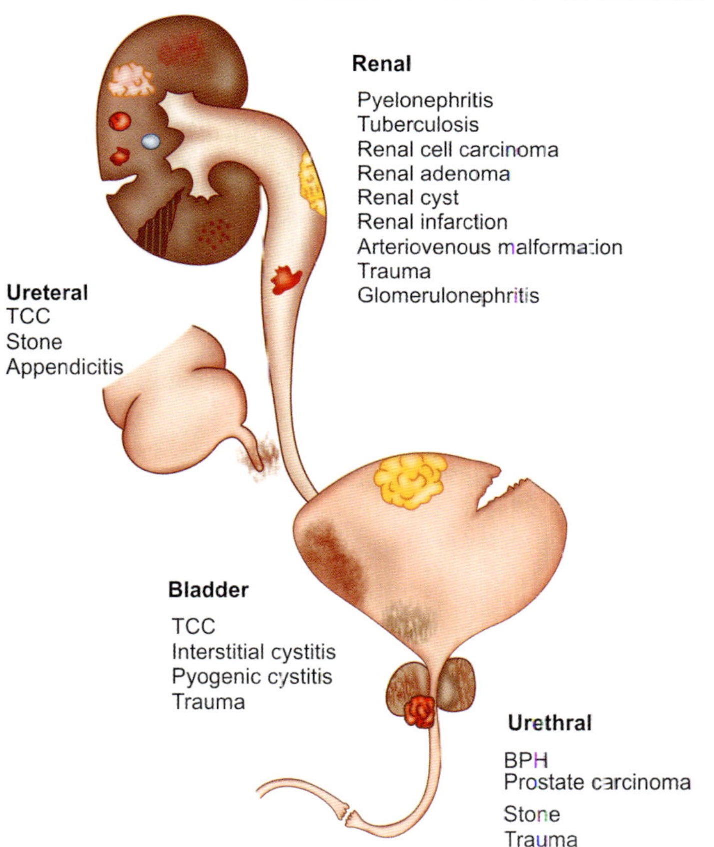

Fig. 10.2: Local causes of hematuria

Amount of Blood in Urine:

Microscopic (smoky urine) ... May be due to glomerulonephritis or bilharzial cystitis.

Moderate (> smoky urine) .... May be due to renal or vesical calculi.

Profuse (Severe) .... May be due to renal or vesical tumors, or renal trauma.

Blood Clots ....

- *Dark clots* (= ceased bleeding).
- *Fresh bright red* (= continuous bleeding).
- *Shape of clot* (worm-like = renal or ureteral, rounded = vesical).

Timing of Bleeding:

Continuous Hematuria .... May result from nephritis or bilharzial cystitis.

Intermittent Hematuria .... Sudden bouts of hematuria with free (clear urine) intervals.

Cyclic Hematuria .... Related to menstruation (= endometriosis).

Relation to Micturition:

Total Hematuria .... All urine is bloody from beginning to end (= renal, ureteric, or vesical, or is pre-renal in origin).

Partial Hematuria ....

- *Initial Hematuria:* 1st urine passed is blood-stained, remainder is clear = urethra (papilloma, stricture, trauma, impacted stone) or prostate.
- *Terminal Hematuria:* Blood at the end of micturition = UB neck and trigone (e.g. Tumors or polyps of the UB neck or senile prostatic hyperplasia, or late in cancer prostate).

Pain: Present or Absent?

Painful Hematuria:

Total hematuria ....
- *Site*: Kidney - ureter - UB.
- *Causes*: Renal stone or trauma - stone or stricture ureter.

Initial hematuria ....
- *Site*: Anterior urethra
- *Causes*: Anterior urethritis - rupture urethra.

Terminal hematuria ....
- *Site*: UB
- *Causes*: Cystitis (especially bilharzial) - UB ulcers or stone - cancer UB especially with superadded cystitis.

Painless Hematuria:

Total hematuria ....
- *Site*: Kidney - ureter - UB.
- *Causes*: *Pre-renal* (bleeding disorders, SABE, hypertension, drugs, e.g. sulfa and corticosteroids and anticoagulants), *Renal* (Acute G.N, tumors, TB, big stones "staghorn", polycystic kidney, solitary cyst), or *Ureter*: (tumors).

Initial hematuria ....
- *Site*: Anterior urethra.
- *Causes*: Tumors (papilloma).

Terminal hematuria ....
- *Site*: UB.
- *Causes*: Papilloma of UB - senile prostatic hyperplasia.

DIFFERENTIAL DIAGNOSIS OF HEMATURIA - CLINICAL KEY POINTS

It is essential to answer 3 questions:

1. **Is it Hematuria or Not?**

2. Where is the Source of Hematuria ?

Renal Hematuria .... Urine is smoky and blood is well mixed.

Vesical Hematuria .... Urine is mixed with blood which may be in the form of clots, and is usually dark in color (remains in the UB for some time). It may be terminal as in bilharzial cystitis.

Urethral Hematuria............ It is bright red and is either initial or not related to micturition.

3. What is the Cause of Hematuria?

The following approach should be adopted to determine the *site and cause* of hematuria:

History-Taking

Personal Data

Age:

- Adolescents and young adults .... Bilharziasis and papilloma.
- Adults....................... Trauma, stone and hypernephroma.
- Elderly....................... Senile prostatic hyperplasia and cancer.

Sex:

- Females .... UTI.
- Males .... Vesical papilloma - cancer bladder.
- Both ....UTI and stones (1st 4 decades) - tumors (5th decade).

Symptoms

1. Hematuria:

- Bright red or dark? - Continuous or intermittent?
- Relation to urine stream; early or late or mixed?
- Painless (tumor) or painful (trauma, stone, inflammation)?

2. Associated Symptoms

- Renal pain and colic..............Kidney or ureter (e.g. stone).
- Pain referring to glans penis.......................UB base, prostatic urethra.
- Pelvic pain + headache............ Secondaries (kidney - UB - prostate).
- Frequency ....UB or prostatic urethra.
- Hesitancy and urgency.................BNO (prostatic hyperplasia or cancer).
- Fever ....Kidney tumor or infection (UTI).
- Loin swelling.................................Neuroblastoma (child) - Adenocarcinoma.
- Pneumaturia and fecaluria.........................Vesico-colic fistula (cancer colon).

Past History

1. History of recent sore throat is suggestive of nephritis.
2. Trauma - Bleeding tendency - Drugs: e.g. anticoagulants.

Clinical Examination

General Examination:

- Signs of anemia, uremia or infection are searched for.

Abdominal Examination

- A swelling in the loin may be felt. It may be a hypernephroma, or hydronephrosis secondary to a carcinoma of the bladder. Cancer bladder may be felt as a suprapubic mass.
- The external genitalia are examined for inflammatory masses, e.g. TB, epididymitis.

Rectal Examination

- Prostatic enlargement (benign or malignant), or a bladder tumor may be felt.

Investigations

Laboratory Investigations

A. *Blood Examinations:*

- Full blood count (FBC): Infection, chronic blood loss. "Rouleaux" suggest glomerulonephritis.
- Clotting: To exclude an underlying bleeding disorder.
- Urea and creatinine: To assess renal function.
- Autoimmune screen: For glomerulonephritis.

B. *Urine Analysis:*

- The presence of red cells excludes hemoglobinuria and beeturia.
- Bilharzial ova denote urinary bilharziasis (S. hematobium).
- Casts indicate nephritis.
- Pus cells indicate infection.
- Sterile cystitis is either due to TB or tumor.
- Papanicolaou smear may reveal malignant cells.

Radiography

A. *Plain and IVU*......May show stone, tumor filling defect + assess renal function.
B. *Chest X-ray*.......... May show pulmonary metastases.
C. *Skeletal survey*.... May show bone metastases.
D. *CT Scan*............... Renal lesion - renal tumors or cysts.

Cystoscopy

1. Detection of bladder tumors, interstitial cystitis.
2. The site of bleeding if in the bladder or prostate could be visualized.
3. Pathologic areas are biopsied.
4. Blood may be seen coming from one ureter.

Selective Renal Angiography

Renal arteriovenous malformations (AVM).

5. MENORRHAGIA

DEFINITIONS

- **Menorrhagia:** Excessive menstrual flow or undue prolongation of the "period" time.
- **Metrorrhagia (irregular uterine bleeding):** Bleeding which occurs between the periods.
- **Polymenorrhea:** Irregular excessive menstruation in which the cycle is shortened from the usual 28 days to 21 days or even less due to disturbed balance of internal secretions, causing ovulation to occur too early in the cycles.

DIAGNOSIS

The diagnosis of menorrhagia has to be accepted when the patient is having to use more than a dozen and half pads per menstrual period, or when she loses clots, or has flooding.

CAUSES OF MENORRHAGIA

Of endocrine origin	1. At puberty: Mainly due to hypofunction of the anterior pituitary. 2. At maturity without obvious lesions. 3. In relation to the menopause, and in the years preceding.
In the generative system	1. Fibromyomata – Adenomyoma. 2. Chronic salpingo-oophoritis – Tuberculous endometritis. 3. Endometriosis. 4. Intrauterine contraceptive device (ICD). 5. Acute infectious diseases: Influenza, enteric, cholera, variola, malaria, diphtheria and measles.
In the circulatory system	1. Uncompensated valvular heart disease. 2. Liver cirrhosis. 3. Pulmonary emphysema.

Contd..

Contd..

	4. Hyperthyroidism – hypothyroidism. 5. Chronic alcoholism. 6. The blood itself: Deficient coagulability, purpura, hemophilia, leukemia. 7. High blood pressure: Arteriosclerosis.
In the nervous system	1. Excessive coitus. 2. Prevention of conception. 3. A single excessive period: Fright, violent emotion, sudden changes of temp., cold bath, dancing, hunting, gymnastics, bicycling, etc.

N.B. Details are beyond the scope of this book.

6. HEMOPTYSIS

DEFINITIONS

- Hemoptysis means "*blood spitting*". By a widely accepted convention, it is generally used to refer specially to the "*expectoration of blood from the bronchi or lungs*". The blood, either alone or mixed with sputum, is nearly always produced by *coughing*, but rarely may trickle past the larynx and be spat out without exciting cough.
- Bleeding from the *nose, mouth, throat, pharynx or larynx* may lead to the spitting of blood or blood-stained secretions. This is sometimes called "**spurious hemoptysis**" since the blood is not from the chest and is not in the strict sense expectorated.
- Irrespective of verbal usage, bleeding *from the upper respiratory tract* must be included in the differential diagnosis of hemoptysis.

SOURCES OF HEMOPTYSIS

Mouth (Gums)	***Bleeding gums due to general condition or mouth lesion:*** 1. Blood dyscrasias: Acute leukemia, aplastic anemia, thrombocytopenia, hemophilia, purpura. 2. Syphilis. 3. Febrile states. 4. Hodgkin's disease (rare). ***Bleeding gums due to purely local conditions:*** 1. Injury (e.g. toothbrush). 2. Dental caries. 3. Pyorrhea alveolaris. 4. Actinomycosis. 5. Acute or chronic stomatitis: aphthous stomatitis, ulcerative stomatitis, Vinvent's angina, gangrenous stomatitis (cancrum oris, phagedena oris, noma oris).

Contd...

Contd...

	6. Tuberculous gingivitis. 7. Papilloma. 8. Epulides. 9. Myeloma. 10. Epithelioma. 11. Erythema bullosum. 12. Dermatitis herpetiformis. 13. Pemphigus.
Nose (Epistaxis)	***Epistaxis due to local causes:*** 1. Cardiovascular conditions: Hypertension. 2. High venous pressure: Bronchitis, emphysema, right heart dilatation. 3. Abnormal blood and capillaries: Hemophilia, von Willebrand's disease, vitamin K deficiency, thrombocytopenia, anticoagulants. 4. Acute specific fevers: Enteric, influenza, scarlet fever, small pox. ***Epistaxis due to local causes:*** 1. Spontaneous epistaxis (from dilated blood vessels of nasal septum). 2. Trauma (blow, fist, cricket ball, windscreen of a car). 3. Foreign body and nose picking. 4. Infection (TB, $). 5. Atrophic rhinitis. 6. Neoplasms of the nasal cavities, paranasal sinuses or nasopharynx (septal angioma, nasopharyngeal angiofibroma). 7. Osler-Weber-Rendu disease.
Larynx	Carcinoma.
Trachea	1. Carcinoma 2. Foreign body.
Bronchus	1. Neoplastic: Carcinoma – adenoma. 2. Inflammatory: Bronchiectasis –chronic bronchitis. 3. Foreign body.

Contd...

Contd...

Lungs	1. Infection (TB, other granulomas, pneumonia, lung abscess, parasitic infestations). 2. Infarction. 3. Arteriovenous aneurysm. 4. Idiopathic hemosiderosis. 5. Trauma.
Cardiovascular	1. Mitral stenosis. 2. Left ventricular failure. 3. Aortic aneurysm.
Bleeding states	1. Thrombocytopenia. 2. Henoch-Schonlein purpura. 3. Leukemia. 4. Scurvy.

N.B. Details are beyond the scope of this book.

CHAPTER

11

Differential Diagnosis of Urinary Retention

URINARY RETENTION

DEFINITIONS

Urinary retention is defined as the inability to micturate. It could be acute or chronic, painful or painless, and complete or with overflow incontinence.

- **Acute retention:** Sudden inability to micturate in the presence of a *painful* bladder.
- **Chronic retention:** Presence of an enlarged, full, *painless* bladder with or without difficulty in micturition.
- **Overflow incontinence:** Uncontrollable leakage and dribbling of urine in the presence of a full bladder.

ACUTE URINARY RETENTION

Causes

Mechanical Obstruction (Increased Outlet Resistance)

A. Bladder Neck Obstruction (BNO)	B. Posterior Urethra (straining hinders micturition)	C. Anterior Urethra (straining helps micturition)
1. Stone impaction at internal meatus. 2. Blood clot retention.	1. Congenital urethral valve. 2. Senile prostatic hyperplasia.	1. Congenital pin-hole meatus. 2. Phimosis, and para-phimosis.

Contd...

Contd...

3. Tumor of the urinary bladder protruding into the urinary bladder neck or infiltrating it. 4. Fibrosis (e.g. bilharziasis). 5. Pressure from outside. 6. Gravid uterus. 7. Fibroid. 8. Ovarian cyst. 9. Fecal impaction.	3. Cancer prostate. 4. Prostatic abscess 5. Prostatitis. 6. Stone.	3. Stricture urethra. 4. Rupture urethra. 5. Cancer urethra (rare). 6. Stone. 7. Foreign body.

Neurogenic Causes (Weak Detrusor Contraction)

1. *Postoperative:* Due to pain, drugs, pelvic nerve disturbance (or after painful conditions).
2. *Pressure on the spinal cord* by injury (e.g. fracture or dislocation) or disease (e.g. Pott's) of the *spine.*
3. *Spinal cord* and *nerve root* diseases, e.g. transverse myelitis, disseminated sclerosis and tabes dorsalis.
4. *Diabetes*: Progressive lower motor neuron (LMN) pattern.
5. *Hysterical* (psychological).
6. *Drugs*: Anticholinergics, antihistaminic, muscle relaxants, and some tranquilizers.
7. *Idiopathic*: Detrusor sphincter dyssynergia? bladder neuron degeneration?

Differential Diagnosis

A useful clinical approach is to answer three main questions:

1. Is it "retention" or anuria? .... (Anuria = failure of the kidney to form urine).
2. Is it obstructive or not?.................. i.e. obstructive or neurological.
3. If obstructive.................................. What and where is the obstruction?

Retention or Not?

Point of Difference	Acute Retention	Anuria
1. Desire to pass urine:	+	-
2. History or lower urinary tract manifestations:	+	-
3. History of upper urinary tract manifestations:	+	-
4. Renal swelling and tenderness:	±	-
5. Full U.B (dull - empties by catheterization):	+	-
6. General condition:	Good !	Bad (Uremic)

Obstructive or Not?

- Obstructive: History of operation, drugs, injury, nerve disease, psychological trouble.
- If not, it must be .... obstructive!

What and Where is the Obstruction?

History-Taking

Age:

- Children.................Phimosis, meatal ulcer with scab formation.
- Young Adults......... Paraphimosis, prostatitis and urethritis.
- Adult.......................Stricture and stone impaction.
- Elderly....................Senile prostate.
- Over 60 years......... Cancer prostate.

Sex:

- Male......................Prostatic hyperplasia (old), urethral stricture (adult), postoperative.
- Females................ RVF, other gynecological disorders, hysterical and disseminated sclerosis.

Symptoms

- Inability to pass urine.
- Pain which is spasmodic and occurs periodically as the muscle of the bladder contracts.

Past History:

1. Pelvic or renal operations.
2. Symptoms of bladder neck obstruction suggest benign or malignant prostate.
3. History of injection of hemorrhoids suggest prostatic abscess.
4. Drug intake.
5. Diseases: Bilharziasis, gonorrhea.

Clinical Examination:

A. *General examination:* Look for evidence of dehydration or uremia (chronic retention).
B. *Local examination:*
    1. *Full urinary bladder* as evidenced by:
        a. Abdominal Examination:
            - A fluctuant, tense cystic swelling in the suprapubic area.
            - It is pelvi-abdominal (arises from pelvis), i.e. you can not reach its lower border.
            - Globular in shape and variable in size.
            - Manual mobility (side-to-side and antero-posterior).
            - No mobility with respiration (extraperitoneal and has no relation to the diaphragm).
            - Slightly tender on deep pressure which initiates and exaggerates desire to micturate.
            - It is dull on percussion (urine).
        b. PR Examination:
            - A boggy cystic swelling may be felt by PR (full bladder base).
            - It initiates the desire for micturition.

c. Bimanual Examination:
   - UB base is felt by PR while a swelling is felt with the hand on suprapubic area.
2. Both loins are palpated for the presence of kidney swelling.
3. The penis is examined for evidence of scars, phimosis, pin-hole meatus, stricture, etc.
4. Rectal examination:
   a. The bladder is felt as a cystic mass above the prostate.
   b. The prostate is difficult to assess properly while the bladder is full. However, cancer prostate or senile enlargement could be suspected.

Investigations:

1. *Laboratory:* Blood and urine analysis (for infection and cytology if tumor is suspected).
2. *Radiological*:
   a. Plain X-ray: A stone may be seen.
   b. IVU: Cancer UB (filling defect), impression of enlarged prostate, stone.
   c. Urethrogram: Urethral valve or stricture, enlarged prostate.
   d. Cystography: Cancer UB.
3. *Endoscopic*: Urethroscopy and cystoscopy.
4. *Urodynamics:* Allows identification and assessment of neurological problems, assesses benign hyperplasia of the prostate (BHP).

Differential Diagnosis:

1. **Stricture of Urethra:** Usually a young patient, with a history of gonorrhea or urethral injury, gradually increasing difficulty in micturition, narrowing of the stream, and inability to finish the flow completely without some dribbling of urine. Urethroscopy is diagnostic.

2. **Prostatic Enlargement:** The patient is usually above 55 years, has been troubled with increasing frequency in micturition, especially at night, with straining and loss of force in the stream of urine. The prostate is found to be enlarged by PR; it may be smooth, uniform in consistency, elastic and movable in the pelvic space in case of ***adenomatous enlargement***, or nodular, hard irregular and fixed in case of ***carcinoma.*** In case of retention from ***acute prostatitis*** or ***prostatic abscess***, the patient gives a history of recent urethral discharge.
3. **A Small Calculus:** It may be passed into the urethra and become arrested at a narrow part, usually at the meatus or membranous urethra. It may occur at any age, causing pain with cessation of flow of urine and dribbling of a few drops of blood. The stone may be palpated if it lies in the penile urethra or perineum, or will be felt on passing an instrument into the urethra.
4. **Pedunculated Vesical Tumor:** Its free portion may block the internal urethral orifice. On any attempt of micturition the growth is forced into the orifice and obstructs it. It is rare and can be detected by cystoscopy.
5. **Traumatic Rupture of Urethra:** It is often associated with fracture pelvis. The history of injury and appearance of blood at the external urethral orifice and a hematoma in the perineum will point to the diagnosis.

CHRONIC URINARY RETENTION

The bladder is full with large volumes of residual urine and the patient voids infrequent small amounts. At start voiding occurs voluntary with noticeable urgency. By time precipitance occurs and voiding becomes involuntary on the first desire, or more worse occurs in continuous dribbling *"chronic retention with overflow"*.

Clinical Features

A. *General Examination:* It is almost always associated with a varying degree of renal failure.

B. *Local Examination:*

- The bladder is hugely distended. There is mild or no suprapubic discomfort.
- Passage of catheter (diagnostic test) → passage of urine (residual) and ↓ in size of abdominal swelling.

Investigations

- *Ultrasound or IVU* may reveal chronic retention not detected clinically. Furthermore, US will show dilatation of the upper tracts even when there is renal impairment.
- *Cauterization* is required to confirm the diagnosis only when there is clinical doubt and when scanning facilities are unavailable.
- *Blood tests* are taken to assess renal function.

Clinical Key Points — Retention of Urine

Commonest causes of acute urinary retention:

1. Urethral stricture.
2. Prostatic enlargement.

Factors that may precipitate acute retention:

1. Surgery.
2. Drug therapy (e.g. diuretics, anticholinergics, antidepressants and sympathomimetics).
3. Alcohol.
4. Cerebrovacular accident.
5. Constipation.
6. Painful conditions of the perianal region (e.g. hemorrhoids).
7. Prolonged recumbence.
8. Acute urinary infection.

Complications of Urinary Retention:

- Renal: Hydroureter, bilateral hydronephrosis, renal hypertension, renal failure (uremia).
- Extra-renal (straining): Hernia, secondary piles rectal prolapse, uterine prolapse (in females).

Urinary Retention may be due to Mechanical or Neurological Causes:

1. Mechanical causes are either in the lumen of the urethra (intraluminal), in the wall of the urethra (intramural) or outside the wall of the urethra (external).
2. Neurological causes may be upper motor neuron (UMN) or lower motor neuron (LMN):
   a. UMN causes produce chronic retention with reflex incontinence.
   b. LMN causes produce chronic retention with overflow incontinence.

Urinary Retention may be Acute or Chronic:

1. Acute retention is characterized by pain, sensation of bladder fullness and a mildly distended UB.
2. Chronic retention is characterized by symptoms of bladder irritation (frequency, dysuria, small volume), painless, marked distention, overflow incontinence. Often associated with secondary UTI.

CHAPTER

12

Differential Diagnosis of Swollen Limb

SWOLLEN LIMB

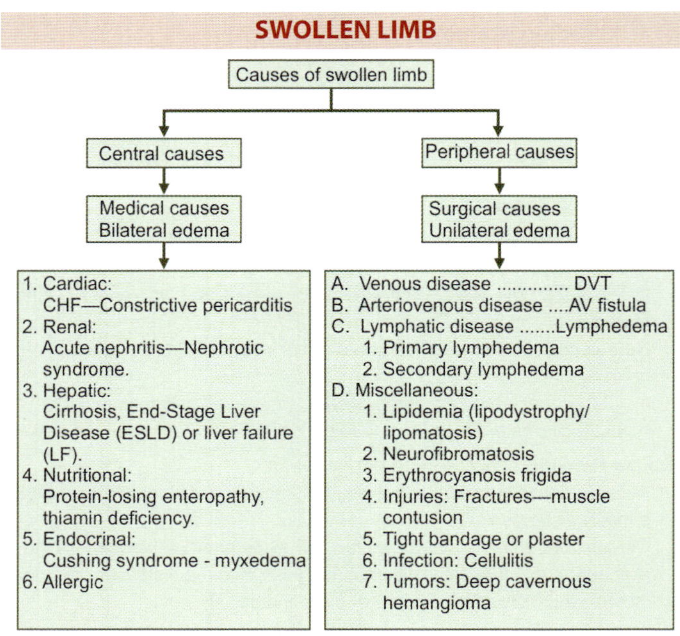

DIFFERENTIAL DIAGNOSIS

1. Is it Central?

It is usually *bilateral and accompanied by generalized edema.* The C/P of heart failure, renal failure or liver failure, etc. can be easily diagnosed by history-taking and physical examination and appropriate investigations.

2. Is it Unilateral?

Is it due to a *local cause* (Arteriovenous, venous, lymphatic or others)?

3. Is it A-V Fistula?

A. *Local Manifestations:*
   a. There is a pulsating swelling characterized by being:
      - Soft and empties on pressure.
      - Pulsatile (less marked than that of arterial aneurysm because the vein acts as a safety valve).
      - Classical continuous machinery murmur (louder than in aneurysms).
      - Thrill which is maximum in systole (stronger than that of aneurysm).
   b. Warming of the skin in the region of - and distal to - the fistula.

B. *Distal Manifestations:*
   a. Effects of "*Ischemia*": Pallor, absent pulse, digital gangrene, etc.
   b. Effects of "*Chronic Venous Congestion*":
      - Secondary varicose veins which are pulsatile and do not empty on elevation.
      - Venous hypertension leading to congestion, edema, ulceration, pigmentation chronic eczema, as well as local gigantism in children.

C. *Central Effects:*
   a. Cardiac enlargement due to shunting of arterial blood and VR (cardiac hypertrophy).
   b. Branham's bradycardia reaction.

4. Is it Venous?

DVT: Phlegmasia Alba Dolens (PAD), Phlegmasia Cerula Dolens (PCD), secondary V.V. ,etc.

- Venous edema is a non-inflammatory, soft, pitting edema.
- Its extent varies, and it is exacerbated by prolonged standing and heat.
- It is accompanied by or is complicated by pain, heaviness, hyperpigmentation, dermatitis, often varicose veins, and sometimes ulcerations and scleroderma-like involvement of the dorsal and malleolar aspects of the foot.
- It starts at and involves mainly the calves and ankles.

Criteria	Phlegmasia Alba Dolens	Phlegmasia Cerula Dolens
Severity:	Less severe	More severe
Pathology:	Partial vein occlusion + moderate arterial spasm.	Complete vein occlusion + obstruction of arterial blood.
Arterial pulse:	Felt (↓)	Not felt (often misdiagnosed as arterial embolism; however, absent pulse in a greatly swollen limb suggests that the main vein and not the main artery is blocked).
Color:	White	Blue (cyanotic, mottled) and cold.
Fluid loss:	Less marked (no shock)	More marked (shock always present).
Toxic face:	-ve	+ve

5. Is it Lymphatic?

Lymphedema (Is it primary or secondary?).

- *Lymphedema is mainly a clinical diagnosis.* It has a different presentation than venous edema. It is usually firm, sometimes sclerotic, but with *no* gaiter aspect. It is sometimes soft, but is *not* a pitting type of edema.

- It has a painless white appearance, and is frequently complicated by lymphangitis or erysipelas. It is also often accompanied by inflammatory erythematous plaques.
- Improvement with bed rest is inconsistent and often incomplete.
- Lymphedema affects mainly the ankle and dorsal aspect of foot. When it affects the leg, it does *not* leave the contour of the calf intact, but produces a post-like aspect. Involvement of the dorsal aspect of the toes of the foot includes edema with thickening of the skin, which can not be pinched between 2 fingers. This sign (*Stemmer's sign*) is specific for lymphedema, and thus enables its clinical confirmation.
- Lymphedema is not complicated by ulceration, but rather by an elephantiasis-like presentation with sclerosis and vegetation (hyperpapillomatosis).

Point of Difference	Primary Lymphedema	Secondary Lymphedema	Acute Lymphangitis
Context	Familial	Neoplasia	Portal of entry
Onset	Insidious	Insidious	Acute
Localization	Distal	Proximal	Distal
Fever, chills	-	-	+
Color	White	White	Red
Warmth	-	-	+
Lymph Nodes	-	+	+
Red cord-like appearance	-	-	+

Differences between Venous, Lymphatic and A-V Fistula as Causes of Swollen Leg

Venous	Lymphatic	A-V Fistula
1. Early, there is edema which pits. Later, it becomes non-pitting. 2. There may be varicose veins, skin pigmentation and ulceration. 3. History of DVT and pain.	1. Lymphedema usually pits, but later becomes harder and non-pitting. 2. The skin is thicker and hyperkeratotic, but there is no pigmentation or ulceration	1. Gigantism of the limb. 2. Distended superficial veins and leg ulcers. 3. Superficial angiomata. 4. To-and-fro murmur. 5. Increased local warmth.

6. Is it *Otherwise*?

1. *Lipidemia*..................... Soft consistency, never affects the foot.
2. *Neurofibromatosis*........ Café au-lait pigmentation + pressure effects.
3. *Deep Cavernous Hemangioma* .... Birth marks, reduction in size on elevation.

HISTORY TAKING

Personal Data

Sex, occupation, and residence, e.g. a male farmer from an endemic area (filarial district).

Complaints

Leg swelling, pain, disturbed body function.

Present History

Analysis of complaints and associated symptoms e.g. attacks of fever, rigors, with diffuse redness and hotness of the skin (lymphangitis) or progressive in the size of the scrotum (filarial hydrocele).

Past History

It is essential to exclude other causes of edema.

Family History

It is *relevant* as the cause may be an endemic or familial disease.

CLINICAL EXAMINATION

General Examination

Careful general systematic examination is necessary for evidence of:

1. Central cause in the heart, liver or kidney, in *bilateral edema*.
2. Abdominal, pelvic or femoral swellings, in *venous edema* due to compression of large veins.
3. Generalized malignant lymph nodes (e.g. malignant inguinal lymph nodes infiltrating the lymphatics).
4. Other filarial lesions in the scrotum (filarial hydrocele or chylocele, lymphoscrotum or elephantiasis of the scrotum, matting of the contents of the spermatic cord).

Local Examination of the Swollen Limb

You should comment on the following:

Skin

For evidence of:

- Venous manifestations........ Varicose veins, ulcerations, pigmentations, etc.
- Lymphatic manifestations...... Hyperkeratosis and wart-like projections, or lymphangitis.
- Arterial manifestations....... Evidence of ischemia or A-V fistula.

Consistency

For "pitting on pressure":
- Pitting edema .... Soft and pits on pressure.
- Non-pitting edema .... Hard and does not pit on pressure.
- Brawny edema .... Indurated but pits on pressure.

Regional Lymph Nodes

- Enlarged and firm ....Filarial or chronic lymphedema.
- Enlarged and hard ....Malignancy.

SPECIAL INVESTIGATIONS

Laboratory Tests

- Complete blood picture.
- Analysis of protein content.

Biopsy

- A lymph node biopsy is indicated in case of presence of enlarged lymph nodes.

Non-invasive Radiological Tests

- Lymphoscintigraphy.
- Ultrasonography (US).
- Computerized tomography (CT).
- Magnetic resonance imaging (MRI).
- Non-invasive venous investigations:
  a. Doppler ultrasound.
  b. Plethysmography.

Invasive Investigations

- Venography.
- Arteriography.
- Contrast lymphangiography.

CHAPTER

13

Differential Diagnosis of Gangrene

GANGRENE

DEFINITION

It means death in bulk of the *macroscopic portions* of the body and usually associated with *putrefaction* (i.e. putrefaction necrosis).

CARDINAL SIGNS OF GANGRENE

1. Loss of pulsations.
2. Loss of sensation.
3. Loss of heat.
4. Loss of color.
5. Loss of function.

TYPES OF GANGRENE

A. Dry gangrene.
B. Wet gangrene.
    1. Non-infective (aseptic)
    2. Infective (septic):
        - Primary: Clostridia of gas gangrene.
        - Secondary: Infection of aseptic gangrene.

CLASSIFICATION OF GANGRENE ACCORDING TO ETIOLOGY

1. Cardiovascular gangrene:
   a. Thrombotic.
   b. Embolic.
   c. Vasospastic.
2. Neuropathic gangrene.
3. Traumatic gangrene.
4. Physico-chemical gangrene.
5. Infective gangrene.
   a. Specific.
   b. Non-specific.
6. Circulatory gangrene.
7. Gangrene complicating certain diseases.
8. Gangrene after slight trauma.

CAUSES OF GANGRENE

1. Cardiovascular Gangrene a. Thrombotic Gangrene: b. Embolic Gangrene. c. Vasospastic Disorders:	1. Senile gangrene (Atherosclerosis). 2. Presenile gangrene (Burger's disease). 3. Diabetic gangrene. Raynaud's disease - Ergot poisoning - Scalene syndrome.
2. Neuropathic Gangrene	1. Leprosy. 2. Syringomyelia. 3. Myelitis, meningomyelitis. 4. Tabes dorsalis. 5. Lesions of the medulla spinalis. 6. Peripheral neuritis.
3. Traumatic Gangrene	1. *Direct*: Crushing or pressure. 2. *Indirect*: Rupture or occlusion of the main artery.
4. Physico-chemical Gangrene	1. Deep burns: Thermal, chemical, electrical, radiation. 2. Frost bite. 3. Trench foot.

Contd...

Contd...

5. Infective Gangrene	1. Non-specific infections: Furuncle, carbuncle, cancrum oris, noma vulvae, phagedena, Meleney's ulcer. 2. Specific Infections: Gas gangrene.
6. Circulatory	1. Rheumatoid arteritis. 2. Syphilitic end arteritis obliterans. 3. Polyarteritis nodosa (PAN). 4. Systemic lupus erythematosis (SLE). 5. Intra-arterial injection of pentothal sodium. 6. Obstruction by new-growth. 7. Following carbon monoxide poisoning.
7. Complicating the following disease and due to slight trauma	1. Febrile diseases: Typhoid, typhus, small pox, measles, cholera, plague, yellow fever, malaria. 2. Marasmus. 3. Poisoning by snake-venom. 4. Leukemia.

CARDIOVASCULAR GANGRENE

Thrombotic Gangrene

Senile (Atherosclerotic) Gangrene

- *Incidence:* It is the most common variety in civil practice.
- *Age:* >50 years; *Sex:* Men > women; *Site:* Lower limb (usually).
- Caused mainly by *senile atherosclerosis,* often supplemented by secondary thrombosis in the main vessels and precipitated by *trauma.* The process is *slow* causing mostly, *dry gangrene.*
- *The onset* is usually preceded by manifestations of *chronic ischemia,* e.g. numbness and tingling, persistent coldness, pallor, intermittent claudication, and rest pain.
- *Gangrene* starts as an area of painful redness in the center of which, a dry black slough appears which may separate slowly leaving an ulcer which may heal and breakdown

again. More often the process spreads gradually till the whole *toe* or even the *foot* is dry, black and dead. The commonest site for the onset is the big toe (**Figure 13.1**) and other toes are affected successively. However, other toes may be affected first (**Figure 13.2**).

- *Pain* is always marked causing exhaustion and insomnia.
- *Toxic manifestations* are common such as fever, anorexia and toxic glycosuria.

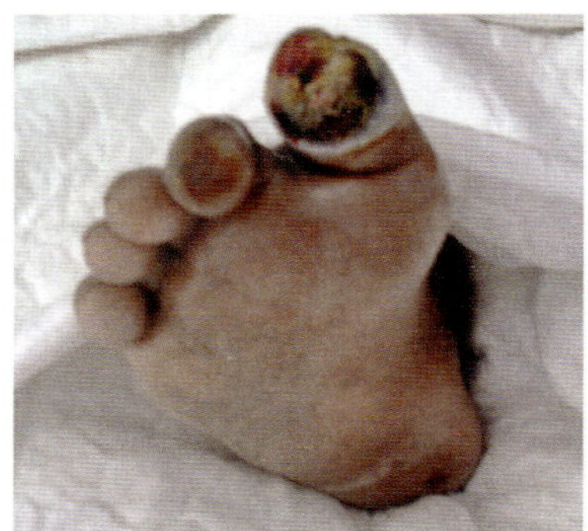

Fig. 13.1: Gangrene of the big toe

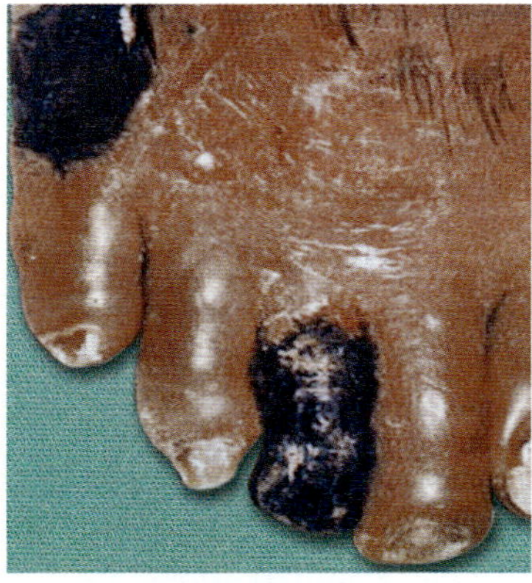

Fig. 13.2: Gangrene of the third toe

Buerger's Disease (Thrombangitis Obliterans or Presenile Gangrene)

- It is an *inflammatory and thrombotic* process of arteries and veins, affecting vessels of limbs and rarely visceral or superficial ones. Characteristically, calcification and deposition of lipids *never occur.*
- It is due to irreversible changes in the walls of affected vessels, and an abnormal degree of sympathetic stimulation (overactivity) that gives rise to spasm of the collaterals.
- It mainly affects the "*medium-sized arteries*" especially the posterior tibial and popliteal arteries (i.e. lower limb). It may also affect "distal arteries" of the upper limb.
- The *distal (usual) type* affects distal vessels (digital) → ulcer and gangrene of toes. Pulses are palpable at the ankle; while the *proximal (rare) type* affects larger vessels (popliteal → calf claudication). Pulses are absent at the ankle or knee.
- *Age* < 40 years (*Presenile gangrene*); *Sex*: Males (almost always) - chronic *heavy smoker.*
- The symptoms are primarily due to *ischemia*. The disease usually progresses in 4 stages: (1) *Phlebitis migrans* (recurrent attacks of superficial phlebitis with swelling of joints and legs), (2) *Claudication* (occurs only in the proximal type. Slowly progressive pain with pallor, coldness and loss of pulsation at the ankle and knee + ischemic neuropathy, e.g. numbness and burning), (3) *Rest pain*: Usually ↓ by dependency and exposure, and (4) *Trophic (nutritional changes),* e.g. ulcers, fissures and finally *Dry Gangrene* which develops early in the distal type and delayed (within years) in the proximal type.
- *Plain X-ray* → *No* calcifications. *Arteriography* → Segment obliteration of arteries. Collateral circulation in chronic cases is well developed and appears as "tree roots" or "spider legs". Recanalized thrombosed arteries give a

"corkscrew" appearance of the vessel, extensive abrupt occlusions in small arteries while large vessels are normal + extensive collaterals.

Differences between Atherosclerosis and Buerger's Disease

Criteria	Atherosclerosis	Buerger's Disease
Incidence	More common	Less common
Etiology	A degenerative disease	Immunological ↑ by smoking.
Pathology * Artery * Veins * Nerve	 Proximal - no recanalization No migratory thrombophlebitis Not affected	 Distal - followed by recanalization Positive Peripheral nerve affection
Age	Old	Around 40 years
Smoking	May be smoker	Heavy smoker
Course	Progressive	Progressive episodes
Gangrene	Can be extensive	Usually limited
Plain X-ray	Calcification	No calcification
Arteriography	Large vessels ± collaterals, plaque (irregular lining)	Small vessels, good collaterals, smooth intimal lining

Diabetic Gangrene

- It results from:
    1. *Impaired glucose metabolism favoring sepsis (*due to ↓ vitality of the tissues, impaired defensive mechanisms and ↑ bacterial growth).
    2. *Diabetic angiopathy* (atherosclerosis occurs earlier in diabetic patients and spreads > the senile type).
    3. *Diabetic neuropathy* (anesthesia of the toes and distal foot predisposes to injury resulting in trophic changes in the tissues).

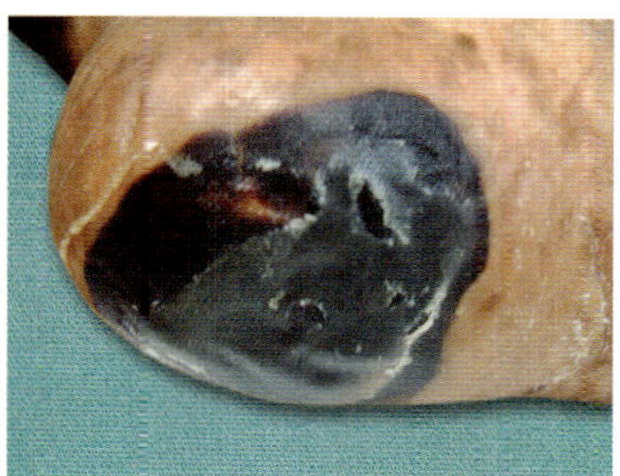

Fig. 13.3: Gangrene of the heel

4. *Diabetic retinopathy* (it makes care of the feet more difficult and injury more likely due to visual defects).

- Mostly precipitated by *trauma*, but may be associated with sepsis. Therefore, it tends to be of the *wet type*.
- *Sites*: The *toes* are affected most; however, any part of the *sole, particularly the heel* (**Figure 13.3**), even the *whole leg* may be affected, thus necessitating amputation.
- *Age:* It is rare below the age of 40 years
- *Sex:* Men are equally affected as women.
- *Infective type*: It is commoner in young diabetic patients with *neuropathy,* but little or *no* ischemia. It is a *moist infective gangrene* due to infection with pyogenic organisms especially anaerobic streptococci. A patch of infection develops in one of the toes or heel and extends as a dissecting cellulitis and tenosynovitis, with extensive sloughing and severe toxemia. Severe edema may obscure the ankle pulse, but the foot is warm and popliteal pulse can be felt.
- *Ischemic type*: It is commoner in "old" diabetics, with progressive ischemia (= senile gangrene in a diabetic patient !!!). It starts dry, but may turn moist or multicentric, affecting patches of skin at a distance from the primary lesion. The limb is ischemic with absent pulse at the ankle and even at the knee.

Embolic Gangrene

- It results from occlusion of the main artery, by an *embolus* derived from left atrium (atrial fibrillation or CHF), mural thrombus (myocardial infarction), mitral valve (endocarditis), atheromatous plaque (in the aorta), mural vegetations (in an aneurysm), or a systemic vein in the presence of a patent septum (paradoxical embolism).
- Arrest of the embolus anywhere mostly at *major bifurcations* (aortoiliac, femoropopliteal and brachial). The *femoral* is affected in > 50% of cases. As the "vis-a-tergo" is suddenly lost, venous return ↓ very much and the gangrene tends to be *moist*.
- *Clinical Features* (**5 Ps**):
    1. ***Pain:*** It is the 1st complaint, usually sudden, severe and cramping. It starts at the site of impaction, shoots downwards, and is often associated with numbness which may proceed to "glove-and-stocking" anesthesia.
    2. ***Progressive ↓ in t°:*** In the distal part of the limb, until it approximates "room t°".
    3. ***Paralysis:*** Skin becomes insensitive and the muscles become weak and flaccid.
    4. ***Pulsation:*** Lost in distal vessels and at the site of occlusion. The artery may be thickened and tender.
    5. ***Pallor***: Soon followed by cyanosis. Some hours later, white patches appear and coalesce to give a mottled appearance which together with the streaking by blood-stained venules → *marbling* of the skin. *Blood blisters* often develop before the onset of the *gangrene* which is usually "*moist and sterile*".
- *Diagnosis of the site of occlusion* can be detected by the site of initial pain, highest non-pulsatile segment, upper limit of ischemia, and by oscillometry and arteriography.

Raynaud's Disease and Phenomenon

Raynaud's Syndrome

It is a condition characterized by episodic attacks of severe vasoconstriction causing closure of *small arteries and arterioles* of the distal part of extremities in response to *cold or emotional stimuli*. Fingers and hands are most frequently involved. It is due to either Raynaud's disease or Raynaud's phenomenon.

Raynaud's Disease

It is the primary form which is *bilateral and symmetrical*, primarily seen in *women* between 20–40 years of age due to sympathetic hyperactivity to cold. It is "idiopathic". There is a definite hereditary factor.

Raynaud's Phenomenon

It is the secondary form associated with several conditions which must be ruled out before diagnosis of Raynaud's disease is made! Examples include thromboangitis, scleroderma, PAN, SLE, intoxication (lead, arsenic), drugs (ergotamin, propranolol), blood abnormalities (cryoglobulin, macroglobulin), and neurologic disorders (thoracic outlet syndromes).

Clinical Picture

Raynaud's disease is almost confined to "women" between the age of 20–40 years.

- *Recurrent attacks:* These attacks are usually "bilateral" affecting the "hands", rarely the feet, but *never* the nose or ears. They are precipitated by exposure to cold or emotional stress. Each attack consists of 3 phases:
    1. *Pallor:* Blanching of the digits and diffuse aching pains due to arrest of the blood supply caused by severe vasospasm with cessation of capillary perfusion.

2. *Cyanosis:* As the spasm passes off, a trickle of blood enters the dilated capillaries to be immediately deoxygenated by the starved tissues. Fingers become swollen and congested + numbness and burning pain.
3. *Rubor (unusual redness):* With recovery, the affected part becomes flushed (red and warm) due to reactive hyperemia and capillary dilatation from accumulation of tissue metabolites during the anoxic period. Pain is replaced by tingling and other paresthesias.

Clinical Examination

- As the disease progresses, atrophy of the terminal pulp of the finger or fingers most affected occurs. The nails are often ridged and brittle, and paronychia is common.
- In advanced cases, small areas of painful superficial necrosis, sometimes preceded by cutaneous calcification, occur on the fingertips. Occasionally, ***gangrene*** involves a more substantial part of the finger.
- In longstanding cases, other signs include *scleroderma* (sclerosis of the SC tissue with diffuse contraction) mostly affects skin of the face and hands, especially the fingers, and *telangiectasia* over the face, hands and forearms.
- The following features can help in diagnosis:
  1. *Raynaud's test:* Immersion of the hand in cold, then warm water → an attack.
  2. *During the attack*: Pulses are felt because spasm is in the digital arteries and arterioles.
  3. *Between the attacks*: The skin is normal. In severe cases, there may be trophic changes, and in longstanding cases, scleroderma and telangiectasias.

Investigations

These investigations are especially indicated in *Raynaud's syndrome.*

1. *Laboratory Tests:*
   - CBC and ESR.
   - Direct Coomb's test, anti-nuclear antibody, rheumatoid factor, complement C3 and C4 and cryoglobulins.
   - Systemic erythematosis test.
   - Venereal disease research laboratory studies.
2. *Nerve Conduction Studies.*
3. *Radiological Studies:*
   - Plain X-ray of the hand + Barium swallow.
   - Doppler US (digital).
   - Cryogenic arteriography (arteriography is made at room temperature, then repeated after exposure to cold for 30 seconds, revealing marked vascspasm).
   - Photoplethysmography (a recent noninvasive technique).

NEUROPATHIC GANGRENE

Leprosy

- The gangrene usually affects the *upper limb*. It develops due to partial ulnar nerve lesions in *both hands*. The ulnar nerves become: palpable, thick and nodular.
- Other signs of leprosy may be present: leonine face, loss of eyebrows, and destruction of nasal cartilage.
- *Diagnosis* is made sure by examination of the nasal discharge for "B. leprae".

Syringomyelia

- It usually affects *upper limbs*. Gangrene starts as a painless "whitlow" affecting both hands symmetrically.
- Examination reveals: Bilateral claw hand with muscle atrophy and dissociated sensory loss, i.e. loss of pain and temperature sensations, but *not* touch and muscle sensations. Other signs of syringomyelia include scoliosis,

unequal miotic pupils, Charcot's disease of the shoulder joint, and spastic paralysis of the lower limb.

TRAUMATIC GANGRENE

Direct Trauma

Crush Injuries

Crush injuries → tissue destruction → severe infection → wet (moist) gangrene.

Bed Sores (Decubitus Ulcers)

- It occurs in "bed-ridden patients" such as paraplegic patients. *Predisposing factors* are: Pressure - Injury - Malnutrition - Anemia - Moisture.
- *Common sites:* Pressure points, e.g. over sacrum (**Figure 13.4**), ischial tuberosity, greater trochanter, scapula.
- A bed sore is to be expected if "erythema", which does *not* change color on pressure, appears. The skin becomes swollen, shiny, congested and soon sloughs away leaving a spreading ulcer which may penetrate deeply to involve the muscles and bone.
- The acute or trophic type of bed sores is associated with disease or injury of the spinal cord and often progresses with alarming rapidity in spite of every care and attention .

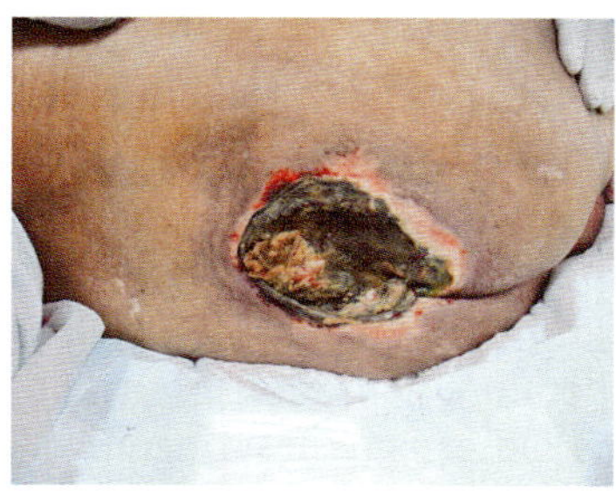

Fig. 13.4: Gangrene at the sacrum of a bedridden old patient

Indirect Trauma

- *Etiology:* Rupture, spasm, thrombosis, or ligation of the main artery. Constriction of the limb by tourniquet, bandages, plasters or splints.
- *Clinical picture: "sterile wet gangrene"*, similar to embolic gangrene (refer back).

Physico-Chemical Gangrene

Frost Bite

- *Etiology:* Severe cold exposure → freezing of tissues, which may be injured by the formation of "ice crystals" in the cell, or mostly, they are damaged during "thawing", which causes severe vasodilatation with leakage of plasma into the tissues and thrombosis in the blood vessels.
- *Clinical picture:* There is severe burning pain in the affected part, which becomes waxy, shrunken and painless. Rapid warming causes severe congestion, which may end in gangrene.

Trench Foot

- *Etiology:* It is due to exposure of the foot to "cold and damp" as occurs in: Life boat (Immersion Foot), Trenches (Trench Foot), and Dug-outs (Shelter Foot).
- *Clinical picture:* It results from *arterial spasm* which causes pain and numbness in the foot followed by: Swelling, congestion, mottling, blistering, and moist gangrene occur in severe cases.

INFECTIVE GANGRENE

Specific Infection

Gas Gangrene

- It is an acute spreading gangrene associated with gas formation and profound toxemia due to infection of extensive deep wounds by anaerobic spore-bearing bacilli of the clostridium group (mainly *Clostridium welchii*).

- *General Examination:*
  1. Anxiety, pallor, fever, tachycardia.
  2. In severe cases, there is shock and cyanosis.
- *Local Manifestations*:
  1. Wound....... Pain + numbness, swollen + crepitus with gas bubbles.
  2. Exudate...... Mousy odor and later, it becomes dark, copious and offensive.
  3. Muscles...... Lose contractility and become brick red, then greenish and finally black.
  4. Skin............. Mottled with greenish patches, with or without large blebs.
- *Investigations:*
  1. Laboratory tests show no leukocytosis (characteristic).
  2. X-ray films show the gas.

Non-specific Infection

Cancrum Oris

- It is a *gangrenous infection of the cheek in young children,* caused by mixed infection with streptococci, Vincent's spirillum and bacilli which enter via mucosal abrasions.
- It starts on the inside of the cheek as an indurated black patch which ulcerates and extends widely, eating up the cheek, lips and palate, and exposing the bones of the face.
- The general condition is poor and death may occur due to severe toxemia, septicemia, bronchopneumonia, sinus thrombosis and meningitis.

Noma Vulvae

- It is a similar condition affecting the *vulvae and perineum of "marasmic children".*

Phagedena (Hospital Gangrene)

- It was formerly common as a rapidly spreading cellulitis which attacked operation wounds and was followed by rapid *death*.
- Nowadays, the term may be used to describe a *"sloughing ulceration of the penis"* (which may occur as a complication of chancre and soft sore).

Meleney's Ulcer (Progressive Postoperative Gangrene)

- It is a spreading gangrene of skin which may follow drainage of empyema, liver or appendicular abscess.
- It is caused by mixed infection with nonhemolytic streptococci (from lungs or bowel) and staphylococci (from the skin).
- It starts 4 weeks after operation and spreads slowly until extensive areas are involved, the edges become raised, edematous, undermined and very tender, and the floor shows extensive sloughing and fever, tachycardia and insomnia, but marked toxemia develops only after several weeks.

CHAPTER

14

Differential Diagnosis of Testicular Atrophy and Impotence

1. TESTICULAR ATROPHY

DEFINITION

When one testis is smaller than the other, it is first necessary to determine which is the normal one. Some inequality may be *physiological,* as is the case with paired organs generally. **Physiological atrophy** of the testes is apt to occur in advanced life; it may begin as early as 50, though many older men have testicles of normal size.

A testis in an **abnormal position**, as in the inguinal canal, is subject not only to such causes of atrophy, but may also be inhibited in growth from pressure by surrounding parts.

CAUSES OF ATROPHY OF A NORMALLY SITUATED TESTIS

Interference with the Blood Supply

1. *Compression of the spermatic cord,* e.g. by inguinal hernia, spermatocele, or ill-fitting truss.
2. *Compression of the testicle* by affections of the tunica vaginalis, such as hydrocele or hematocele.
3. *Venous stasis*; the result of varicocele.

4. *As a sequel of operation in the region of the spermatic cord,* e.g. for cure of varicocele, spermatocele, hernia, or most commonly imperfectly descended testis (usually not very well developed and dissection may damage its blood supply).
5. *Elephantiasis.*
6. *Torsion* due to repeated attacks or rotation and derotation.
7. *Injury,* e.g. direct blow or falling astride. It causes hematoma within the tunica albuginea, with pressure atrophy of the seminiferous tubules and a gradual fibroblastic replacement, which eventually leaves the testicle a small dense node of functionless fibrous tissue.

Atrophy after Orchitis or Epididymitis, Due to

1. Gonorrhea
2. Tubercle
3. Mumps
4. Typhoid fever
5. Syphilis
6. *X-rays:* Radiologists are now careful to use protecting lead shield
7. *Klinefelter's syndrome (seminiferous tubule dysgenesis)* becomes apparent about puberty, with a varying degree of eunuchoidism, gynecomastia, azoospermia, and small testes.

Disturbance of the Endocrine System

1. *Destruction, disease or atrophy of the anterior pituitary* as in:
   - Simmond's disease.
   - Progeria.
   - Fracture of the base of the skull.

2. *Dystrophia myotonia:* Bilateral testicular atrophy + wasting of sternomastoid, facial muscles, muscles of mastication, muscles of forearm, the vasti, dorsiflexors of the feet and peroneii. There is a great difficulty in relaxing muscles. A smile tends to persist ! Cataract, baldness, general loss of weight and sexual impotence complete the picture.
3. *Advanced hepatic cirrhosis.*
4. *Advanced hemochromatosis.*

2. IMPOTENCE

DEFINITIONS

Impotence

It is the inability to perform the sexual act. It may be complete or partial, temporary or permanent.

Sterility

It is the inability to reproduce. Sterility may exist without impotence and an impotent man may be fertile.

Premature Ejaculation (Ejaculatio Praecox)

It is the emission of semen before penetration has taken place. It is merely a variety of impotence, having the same etiology.

TEMPORARY IMPOTENCE

In ***healthy men***, temporary impotence may occur in states of *fatigue, anxiety, worry* over personal affairs, in the first weeks of married life due to *emotional tension*, the first act of intercourse with a virgin from apprehension of inflicting pain upon her, and from apprehension in case of marriage without a prior experience of sexual intercourse.

CAUSES OF IMPOTENCE

Impotence Secondary to Physical Abnormality

1. *Deformation of the penis:* Congenital or acquired.
2. *Severely or chronically physically ill patients.*
3. *Endocrine disorders* (e.g. congenital eunuchoidism, sexual infantilism, Frolich's syndrome): Patients also lack the sexual desire!
4. *Men given estrogens* (e.g. for R/ of cancer prostate), or some *anti-hypertensives* (e.g. methyl dopa). Patients may also lack the sexual desire!

5. *Diabetes mellitus* (the most important).
6. *Spinal cord disorders* (compression, paraplegia, tabes dorsalis, disseminated sclerosis, etc).
7. *Leriche syndrome.*
8. *Alcohol,* though increases the desire, it tends to reduce potency.
9. *Advancing age*: Impotence occurs as part of the aging process.

Primary Impotence (Abnormal Psychological Influences)

1. *Anxiety*: Chronic anxiety is likely to be inhibitory to erection.
2. *Depression*: It is the easiest cause to R/; however, antidepressants may themselves cause impotence in some patients, though not permanently.
3. *Abnormalities of sexual inclination:* It may be associated with incapacity to perform the sexual act under conventional conditions, e.g. either suffering or inflicting pain may be necessary to achieve erection.
4. *Homosexuality,* latent or overt.
5. *Relative impotence:* The patient cannot effect coitus with one woman but is potent with others.
6. *Absence of ejaculation* (*Coitus reservatus*): It is the rarest form of impotence. Its origin is obscure. It has been claimed that patients are either "narcissistic" and incapable of "giving" of themselves, or have only feeble sexual desire and do not arrive at a sufficient intensity of excitement to attain ejaculation.
7. *Marital disturbance:* A wife can, by nagging or some other untoward behavior, render her husband impotent!!!! Similarly if she fears pregnancy, and the husband in turn, fears of making her pregnant !! The implication is that treatment is likely to be much more successful if both husband and wife are involved.

CHAPTER

15

Differential Diagnosis of Gynecomastia

GYNECOMASTIA

DEFINITIONS

Gynecomastia

Gynecomastia means generalized enlargement of the male breast due to development of its glandular components (**Figure 15.1**).

Pseudogynecomastia

It means predominance of mammary tissue due to deposition of fat.

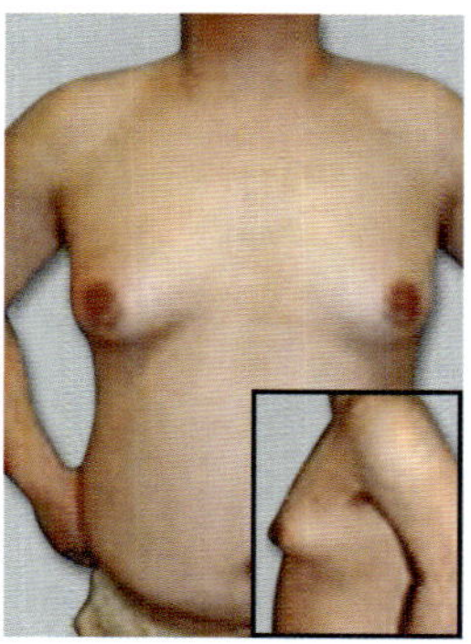

Fig. 15.1: Gynecomastia

CAUSES OF GYNECOMASTIA

I. Physiological	1. Neonatal. 2. Pubertal. 3. Involutional.
II. Pathological	*Endocrine:* 1. *Testis*: Pubertal testicular failure - tumors - leprosy - mumps orchitis. 2. *Thyroid*: Hyperthyroidism. 3. *Adrenal*: Adrenocortical tumor. 4. *Disorders of sex*: True hermaphroditism - testicular feminization. 5. *Pituitary*: Acromegaly - Chromophobe adenoma. 6. *Other endocrine disorders*: After prostatectomy - Albright's syndrome 7. *Diseases of the liver.* 8. *Renutrition.* *Chromosomal anomaly:* Klinefelter's syndrome. *Diseases of the CNS:* 1. Traumatic paraplegia. 2. Friedreich's ataxia. 3. Syringomyelia, 4. Myotonica congenita. *Diseases of the respiratory system:* Bronchogenic carcinoma. *Drugs:* • Estrogens, androgens, chorionic gonadotropins. • Digitalis. • Chlorpromazine. • Isoniazid. • Tricyclic antidepressants. • Spironolactone, cimetidine (testosterone inhibitors). • Methyldopa, reserpine. • Radioactive iodine.

PHYSIOLOGICAL GYNECOMASTIA

Neonatal Gynecomastia

- It is characterized by being *transient* and the possibility of expressing fluid from them (*witch's milk*).

- It may be *caused* by:
  1. Maternal chorionic gonadotropins stimulating the Leydig cells of the testis (which immediately after birth are found to be relatively abundant) to secrete estrogen which produces the gynecomastia.
  2. Hang-over influence of the high concentration of maternal estrogen.
  3. Prolactin (though prolactin is not found in adults unless associated with galactorrhea).
- *Histologically*, these breasts are found to be miniature lactating glands.

Pubertal Gynecomastia

- It results from increased serum estradiol:testosterone ratio.
- The breast enlarges at puberty and may simulate the female breast.
- It may be unilateral or bilateral with or without pseudolactation.
- It usually regresses as adult testosterone levels are produced, if not, removal of excessive mammary tissue should be removed by plastic surgery that should not be delayed to save the boy from embarrassment.

Involutional (Senescent) Gynecomastia

- Very rarely, gynecomastia develops in men in the 6th decade or later due to ↓ testosterone levels. It is associated with loss of libido and ↑ urinary output of gonadotropins, and sometimes with hot flushes.
- It is essential that organic conditions (e.g. liver disease, bronchogenic carcinoma, etc.), should be excluded before assuming the gynecomastia to be due to the male climacteric.

PATHOLOGICAL GYNECOMASTIA

Endocrine Causes

Disorders of the Testes

Hypogonadism: Gynecomastia does *not* develop in hypogonadism due to pituitary deficiency and is not seen in testicular failure that occurs in adult men. It is only seen in Klinefelter's syndrome and prepubertal testicular failure in which no testicular tissue can be found in the scrotum, and gynecomastia may be evident even before the age of puberty. It is assumed to result from estrogens secreted by the adrenal cortex.

Tumors

1. *Chorionic carcinoma:* It is the commonest tumor to produce gynecomastia. Chorionic gonadotropins are present in large quantities in urine and stimulate the production of estrogen by the interstitial cells. Besides gynecomastia, there may be pigmentation of nipple and areola, often with nipple secretion of a white fluid.
2. *Seminoma*: It is rare for seminoma to be associated with gynecomastia, but it has been recorded.
3. *Interstitial-cell tumor*: It is very rare before puberty. Gynecomastia may be due to excessive production of estrogen, as well as androgen. It regresses when the tumor is removed.
4. *Sertoli cell tumor:* It is the rarest testicular tumor and very rarely is associated with gynecomastia, which results from conversion of testicular androgen to estrogen. It may associated with loss of libido and impotence.

Leprous orchitis: The histological picture of the testis simulates that seen in Klinefelter's syndrome, i.e. clumps of Leydig cells, absence of spermatogenesis, intact Sertoli cells and peritubular fibrosis. This picture is accompanied by raised urinary gonadotropin levels and sometimes by gynecomastia.

Mumps orchitis: Rarely gynecomastia develops 6-12 months after an attack of mumps orchitis which has caused atrophy of the testicles.

Disorders of the Thyroid

A few cases of thyrotoxicosis have been described in association with gynecomastia. Testicular biopsy and hormone assays were normal, though the gynecomastia, which was accompanied by loss of libido and potency, subsided when thyrotoxicosis was treated.

Diseases of the Adrenal Cortex

Adrenal cortical tumors (usually malignant) or hyperplasia are rare in males. They produce excessive estrogen and interstitial cells of the testis undergo hypoplasia. The typical picture is one of feminization, with gynecomastia and pigmentation of nipples. Occasionally, clear or milky fluid can be expressed from the nipples. Libido and potency progressively ↓. Aspermia is usually and the testes may be palpably atrophied.

Disorders of Sex

1. *True Hermaphroditism:*
   In this rare condition, gynecomastia frequently develops.
2. *Testicular Feminization:*
   A type of *male* pseudohermaphroditism (proved genetically) in which gonads (testes) contain Sertoli cells but no germinal elements. They secrete normal amounts of androgen and estrogen but all the tissues of the body are unable to respond to androgen and therefore assume female physical characters including large breasts (*not exactly gynecomastia*). External genitalia are those of a normal female but the vagina ends as a blind pouch and the uterus is vestigial or absent.

Diseases of the Pituitary Gland

1. *Acromegaly*: Gynecomastia has been rarely reported in association with acromegaly. Galactorrhea has been described more since prolactin and growth hormone are secreted by the eosinophil cells of the pituitary.
2. *Chromophobe adenoma*: Certain chromophobe cells are pre-eosinophil cells. Very occasionally a case of chromophobe adenoma accompanied by impotence, testicular atrophy and gynecomastia has been described.

Miscellaneous Endocrine Disorders

- *Following prostatectomy:* A few cases have been reported and in some instances subsequently subsiding. The pathogenesis is not clearly defined and it may be just coincidental.
- *Albright's syndrome:* It usually occurs in girls but has been described in boys and occasionally gynecomastia occurs. It consists of:
  1. Precocious puberty.
  2. Polyostotic fibrous dysplasia.
  3. Patchy pigmentation of the skin.

Disease of the Liver (Cirrhosis)

Gynecomastia occurs in many cases of cirrhosis with severe liver damage due to failure to inactivate estrogen. It is interesting that hemochromatosis has not so far been accompanied by gynecomastia.

Renutrition

It is probably associated with a resurgence of pituitary activity with secretion and release of gonadotropins.

Klinefelter's Syndrome

General Characteristics

- It is due to abnormal sex chromosome pattern **47-XXY**.
- The testes are small; however, interstitial cells are increased in number and presumably produce androgens and estrogens in varying proportions.
- If the conversion of androgen to estrogen is abnormally high, gynecomastia may develop, and in some cases signs of androgenic insufficiency may be evident.

Diseases of the Central Nervous System

Traumatic Paraplegia

About 20% of such patients develop gynecomastia. The testicular biopsy shows a picture similar to that found in Klinefelter's syndrome (no germinal epithelium). It is possible that the phase of malnutrition and mild liver deficiency that occur in paraplegic patients may account for the testicular changes.

Syringomyelia and Friedreich's Ataxia

They are also sometimes associated with gynecomastia when disturbances of metabolism and nutrition have been recorded. Testicular histology resembles that found in Klinefelter's syndrome.

Dystrophia Myotonica

Gynecomastia has rarely been described, sometimes associated with extreme debility. Testicular histology resembles that found in Klinefelter's syndrome.

Diseases of the Respiratory System

Bronchogenic Carcinoma

Gynecomastia results from estrogen secretion by the tumor and the nipples may be deeply pigmented. Most cases have also shown *osteoarthropathy*. In some cases, the gynecomastia disappeared rapidly on removal of the tumor.

Drugs

- **Estrogens:** When estrogens are administered therapeutically to men, one must expect gynecomastia.
- **Androgens:** These very rarely give rise to gynecomastia. It seems possible that methyl testosterone may lead to gynecomastia, whereas other androgens do not.
- **Chorionic gonadotropins:** Their administration to normal adult men leads to an increased production of estrogen and the Klinefelter picture of testicular histology. Gynecomastia occasionally develops when chorionic gonadotropin is administered in the treatment of undescended testis.
- **Digitalis:** The occurrence of gynecomastia in patients treated with digitalis is occasionally reported though the mechanism is not exactly identified.
- **Chlorpromazine and reserpine:** They have been reported as giving rise to gynecomastia on rare occasions.
- **Other drugs:** Isoniazid, tricyclic antidepressants, spironolactone, methyl dopa and meprobamate are other drugs which occasionally give rise to gynecomastia.

Bibliography

1. Al-Falouji, McBrien M (Eds). Postgraduate Surgery: The Candidate Guide. William Heinemann Medical Books, London, 1986.
2. Beshara FM. Principles of Clinical Surgery. Dar Nashr El-Sakafa, Alexandria, 1988.
3. Browse NL. An Introduction to the Signs and Symptoms of Surgical Disease. Butler and Tanner, Ltd) ELBS, London, 1986.
4. Clair A (Ed). Hamilton Bailey's Demonstration of Physical Signs in Clinical Surgery. ELBS, London, 1980.
5. Das S (Ed). A Manual on Clinical Surgery (9th edn). Mayor's Court, Kolkata, 2011.
6. Davis JH. Clinical Surgery. Mosby CV Co, USA-Toronto, 1987.
7. Gamal Saleh. Clinical Surgery. Notes and Atlas (5th edn).University Book Center, M. Antar Press, Cairo, 1997.
8. Hart FD (Ed). French's Index of Differential Diagnosis (11th edn). John Wright & Sons Ltd, Bristol, United Kingdom, 1979.
9. Ibrahim Amin Ali. An Approach to Clinical Diagnosis Dar Nafeh Press, Cairo, 1980.
10. Magdy El-Saied. Differential Diagnosis and Case Studies in Clinical Surgery. Madina Egyptian Press, Cairo, 1981
11. Mahmoud Sakr. Principles of Surgery (Clinical Surgery), Volume X (A-C). Alexandria, 2000.
12. Majid AA, Kingsnorth N (Eds). Fundamental of Surgical Practice. Greenwich Medical Media, London, 1998.
13. Thorek P. Surgical Diagnosis. JB Lippincott Company, Philadelphia USA, 1977.

Index

Page numbers followed by *f* refer to figure

A

Abdomen 131
Abdominal
- aneurysm 370
- angina 370
- aorta 370
- injury 457
- mass 144, 184, 463
- migraine and epilepsy 352, 365

Abnormal
- protrusion of eyeball 77
- pulsation of retinal vessels 77

Abnormalities of
- colonic motility 428
- sexual inclination 530

Abscess 55, 194
Abuse of laxatives 435
Accessory breast 118
Achalasia 418
- of cardia 422, 423*f*

Acholuric jaundice 342
Acinar cysts 133
Acquired swellings 5
Actinomycosis 81, 151, 155, 277, 300, 305, 312
- of appendix 195

Acute
- abscess 115, 123, 194
- appendicitis 351, 352, 366, 397, 483
- back pain 376
- breast abscess 123*f*
- cancer of pregnancy and lactation 349
- cervical lymphadenitis 60
- cholecystitis 351, 353
- cystitis 395, 482
- diffuse swellings 13
- encephalitis lethargica 425
- epididymitis 388
- epididymo-orchitis 217, 218
- febrile diseases 457, 467
- fevers 484
- gastritis 461
- gastroenteritis 352, 364
- glaucoma 409
- hepatocellular damage 441
- infection of upper jaws 13
- inflammation 395
- intestinal obstruction 367
- intussusception 478
- ischemia 402
- lactational carcinoma 123
- laryngitis 426
- lump 139
- lymphadenitis 55
- massive liver necrosis 468
- mastitis 122, 348
- mesenteric lymphadenitis 352, 364
- non-specific
  - lymphadenitis 153, 289
  - mesenteric lymphadenitis 152
- orchitis 218, 388
- osteomyelitis 259
- pancreatitis 351, 353, 374
- parotitis 45
- pericarditis 367

pneumococcal peritonitis 355
porphyria 367
primary pneumococcal peritonitis 351
prostatitis 395, 501
pyelitis 351, 354
regional ileitis 351, 354
retention 496
salpingitis 354, 483
solid swellings 215
submandibular sialadenitis 55
suppurative mastitis 348
swellings 122
in parotid region 45
thyroiditis 80
tonsillitis 352
urinary retention 496
venous ulcer 330*f*
Adamantinoma 33
Adenocarcinoma 419
Adenolymphoma 47, 48, 52
Adenomatous enlargement 501
Aganglionosis 429
Aird's test 380
Albright's syndrome 536
Alopecia neoplastica 250
Alveolar abscess 36
Amebic
abscess 160
dysentery 476
hepatitis and abscess 277
liver abscess 280
Ameboma 150, 155
Ameloblastoma 33
of mandible 53
Amount of blood in urine 486
Ampulla of Vater 473
Amyloidosis 286, 429, 457
Anal
carcinoma 385, 385*f*
disorders 430
fissure 382
Anemia 456, 463
Aneurysm of
axillary artery 117
following trauma 117*f*
external iliac artery 154, 196
popliteal artery 226
thoracic aorta 460
upper abdominal aorta 173
Aneurysmal bone cyst 266
of radius 267*f*
Angina pectoris 406, 409
Angioneurotic edema of face 13
Ankylosing spondylitis 374, 377
Anthrax 312, 457
Antibiotic glossitis 346
Anxiety 350, 397, 530
Aortic aneurysm 420
rupturing into esophagus 456
Aphthous ulcers 315, 320
Appendiceal inflammation 394
Appendicitis 372, 379
Appendicular
abscess 148, 149
mass 148, 155
Areolar tissue 115, 147
Arterial ulcer 333, 334
Arteries 18
Arteriosclerosis 483
Arteriovenous fistula 200
Artifact ulcer 343
Aspiration 104
Atherosclerosis 405, 484, 516
Atresia 445
Atrophy 231, 527
Autoimmune
diseases 52
thyroiditis 82
Automutilation ulcer 343
Autonomic neuropathy 429
Axillary
lymph nodes 118, 125
nerves 115

tail of
breast 118
Spence 118

B

Bacillary dysentery 477
Bacillus botulinus 425
Backer's sign 77
Bacterial endocarditis 283, 457
Baker's cyst 225*f*, 226
Balance's sign 363
Balanitis 325, 396
Barium
enema 156, 169, 183, 477
swallow 418, 423, 459
Basal
cell carcinoma 243, 300, 306, 312, 320, 341
pleurisy 352
Bed sores 522
Behcet's syndrome 325
Benign
breast 136
eczema of nipple and areola 137*f*
gastric ulcer 368
lymphogranulomatosis 297
mucoepidermoid tumor 48
neoplasms 138
tumors of
parotid gland 47
skin adnexa 239
skin dermis 240
skin epidermis 236
thyroid gland 83
Bilateral
accessory breasts 118*f*
breast lesions 139
lesions of parotid gland 52
post-phlebitic ulcers 332*f*
Bilharzial
dysentery 476
mass 208
splenomegaly 285
Biliary colic 351, 358
Bilocular hydrocele 205
Biopsy 510
Bitten tongue 345
Black
measles 457
water fever 457
Bladder carcinoma 176
Bleeding
disorders 484
per rectum 472
Blood
borne infection 295
cyst 96
diseases 457, 466
disorders 379
dyscrasias 470
vessels 115
Blue nevus 238
Body of
epididymis 214
testis 214
Boeck's sarcoid 67, 297
Bone 131
cysts 266
swellings 111, 259, 276
tumor 405
Bony swellings 10, 12
Bowel
disorders 430
pseudo-obstruction 428
Bowen's disease 237
Branchial cyst 103
Breast
abscesses 138, 348
cancer 136
hypertrophy 121
lesions in children and adolescents 137

Brodie's
  abscess 260, 261*f*
  disease 377
Bronchial carcinoma 378
Bronchogenic carcinoma 538
Buerger's disease 405, 515
Bulbar paralysis 424
Burkitt's lymphoma 39, 40*f*
Bursa 224
  of Adam's apple 95

C

Cachexia 463
Calcular obstructive jaundice 447, 451
Calculus in duct of submandibular salivary gland 345
Cancellous exostosis 228
Cancer
  cecum 149, 155
  colon 408
  esophagus 419*f*
  head of pancreas causing CBD obstruction 449*f*
  of breast 11
  of hepatic flexure 168
  thyroid 83
Cancrum oris 524
Carbon tetrachloride 442
Carcinoma of
  breast 127
  esophagus 418
  head of pancreas 165
  maxilla 38
  maxillary sinus 27
  parotid gland 50
  sigmoid colon 180*f*
  stomach 171
  thyroid gland 422
  upper parts of colon 475
  uterus, vagina or colon 483
Carcinomatous
  epulides 31
  ulcer 305
  ulceration of larynx 426
Cardiovascular
  gangrene 512, 513
  system 76
Carotid
  and subclavian aneurysms 108
  body tumor 98, 99*f*
Cat scratch disease 65, 291
Cauda equina 398
Causes of
  acute swellings of tongue 21
  atrophy of normally situated testis 526
  cervical lymphadenopathy 60
  chronic
    leg ulcer 328
    or persistent swelling of tongue 21
    peritonitis 188
  chylous ascites 188
  death 321
  dysphagia 416
  dyspnea in thyroid patient 90
  early spread of carcinoma of tongue 321
  functional dyspepsia 414
  gangrene 512
  gynecomastia 532
  hematemesis 456
  hematuria 480, 488
  huge
    abdominal distention 186
    cysts of abdomen 184
  hypoproteinemia 187
  mastitis 348
  menorrhagia 491
  organic dyspepsia 410
  pain in penis during micturition 395
  red coloration of urine 480

sudden enlargement of thyroid gland with pain 90
swelling 43
tender spleen 286
thyroid enlargement 69
tongue ulcers 317
Cavernous hemangioma 255
Cellulitis 7, 405
Cephalhematoma 5
Cerebral vomiting 407
Cerebrospinal fluid 2
Cervical
lymphadenopathy 60, 67
rib 406
syndrome 101
Cervicofacial actinomycosis 36
Chaga's disease 429
Chancroids of penis 325
Characteristic of hepatic swelling 278
Charcot's
disease 522
triad 447
Chicken pox 283, 320
Cholangiocarcinoma 163, 444
Cholangitis 445
Cholecystitis 379, 408
Choledochal cyst 165, 185
Cholelisthiasis 379
Cholera 457, 468
Chondroma 134
Chondrosarcoma 154, 261 265
Chorionic
carcinoma 534
gonadotropins 538
Chromophobe adenoma 536
Chronic
abdominal infections 372
abscess 115, 194
back pain 376
bronchitis 409
cervicitis 379
cystic swellings 224, 226
diffuse swellings 14
gastritis 462
hematoma 124
hepatocellular damage 443
indurative cavernositis 396
intestinal obstruction 408
intracranial abscess 11
ischemia 402, 513
lump 139
lymphatic leukemia 66
mastitis 348
meningitis 378
nephritis 457, 468
non-specific
breast abscess 124
lymphadenitis 61, 289
ulcer 310
osteomyelitis 260*f*
parotitis 47
phagedenic ulcer 338
retention 496
salpingitis 379
solid swellings 219, 227
specific lymphadenitis 61
submandibular sialadenitis 56
superficial glossitis 319
swellings 124
in parotid region 46
thyroiditis 81
torsion 216
uremia 457
urinary retention 501
venous congestion 505
Circoid aneurysm 4, 4*f*
Cirrhosis 164, 277, 536
of liver 457
Clamydial lymphadenitis 65
Classification of
goiter 69
mass in right hypochondrium 157
swellings of scalp 1
ulcers 299

- Cleft palate 416
- Clergyman's knee 234
- *Clostridium welchii* 524
- Cock's peculiar tumor 7, 231
- Codmann's triangle 264
- Coitus reservatus 530
- Cold abscess 95, 107, 110, 115, 156, 199
- Colloid goiter 70, 82
- Colonic
  - disorders 430
  - inertia 428
  - tumors 156
- Colonoscopy 156, 169, 175, 478
- Color of urine 484
- Complications of urinary retention 503
- Compressing esophagus 420
- Compression of
  - spermatic cord 526
  - testicle 526
- Condylomata acuminata 327
- Congenital
  - biliary atresia 443
  - fissured tongue 346
  - hydrocele 204
  - stricture of esophagus 419
  - swellings 2
  - toxoplasmosis 442
- Congestive heart failure 76, 282
- Conjugated hyperbilirubinemia 441, 445
- Conjugation of bilirubin 441
- Connective tissue tumors 48
- Constipation 427
- Core-needle biopsy 86
- Cornu cutaneum 237
- Coronary thrombosis 352, 364, 367, 406
- *Corynebacterium diphtheriae* 337
- Costoclavicular compression 406
- Courvoisier's law 165, 447, 448
- Coxsackie B virus 442
- Crab's claw 240
- Cracked
  - corner of mouth 314
  - lips 314
  - nipple 347
- Crohn's
  - disease 152, 351, 354, 377, 473, 477
  - mass 156
- Crush
  - fractures 374
  - injuries 522
- Cruveilhier's sign 199
- Cullen's sign 353
- Curling's ulcer 469
- Cutaneous
  - and subcutaneous swellings 110
  - horn 237
- Cyanosis 520
- Cylindroma 239, 239*f*
- Cyst
  - formation 73
  - of jaw 27
- Cystadenoma of thyroid gland 96
- Cystic
  - and pseudocystic swellings 92
  - hygroma 107, 108*f*, 119
  - swellings 12, 14, 21, 96, 97, 103, 110, 215
    - of breast 133
    - of parotid gland 14
    - of skin and SC tissues 230
- Cystosarcoma phylloides 126
- Cysts of
  - floor of mouth 23
  - skin and subcutaneous origin 133
  - testis 391
- Cytomegalovirus 442

D

- Dacryocystitis 15
- Dalrymple's sign 76

De Quervains' disease 80
Decubitus ulcers 522
Deep
- cervical ranula 23
- vein thrombosis 403

Deformation of penis 529
Degeneration cyst 185
Dengue fever 457
Dental
- cysts 32
- granuloma 35
- ulcers 317

Dentigerous cysts 32
Depressed fracture 6
Depression 530
Dermatofibroma 249
Dermatofibrosarcoma protuberans 257, 257*f*
Dermoid cyst 4, 14, 58, 110, 232, 230
Determination of nature of jaundice 455
Diabetes mellitus 530
Diabetic
- angiopathy 516
- gangrene 516
- ketoacidosis 352, 365
- neuropathy 516, 517

Diffuse
- diaphysitis 269
- hemangioma 14
- hydrocele of cord 208
- lytic destruction of proximal humerus 269*f*
- macroglossia 21
- osteomyelitis 269
- swellings 13, 21

Digestive system 75
Diphtheric desert sore 337
Direct
- abdominal injury 470
- inguinal hernia 190

Diseases of
- adrenal cortex 535
- bladder 395
- body of testis or epididymis 387
- central nervous system 537
- coverings of testis 392
- duodenum 457, 464
- esophagus 456, 459
- liver 536
- pituitary gland 536
- prostate 395
- respiratory system 538
- spermatic cord 393
- stomach 457, 461
- urethra 395

Disorders of
- sex 535
- testes 534
- thyroid 535

Disseminated lymphoma 84
Disturbance of endocrine system 527
Diverticular disease 156
Diverticulitis 351, 353
- colon 483

Donovan bodies 326
Dorsum of wrist 233*f*
Draining lymph nodes 300
Drug-induced
- cholestasis 443
- constipation 429
- gastritis 462

Dry gangrene 513
Dubin-Johnson syndrome 444
Duct
- papilloma 125
- system 133

Duodenal
- carcinoma 465
- diverticulum 464
- ulcer 457, 458, 464

Duodenum 369
Dysmenorrhea 351, 359, 379
Dyspepsia 407

Dyspeptic ulcers 315, 320
Dysphagia 416, 420, 422
lusuria 422
Dystrophia myotonica 537

C

Early Hodgkin disease 292
Ectopic
salivary gland tumor 26
testis 196, 200
Effusion of hip joint 201
Ehler-Danlos syndrome 457
Elephantiasis 527
scroti 212
Embolic gangrene 518
Empyema necessitans 112
Encephalocele 2, 2*f*
Encysted
fluid 188
hydrocele of cord 195, 205
Endocrine disorders 529, 536
Endometrioma of round ligament 196
Endoscopic retrograde cholangio-pancreatography 450
End-stage liver disease 279
Enlarged
axillary lymph nodes 136
lymph nodes 192, 200
popliteal lymph nodes 227
Eosinophilic granuloma 378
Epigastric pain 367
Epiphysitis 377
Epistaxis 456, 458
Epithelioma 7, 210, 320, 327, 460
of floor of mouth 26
of penis 396
of scrotum 323
of tongue 346
Epitheliomatous
transformation 245
ulcer 321, 321*f*
Epstein Barr virus 294
Erosive gastritis 458
Eructio nervosa 410
Erysipelas 7
Erythema bullosum of buccal cavity 426
Erythrocytosis 163
Erythromelalgia 401
Esophageal
cancer 418
carcinoma 378, 460
ulcer 460
varices 458, 459, 459*f*
Evidence of retrosternal extension 88
Ewing's
sarcoma 270*f*
tumor 270
Excessive callus formation 259
Exophthalmos 78
External
angular dermoid cyst 14
hernia 361
Extra-abdominal
causes of pain 409
disease 363
Extra-medullary intraspinal tumor 394
Extravasation of urine 222

F

Facial nerve 53
palsy 51*f*
Factitious ulcer 343
Febrile disorder 376
Fecal impaction 437
Felty's syndrome 283, 342
Femoral
artery aneurysm 199
hernia 190, 197, 198
neuroma 200
swellings 197

Fibroadenoma 126, 133, 135
Fibroblastic tumors 240
Fibrocystic disease 125, 349
Fibromyoma 196
Fibrosarcoma 256
Fibrous epulides 29, 29*f*
Filaria sanguinis hominis 212
Filarial
- funiculitis 207
- mass 208
- nodes 154

Filariasis 193, 290
Fine needle aspiration cytology 86
Fistulae 323
Flavaspidic acid 441
Fluctuating jaundice 447
Fluorosis 377
Focal nodular hyperplasia 163
Follicular adenoma 83
Footballer's ulcer 335
Foreign body
- in tongue 345
- in urethra 395
- perforating esophagus and aorta 456, 461
- reaction 349

Frank
- hematuria 479
- red blood 472
  - passed per anus 474
  - per rectum 472

Frei's intradermal test and biopsy 291
Frenulum ulcer 317
Friedreich's ataxia 537
Frolich's syndrome 529
Frost bite 523
Functional
- dyspepsia 407
- grades of dysphagia 416

Fungating
- breast cancer 130*f*
- malignancy 313
- tumors 341

Fungus infections 305
Furunculosis 13
Fused kidneys 166

G

Galactocele 133, 349
Gallbladder swelling 165
Gallstone
- colic 374
- ileus 361

Ganglion 233
Ganglioneuromatosis 429
Gangrene 511, 513
- of big toe 514*f*
- of heel 517*f*
- of third toe 514*f*

Gas gangrene 523
Gastric
- carcinoma 368, 463
- crises of tabes 408
- dilatation 413
- ulcer 412, 457, 458 461

Gastritis 412, 457
Gastrocnemius muscle 225
Gastroscopy 175
Gaucher's disease 67, 283
Generalized
- bone disease 268, 271, 273
- lymph node enlargement 294
- medical diseases 352, 365

Genitourinary system 76
Giant cell epulides 29
Giant
- cell
  - granuloma 357
  - lesions 41
  - tumor 40, 262 263*f*
- soft fibroadenoma 126
  - of left breast 127*f*

Giffod's sign 77
Gilbert's syndrome 441
Globus hystericus 424

Glomerulonephritis 481
Glossitis 346
Goiter 69
Gonorrhea 527
Good-Sall's rule 384
Gouty ulcers 302
Granuloma
 inguinale 326
 venereum 326
Granulomatous
 colitis 477
 epulides 30, 30*f*
Grave's disease 75, 82
Grey-Turner sign 353
Groin
 hernia 190
 swelling 202*f*
Gronblad-Strandberg syndrome 474
Gumma of
 breast 125
 testis 219, 324, 389
Gummatous
 ulcer 303, 319, 336
 ulceration of penis 327
Gynecomastia 122, 134, 135*f*, 136, 531, 531*f*

H

Haemophilus ducreyi 304
Hairy mole 238
Hand-Schuller-Christian disease 68, 283
Hard
 chancre 303
 fibroadenoma 126
 lump 139
 swelling in thyroid 89
Hashimoto's disease 81
Healing ulcer 335
Hemangioma 9, 14, 20, 110, 162, 464
 of upper jejunum 470
Hematemesis 456
Hematocele 214, 392
 of cord 207
Hematoma 110, 156
Hematonephrosis 167
Hematuria 479, 487, 488
Hemoglobinuria 479
Hemolytic
 anemia 283
 disease of newborn 443
 jaundice 452
Hemoptysis 456, 458, 493
Hemorrhage 73
Hemorrhagic erosions 457, 463
Hepatic
 adenoma 162
 amebiasis 442
 cirrhosis 528
 jaundice 451, 452
Hepatocellular carcinoma 163
Hepatoma 164
Hernia 203, 361
 of apex of lung 113
 testis 218
Herpes
 genitalis 325
 simplex 325, 442
 zoster 352, 365
Herpetic ulcers 318
Hiatus hernia 368, 379
Hindgut dysfunction 428
Hirschsprung's disease 429, 436
Hodgkin's disease 63, 65, 193, 277, 295, 466
Honey-comb appearance 459
Hospital gangrene 525
Hour-glass stomach 413
Housemaid's knee 234
Hunger pain 409
Hunterian chancre 303

Hydatid
cyst 161, 171, 185, 268, 281, 281*f*, 283
of Morgagni 215, 216*f*
disease 277
Hydradenitis suppurativa 120, 120*f*
Hydrocele 204, 212, 213, 220, 392.
of cord 195
of femoral hernial sac 198
of hernial sac 195, 205
Hydronephrosis 167, 184
Hydrophobia 424
Hypercalcemia 163
Hypernephroma 167
Hypernephrosis 379
Hyperparathyroidism 37, 377
Hyperphosphatemic rickets 377
Hypertrophic ileocecal TB 150, 155
Hypoglycemia 163
Hypogonadism 534
Hysteria 352

I

Iliac
abscess of pyogenic origin 148
artery 147
bone 147
swellings 154
lymph nodes 147, 153
Iliopsoas cold abscess 148
Immune hemolytic anemia 440
Impacted foreign bodies 422
Implantation dermoid cyst 232
Incisor teeth of lower jaw 29*f*
Inclusion dermoid cyst 3, 231*f*
Indirect inguinal hernia 190, 203
Infected
granuloma 6
hematocele 324
sebaceous cyst 311
Infectious mononucleosis 283, 294, 442
Infective
gangrene 513, 523
hepatitis 277, 281
Inflammatory
arthropathies of spine 377
bowel disease 377
lesions of breast 349
ulcers 318
Inguinal
femoral swellings 201
swellings 190
Inguinoscrotal swellings 203
Injury of urethra 395
Inner angular dermoid cyst 15
Interacinar cysts 133
Internal
hemorrhage 362
hernia 361
Interstitial
cell tumor 534
orchitis 389
Intestinal
colic 351, 358, 372
obstruction 359, 372
Intra-abdominal swellings 147, 148, 156, 171, 175, 176, 178, 181, 184
Intracranial extension 3
Intrahepatic
and extrahepatic obstruction 445
cholestasis 443
Intrathoracic swelling 88
Intussusception 151 168
of small bowel 360*f*
Involutional gynecomastia 533
Iron therapy 471
Irreducible
femoral hernia 200
hernia 203
Irregular uterine bleeding 491
Irritable bowel syndrome 434

Ischemia 361, 505
Ischemic ulcer 300, 328, 334*f*
Ivory osteoma 10

J

Jaundice 439, 441, 443
Jejunojejunal intussusception coiled spring appearance 152*f*
Joffroy's sign 76
Juvenile hypertrophy of breast 138

K

Kala-azar 283
Keloid 16
Keratoacanthoma 239, 251
Kidney and suprarenal gland 166
Klebsiella pneumoniae 442
Klebs-Loeffler bacilli 424
Klinefelter's syndrome 527, 136, 537
Kwashiorkor 210

L

Laceration of esophageal wall 460
Lacrimal sac inflammation 15
Langerhan's cells 68
Laparotomy 450
Large
- breast 139
- lump 139
- multi-nodular goiter 71*f*
- pleomorphic adenoma of left parotid gland 47*f*
- right parotid carcinoma 50*f*

Laryngeal diseases 426
Laryngitis 426
Laryngocele 95, 104, 105*f*
Lead poisoning 375, 424
Left
- cystic hygroma 119*f*
- indirect inguinal hernia 192*f*
- lobe of liver 183
- mixed salivary tumor 57*f*
- submandibular sialadenitis 58*f*
- suprarenal gland 183
- ureteric stone 358*f*

Leg ulcer 343
- complicating blood diseases 342
- in rheumatoid arthritis 342
- in tropics 337

Leiomyoma of upper jejunum 470
Leiomyosarcoma 464
Leishmania donovani bodies 337
Leishmaniasis 312
Leprosy 521
Leprous orchitis 534
Leptospira icterohemorrhagiae 442
Leptospirosis 442, 457, 468
- icterohemorrhagica 378

Leriche syndrome 530
Lesions of brachial plexus 406
Leukemia 66, 277, 296, 466, 483, 484
Leukemic splenomegaly 285
Lid
- lag sign 76
- retraction sign 76

Ligament
- of Treitz 472
- tears 405

Lipoma 8, 16, 102, 196, 200, 228, 253
- in axilla 119
- of cord 220
- of scalp 9

Liposarcoma 256
Liver
- abscess 113
- and gallbladder 369
- cirrhosis 279, 465, 491
- malignancy 279
- swelling 156
- tumors 162

Local
- lesions of penis and urethra 396
- swellings in breast 121

Low gut obstruction 359
Lucey-Driscoll syndrome 441

Lumbar vertebrae 398
Lumbosacral plexus 398
Lump in breast 127
Lumpy axilla 139
Lupoid ulceration of penis 327
Lupus vulgaris 303
Lymph
cysts 107
node 20, 53, 115, 130, 245, 254, 315, 326
swellings 54
varix 208
Lymphadenopathy 102, 173, 287
Lymphangiectasis 208
Lymphangioma 14, 20, 107, 256
Lymphangitis of penis 396
Lymphatic
drainage of lips 18*f*
leukemia 194, 283
Lymphoepithelioma 320
Lymphogranuloma
inguinale 193, 291, 326
venereum 326
Lymphoma 65, 88, 153, 154, 286

M

Mafucci syndrome 273
Magnetic resonance cholangio-pancreatography 444, 450
Magnusonus test 380
Malaria 28*f*, 457
Malarial
cachexia 457, 467
dysentery 477
splenomegaly 285
Male
breast diseases 134
fern extract 441
Malignant
disease 394
of rectum and colon 475
of testis 324
fibrohistiocytic tumors 257
fibrous histiocytoma 258
hypertension 457
measles 457, 467
melanoma 247, 243*f*, 300, 300, 307, 313, 341
obstructive jaundice 448, 451
osteoclastoma 265
scarlet fever 457, 467
skin tumors 16
transformation 231
of pleomorphic adenoma 51
tumors 22, 52, 83, 111, 112, 127, 228, 229, 263
of parotid gland 50
of skin 243
of testis 390
ulcer 305, 314, 320 340
of leg 341*f*
ulceration of left breast carcinoma 130*f*
variola 457, 467
Malingering 456, 459
Mallory-Weiss syndrome 456, 457, 460, 474
Mammary Paget's disease and eczema 140
Mammography 350
Marjolin ulcer 247, 306, 332, 333*f*
Mass in
epigastric region 170, 170*f*
left
hypochondrium 181, 182*f*
iliac fossa 178, 181*f*
lumbar region 183
right
hypochondrium 156, 169*f*
iliac fossa 147, 155*f*
suprapubic region 176
umbilical region 173, 174*f*
Masseter muscle 43, 53
Mastalgia 140

Mastitis 135
  carcinomatosa 349
  of infancy 135
  of puberty 135
Mastodynia 140
McBurney's point 352
Meckel's
  diverticulitis 353, 473
  diverticulum 470
Mediastinal tumor perforating esophagus and aorta 456, 461
Medullary
  carcinoma of thyroid 87
  giant cell tumor 228
Melena 456, 470, 472, 473
Meleney's
  gangrene 336
  ulcer 300, 305, 336, 525
Meningocele 2
Menorrhagia 491
Menstruation 347
Meralgia paresthetica 400
Mesenteric
  cyst 185
  lymph nodes 152
  vascular occlusion 351, 361
Metabolic ulcer 299
Metastatic
  carcinoma 250
  lymph nodes 66
  lymphadenopathy 292
  solid tumors 283
  ulcer 300
Metrorrhagia 491
Mid-gut obstruction 359
Midline cystic swellings of neck 92
Migraine 409
Minor salivary gland 58
  tumors 20, 25
Mirrizi syndrome 448
Mitral stenosis 283
Mittelschmerz pain 362
Mixed salivary
  gland tumor 57
  tumor 47
    of hard palate 26*f*
Moebius sign 76
Molluscum sebaceum 311
Monomorphic adenoma 48
Morrant Baker's cyst 225
Mucocele of
  frontal sinus 15
  GB 185
Mucosa of cheek 43
Mucus
  patches 303
  retention cyst 19
    of lower lip 19*f*
  tubercles 323
Multilocular cyst 33
Multiple
  bone swellings 271
  cavernous hemangiomata 273
  circumoral moles 250
  cylindromata 9
  cysts 215
  diphtheric ulcers 338*f*
  dyspeptic ulcers 320*f*
  enchondromata 271, 273
  exostosis 268, 271, 273
  extrasystoles 76
  furuncles of face 13
  hidradenomata 9
  myeloma 10, 10*f*, 112, 271, 378
    of skull 272*f*
  neurofibromatosis 255
  perianal fistulae 384*f*
  polyps 476
  SC lipomata 253*f*
  sebaceous cysts of scalp 230*f*
Mumps 45, 426, 527
  orchitis 535
Murphy's sign 353, 409

Musculoskeletal system 76
Myasthenia gravis 425
Mycosis fungoides 250
Myeloid leukemia 283
Myelomatous epulides 29, 30*f*
Myocardial infarction 283, 350, 352
Myositis of tongue 345

N

Necrotizing pancreatitis 353
Neonatal
  breast enlargement 122, 137
  gynecomastia 532
  mastitis 138
Neoplastic lymphadenopathy 65
Nervous system 131
Neuralgia testis 394
Neurofibroma 9, 16, 228, 254
Neurogenic
  constipation 429
  ulcer 301
Neuropathic
  gangrene 512, 521
  ulcers 339
Neurosis 352, 365
Nevus araneus 242
Niemann-Pick disease 67, 283
Nipple
  deviation 140
  discharge 136, 141
  distortion 136
  retraction 140
Nodular multiple basal cell carcinoma 9
Non-hairy mole 238
Non-Hodgkin lymphoma 65, 153, 194, 277, 296
Non-immune hemolytic anemia 440
Non-lactational right breast abscess 348*f*
Non-malignant ulceration 476
Non-specific
  acute lymphadenitis 155
  chronic thyroiditis 81
  infection 524
  inflammation 289
  lymphadenitis 60
  ulcers 300, 310

O

Obstructive jaundice 452
Obturator pain 400
Ochronosis 377
Odontomas 32
Olecranon bursa 234*f*
Ollier disease 273
Omental infarction 351, 362
Omentum 173
Onset of
  constipation 430
  puberty 347
Osler-Weber-Rendu disease 474
Osteitis
  deformans 273, 342
  fibrosa 37
    cystica 271, 275
Osteoarthritis 405
Osteoarthropathy 533
Osteoblastic metastases multiple sclerotic lesions 11
Osteochondroma 261
Osteoclastoma 40, 264
Osteogenic sarcoma 229, 264, 264*f*, 405
  and osteoclastoma 264
  and sclerosing osteomyelitis 265
Osteoid osteoma 373
Osteomalacia 377
Osteomyelitis 11, 36, 55, 155, 259, 377, 405
  of iliac bone 352
  of skull bones 7
Osteoporosis 377

Outlet obstruction 428
Ovarian cyst 153, 177, 184
Overflow
- diarrhea 428
- incontinence 496

Oxyuris vermicularis 473

P

Pachymeningitis cervicalis 406
Paget's disease 37, 140, 142, 273, 274*f*
- of bone 377

Pain in
- abdomen 351
- breast 140, 347
- foot 400
- front and sides of thigh 399
- lower limbs 398
- penis 395, 396
- perineum 381
- testicle 387
- tongue 344
- umbilical region 371
- upper limbs 405

Painful lump 139
Painless
- lump 139
- progressive jaundice 449

Palatal paralysis 416
Palmar erythema 279*f*
Pancreas 172, 183, 369
Pancreatic pseudocyst 172*f*
Papillary adenoma 83
Papilloma 20, 26, 236, 236*f*, 395
- of renal pelvis 481
- of scrotum 323

Paralytic radiculitis 406
Para-phimosis 396
Parasitic ulcer 337
Parietal swellings 147, 148, 156, 170, 173, 176, 178, 181, 183
Parotid
- cyst 46
- gland 43

Paroxysmal atrial tachycardia 76
Patchy pigmentation of skin 536
Peau d'orange 140
Pedunculated
- carcinoma 395
- lipoma 253*f*
- vesical tumor 501

Pelvic
- abscess 177, 379, 483
- bone tumors 178
- colon 475
- inflammatory diseases 354

Pemberton's sign 89
Penile ulcers 325
Peptic ulcer 379, 457, 470
Percutaneous transhepatic cholangiography 450
Perforated
- peptic ulcer 351, 355
- typhoid ulcer 351, 356

Perianal
- abscess 383
- disease 478
- fistula 384
- hematoma 382

Peri-appendiceal abscess 149*f*
Periarthritis of shoulder joint 406
Perinephric abscess 379
Periostitis 229
Peri-urethral abscess 220
Pertussis ulcer 317
Peutz-Jegher syndrome 250, 473
Phagedena 525
Pharyngeal pouch 105, 421
Phimosis 396
Phlebitis migrans 515
Phylloides 126
Physico-chemical gangrene 512, 523
Pigmented papilloma 249

Plasma cell myeloma 271
Pleomorphic adenoma 47, 48
Plexiform neurofibroma 9, 14, 239
Plummer-Vinson syndrome 423
Pneumatocele 109, 113
Pneumonia of right lung 364*f*
Pointing empyema 112
Polyarteritis nodosa 457
Polycystic
  disease 277, 283
  kidney 166, 379
  liver 158
Polycythemia rubra vera 283
Polymenorrhea 491
Polymyalgia rheumatica 377
Polymyositis 377
Polyostotic fibrous dysplasia 536
Polyps of rectum and colon 476
Popliteal lymphadenitis 227
Porphyria 410
Portal
  hypertension 283
  obstruction 457, 465
  pyemia 277, 442
  vein thrombosis 457, 465
Port-wine stain 241
Post-auricular dermoid cyst 232*f*
Post-diphtheritic dysphagia 424
Post-hepatic jaundice 451
Post-herpetic neuralgia 406
Post-phlebitic ulcer 301, 331, 331*f*
Post-thrombotic ulcers 331
Potato tumor 99
Pott's
  disease 111, 199, 374, 406
  puffy tumor 2, 11
Poupart's ligament 190
Precocious puberty 533
Prehepatic jaundice 451
Premature ejaculation 529
Presenile gangrene 515
Pressure of subclavian aneurysm 406
Primary
  biliary cirrhosis 445
  chancre 323
  epithelioma of urethra 222
  lymphedema 507
  malignant tumors 163
  syphilis 64
  syphilitic lymphadenitis 290
  thyrotoxicosis 72
  tumors 200, 263, 277
  vaginal hydrocele 212, 392
Probe test 384
Proctalgia fugax 385
Progressive postoperative gangrene 525
Prolapse of anal mucosa 478
Prolonged jaundice 457, 469
Prostatic
  abscess 395, 501
  calculus 395
  carcinoma 395
  enlargement 501
  infections 379
Pruritis ani 385
Pseudogynecomastia 531
Pseudopancreatic cyst 172, 185
Pseudoxanthoma elasticum 474
Psittacosis 283
Psoas
  abscess 199, 352
  bursa 201
Psoriasis 377
Pubertal
  gynecomastia 533
  mastitis 347
Puberty 122
Pubic tubercle test 190
Pulmonary
  emphysema 491
  TB 408
Pulsating
  aneurysm 113

swellings 12
tumors 227
Purpura hemorrhagica 466
Pyelonephritis 351, 354
Pyloric stenosis 171, 368
Pyocele 214, 392
Pyoderma gangrenosum 336
Pyogenic
abscess 106, 110
granuloma 242, 251
liver abscess 158
Pyonephrosis 167
Pyrexia 463

R

Ramus of mandible 43
Ranula 23, 58, 93, 103
Rat tail appearance 419*f*
Raynaud's
disease 401, 519
phenomenon 519
syndrome 519, 520
test 520
Rectal
carcinoma 475
disorders 430
Recurrent
appendicitis 409
epigastric pain 367
erysipelas 13
goiter 74*f*
simple nodular goiter 74
Referred pain 401, 405
Reflux
esophagitis 456, 460
stricture 418
Regional lymph nodes 510
Regions of
abdomen 144, 144*f*
femoral triangle 197
Renal
adenoma 481
arteriovenous malformations 490
carcinoma 379
colic 351, 358, 374, 397
infarction 484
swelling 166
TB 481
trauma 166
tumors 167
Respiratory system 75
Retention
mucus cyst 23, 27
of urine 503
Retromammary abscess 134
Retroperitoneal
sarcoma 154, 183, 184
swellings 147, 153, 168, 173, 175, 178, 180, 183, 184
Retropharyngeal abscess 95
Retrosternal
goiter 88
pain 420
Retroversion of uterus 379
Rheumatic pain in abdominal muscles 352, 365
Rheumatoid arthritis 298
Rib deformities 134
Rickets 268, 274
Riedel's
disease 81
lobe 158, 277, 278
Right ectopic testis 394*f*
Ring test 191
Rodent ulcer 300, 306
Rosenbach's sign 77
Rotor syndrome 444
Rovsing sign 352
Rupture
esophageal varices 456
of ovarian follicle 362
Ruptured
aortic aneurysm 352, 363

ectopic pregnancy 352, 362
graafian follicle 352

S

Sacroiliac joints 398
Salivary
adenocarcinoma 320
gland 22
swellings 54
Salmon pink patches 241
Salpingo-oophoritis 351
Saphena varix 199
Sarcoidosis 67, 297, 457
Sarcoma of 173
breast 131
maxilla 39
Sarcomatous
epulides 31
ulcer 300
Scalenus anterior syndrome 406
Scarpa's triangle 197, 199
Schatzki's ring 417
Scheuermann's disease 377
Schistosomiasis 283
Sciatic nerve 398
Sciatica 398, 399
Scleroderma 429
Sclerosing
cholangitis 444
hemangioma 242
Scrotal
and penile ulcers 323
edema 210
hernia 392
sebaceous cyst 210
swellings 210-212, 222
tongue 346
ulcers 323
Scurvy 466
Sebaceous
cyst 1, 4, 7, 14, 96, 109, 110, 115, 230, 232, 324
horn 231
Seborrheic keratosis 233, 249
Secondary
hydrocele 213, 392
malignant tumors 164
stage of syphilis 295
syphilis 64, 319
TB 295
thyrotoxicosis 78
toxic goiter 79*f*
tumor 164
varicocele 206
Semimembranosus bursa 226, 234
Seminal vesiculitis 379
Seminiferous tubule dysgenesis 527
Seminoma 390, 534
Senile
atherosclerosis 513
gangrene 513
Septic infection 193
Sertoli cell tumor 534
Severe
chronic constipation 430
exercise 434
hepatic destruction 442
Sexual infantilism 529
Sickle cell
anemia 342
crisis 379
disease 484
trait 484
Sigmoidoscopy 179
Simmond's disease 527
Simple
goiter 69
multinodular goiter 70
nevus 241, 241*f*
ulcer 455
Site of
appearance of femoral hernia 197*f*
cystic hygroma in posterior triangle 108*f*

Skin
  nodules 129*f*, 307*f*
  swellings 170, 173, 183
  ulceration 136
Sloughing ulceration of penis 525
Small
  bowel enema 156, 175
  calculus 501
  epigastric hernia 368
  intestinal bleeding 470
  pox 320, 467
  right parotid cyst 46*f*
Soft
  chancres 304
  fibroadenoma 126
  sores 300, 304, 325
    of penis 325
  tissue 399
    sarcoma 256, 258
    swellings 8, 12
Solar keratosis 237
Solid swellings 12, 16, 22, 92, 96, 97, 111
  of floor of mouth 25
  of parotid gland 17
  of SC tissues 253
  of skin 235
Solitary
  adenoma 73
  bone cyst 267
  exostosis 261
  nodule 73
  polyp 476
  thyroid nodule 89
Sore throat 426
Spermatic cord lesions 207
Spermatocele 215, 391
Spider nevus 242
Spinal
  caries 367, 374
  cord 430
    disorders 530
    tumors 352
  nerve root compression 352
  pachymeningitis 378
Splenic
  flexure of colon 183
  swelling 181, 182, 284
  vein thrombosis 283
Spondylitis of Reiter's 377
Spondylosis 405
Spring coil appearance 360
Spurious hemoptysis 493
Squamous cell carcinoma 27, 245, 300, 305, 313, 340, 419
Stellwag's sign 76
Stemmer's sign 507
Sterile wet gangrene 523
Sternomastoid
  muscle 100*f*, 103*f*
  tumor 100, 100*f*
Still's disease 283
Stomach 183, 368
Stomatitis 426
Stone in
  cystic duct 165
  submandibular salivary duct 25
Strangulated hernia 204
Strawberry nevus 241
Stricture of urethra 395, 500
Student's elbow 234
Subacute
  epididymo-orchitis 217
  perforation of peptic ulcer 171
  thyroiditis 80
Subaponeurotic hematoma 5
Subareolar mass 136
Subcapsular hematoma 158, 277, 283
Subcutaneous
  bursa 234
  hematoma 5
  tissue 53, 115
Subhyoid
  bursitis 94
  thryroglossal cyst 94*f*

Sublingual
  dermoid cyst 23, 24, 25f, 93
  salivary gland 58
Submandibular
  gland 54
  lymphadenitis 57
  salivary gland 97
Subperiosteal hematoma 5, 6
Subungual hemorrhage 249
Sudden severe epigastric pain 367
Suppurating cysts of scrotum 324
Suprarenal tumors 167
Swallowed blood 456, 458
Swellings in
  body of testis 221
  breast 122
  floor of mouth 23
  groin 190
  lateral side of neck 97
  lymph node 287
  palate 26
  parotid region 43
  submandibular region 54
Swellings of
  axilla 115
  axillary wall 115
  breast 121
  chest wall 110
  connective tissue coverings 210
  face 13
  jaw 17, 28
  lacrimal
    glands 15
    sac 15
  lips 18
  lower pole of parotid gland 98
  mandible 54
  midline of neck 91
  minor salivary glands 58
  nonsalivary gland origin 53
  oral cavity 23
  popliteal fossa 224
  preauricular lymph nodes 17
  salivary
    glands 43
    origin 45
  scalp 1
  spermatic cord 220
  testicle/epididymis 214
  thyroid gland 69
  tongue 21
  tunica vaginalis 212
  whole breast 121
Swollen limb 504, 509
Symphysis menti and tongue 24f
Syphilis 81, 193, 269, 271, 275, 300, 377, 527
  of scrotum 323
Syphilitic
  aortitis 406
  chancre 326
  degeneration 424
  disease of testis 389
  lymphadenitis 64
  proctitis 478
  sore 303
  ulcer 303, 311, 315, 319
Syringomyelia 406, 521, 537
Systemic lupus erythematosis 298, 429

T

Tabes
  dorsalis 352, 365, 374, 401
  mesenterica 153
Tabetic crisis 352, 365
Teitze's disease 350
Tendonitis of
  long head of biceps 406
  supraspinatus tendon 406
Terminal ileal Crohn's disease 156
Tertiary syphilis 64, 319
Testicular
  abscess 324

atrophy 526
diseases 324
feminization 535
Tetanus 425
Third stage of syphilis 290, 315
Thrombangitis obliterans 515
Thrombocytopenic purpura 283
Thrombophlebitis 283
Thrombotic gangrene 513
Thyroglossal cyst 93
Thyroid
gland 97
origin 22
swelling 69
Thyroiditis 82
Thyrotoxic exophthalmos 77
Torsion of
cord 388
fallopian tube, fimbrial and broad ligament cysts 351, 357
testis 209, 209*f*, 215, 216*f*, 218, 391
Toxic goiter 69
Transitional cell carcinoma 481
Transverse colon 173
Traumatic
fat necrosis 124
gangrene 512, 522
mastitis 135
paraplegia 537
rupture of
spleen, liver, or mesenteric tear 352
urethra 501
ulcer 300, 316, 317, 335
Trench foot 523
Treponema
pallidum 290, 326
pertenue 337
Troisier's sign 412, 463
Tropical ulcer 301, 338, 339*f*
True
hermaphroditism 535
herpes linguis 318
melena 456
pancreatic cyst 185
solitary cyst 283
Tubercle 527
Tuberculosis 193, 377, 379
of breast 348
Tuberculous
abscess 124
epididymo-orchitis 219, 389
funiculitis 207
lymph nodes 194
lymphadenitis 289
ulcer 302, 311, 318, 335
ulceration 478
Tumor of
cord or round ligament 196
GB 166
intra-abdominal viscus 379
meninges and roots 406
pyloric end of stomach, and duodenum 168
retroperitoneal structures 379
scrotum 323
skin 115
spinal cord 406
and compression myelitis 375
spine 406
submandibular gland 56
testis 219
tongue 22
Turban tumor 9, 239
Twisted ovarian cyst 351, 357
Types of
gangrene 511
jaundice 452
swelling 116
thyroid cancer 86
ulcers 308

Typhoid
fever 470, 527
splenomegaly 285
Typical branchial cyst 103*f*

U

Ulcerating
infective lesions 310
sarcoma or carcinoma 307
tumors 310, 312
Ulcerative
colitis 377, 477
infective lesions 310
stomatitis 319
Ulcers 299, 302, 311, 416
of face 310
of leg 328
of lips 314
of tongue 317, 426
Umbilical hernia and paraumbilical hernia 371
Uncompensated valvular heart disease 491
Unconjugated hyperbilirubinemia 439, 441, 455
Undescended testis 195
Unilateral
cystic lesions 46
hypertrophy 122
solid lesions 47
Uremia 365, 408
Uremic
colitis 478
gastritis 408
Urinary
bladder 176
retention 428, 496, 503

V

Vaginal discharge 354
Varicocele 205, 220
Varicose ulcer 301, 330
Vascular
sarcoma 196
swellings 196
Veins 18
Venous
stasis 526
ulcer 301, 328, 330
Ventral surface of wrist 233*f*
Very painful ulcer 300
Vesical calculus 395
Vinyl chloride-induced congestion 283
Viral
hepatitis 442
infection 45
lymphadenitis 64
Virus hepatitis 443
Volvulus of
cecum 357
intestine 357
sigmoid colon 356*f*
von Graefe's sign 76
von Recklinghausen's disease 42, 255, 275
von Willebrand's disease 457

W

Warthin's tumor 43
Warts 242
Wasermann reaction 295
Weil's disease 277 283, 378, 442, 457
Whipple's disease 377
Wilm's tumor 167

Y

Yellow fever 442, 457, 467